991

HEALTH
CARE
ETHICS

HEALTH CARE ETHICS
PRINCIPLES AND PROBLEMS

THOMAS M. GARRETT
HAROLD W. BAILLIE
ROSELLEN M. GARRETT

University of Scranton

PRENTICE HALL, *Englewood Cliffs, New Jersey 07632*

Library of Congress Cataloging-in-Publication Data

GARRETT, THOMAS M., (date)
    Health care ethics: principles and problems / Thomas M. Garrett,
Harold W. Baillie, Rosellen M. Garrett.

    p. cm.
    Bibliography.
    Includes index.
    ISBN 0-13-385063-3
    1. Medical ethics.   2. Medical ethics—Case studies.   3. Medical
care—Moral and ethical aspects.   I. Baillie, Harold W., (date).
II. Garrett, Rosellen M., (date).   III. Title.
R724.G35   1988
174'.2—dc19   88-9920
CIP

Editorial/production supervision and
    interior design: *Mary A. Araneo*
Cover design: *Ben Santora*
Manufacturing buyer: *Peter Havens*

Printed in the United States of America

10 9 8 7 6 5 4 3

ISBN   0-13-385063-3

Prentice-Hall International (UK) Limited, *London*
Prentice-Hall of Australia Pty. Limited, *Sydney*
Prentice-Hall Canada Inc., *Toronto*
Prentice-Hall Hispanoamericana, S.A., *Mexico*
Prentice-Hall of India Private Limited, *New Delhi*
Prentice-Hall of Japan, Inc., *Tokyo*
Simon & Schuster Asia Pte. Ltd., *Singapore*
Editora Prentice-Hall do Brasil, Ltda., *Rio de Janeiro*

For Paula
whom we all love
and
John F. McGeehan, M.D.
who cares for all of us

CONTENTS

Problems of Health Care Ethics

PREFACE

Health Care Ethics: Principles and Problems grew out of 10 years of teaching the subject to premedical, nursing, and physical therapy students as well as medical technicians and majors in human resources administration. The book is rooted in the idea that patients, the consumers of health care, are the central actors in health care and have a set of ethical problems distinct from, though related to, those of the various health care professionals who serve them.

As the subtitle suggests, we have attempted to develop a set of principles that can be applied to a variety of problems. Principles alone, however, do not solve problems. We have, then, presented a set of true problems which show how principles meet reality and attempted to arrive at solutions which, though not ideal, will work in the real world. We have not always succeeded, but believe that even the failure reveals much about the nature of life and of applied ethics.

Not everyone will agree with everything we have said. Indeed, there are points where we disagree among ourselves. This is as it should be. In a complicated and problematic area, no one and no society has had enough experience and time to work out the definitive answers to all questions. We can only hope that our arguments and, more important, our efforts to outline the various dimensions of the problems will advance the dialogue that is the necessary condition for ultimate consensus.

While we have not for obvious reasons attempted to discuss all possible positions on all possible questions in health care ethics, we have touched briefly on a large number of topics. Careful use of the index and of cross references in the text should enable the reader to fill out those brief treatments. The references supply leads to further developments.

We have included cases at the end of most chapters since our experience shows that the principles become alive only when applied to the complexities of the concrete world. Some of the cases have been simplified for beginners. Others appear in all their complexity. It is our hope that most of them will challenge those who would like to have simple answers to all problems.

The parenthetical references in the text indicate where the reader may find a fuller or even an opposing development of the point under consideration. The numbered notes refer to brief, largely technical remarks at the end of the chapter.

The authors wish to thank all those students who have challenged them and called for greater clarity and consistency. We also owe a debt of gratitude to the following colleagues and friends who read and criticized one or more chapters: John Carlson, Jean P. Gilbert, Richard Klonoski, Ron McKinney, John F. McGeehan, and David C. Thomasma. Since we have not always followed their excellent advice, they should be held blameless. Many people, nurses and medical social workers in particular, contributed case material or the outlines of cases. Special thanks for this service are due to Katherine Skinner, Shirley Wilson, and Constance Brown. Mrs. Katie Duke of the University of Scranton Library gave us bibliographical assistance beyond the call of duty. Richard Passon, Provost of the University of Scranton, provided us not only with encouragement, but with more tangible resources as well. The typing, mailing, and damage control done by Eleanore Wentland of the University of Scranton made writing this book a livable, even enjoyable, experience.

Finally, we wish to thank all the copyright holders who have graciously allowed us to reproduce their material. Specific acknowledgments are provided in the notes and the references.

Thomas M. Garrett, Ph.D.
Harold W. Baillie, Ph.D.
Rosellen M. Garrett, R.N., Ph.D.

Chapter One
ETHICS, PROFESSIONAL ETHICS, AND HEALTH CARE ETHICS

This is a book about health care ethics, that is, a book about applied ethics in various professional health care fields. It is also about the ethics of the consumer of health care, since the patient must make the most serious ethical decisions of all.

Ethics is that branch of philosophy that seeks to determine how human actions may be judged right or wrong. When the study of ethics is applied to a professional field, it becomes necessary to discuss not only basic ethical positions, but also the nature of the profession and the conditions under which that profession operates.

The study of ethics implies that the human mind is the fundamental means by which actions may be judged. Thus, ethics is not the same as moral theology or religious ethics, since ethics uses reason alone and does not, or at least should not, invoke religious belief as a source of its conclusions. At the same time, ethics need not be taken as an attack on religiously founded morality, which for the believer has a superior validity. Ethics is not, after all, capable of judging the claims of divine revelation.

Nor is ethics the same as law, though, as we will see in the course of this book, the law is an important expression of social judgment about the rightness or wrongness of actions that seriously affect the public good. While law is largely concerned with the public good and the protection of individual rights, ethics goes beyond this to look at the obligations of individuals to themselves as well as to others and to society.

Because it attempts to look beyond the opinions of the group to more fundamental issues about human nature and the nature of human activity in general, ethics is not sociology or a mere description of what a given group thinks is right or wrong. At the same time, ethics must recognize that public beliefs may point to very important insights about the rightness or wrongness of particular activities. In the context of professional ethics, public opinion has a great deal to do with defining the role of the professional and in setting up expectations of the profession. In Chapter Four on Justice we will even see how public opinion has a decisive role to play in the fair distribution of health care.

THEORIES OF ETHICS

Ethical theories, that is, theories about the characteristics of human activity, can be divided into three broad classes.

Consequentialism

The first class, *consequentialism*, sees the rightness or the wrongness of an action in terms of the consequences brought about by that action. These consequences are generally evaluated according to the extent to which they serve some intrinsic good, that is, a good that is good in and of itself independent of any further consequences.

The most common, but not the only, form of consequentialism is utilitarianism. Utilitarianism, or social consequentialism, holds that you should act so as to do the greatest good for the greatest number. For the most part, utilitarianism involves adding up the aggregate of pleasures and pains suffered by the members of the community. The state of affairs that yields the greatest amount of pleasure and the least amount of pain is taken to be the best.

We do not follow this as a general principle since the utilitarian principle tends to overlook the good of the individual and to concentrate on the aggregate of individual goods. Also, utilitarianism is tied to a claim that the consequences of an action are clear enough to be accurately measured and tallied in some way. This dependence on the clarity of the consequences of an action strikes us as largely unsupportable. As will be shown throughout this book, many ethical dilemmas are dilemmas precisely because the consequences of actions are not clear at all. We will, however, encounter many areas in health care ethics where society may rightfully judge that the utilitarian approach is the most reasonable approach available. In any event, as we shall see a little later, we do consider consequences, though in terms of the individual human person rather than in terms of the aggregates.

Deontologism

The second class of ethical theory, *deontologism*, determines the rightness or wrongness of an action by analyzing certain formal properties of the statement of the action. These formal properties reveal characteristics of the action, such as duty or justice or respect for an individual's autonomy. As a result, the deontologist considers the rightness or wrongness of at least some acts to be independent of their consequences; that is, some acts are good or evil in and of themselves. Unlike utilitarians, deontologists, such as Kantians and some natural law theorists, would hold that lying is wrong even if a lie would accomplish great goods for individuals and society. They use formal rules in judging the rightness of an act, such as: "Do unto others as you would have them do unto you," or "Act in such a way that you always treat humanity, whether in your own person or in the person of any other, never simply as a means, but always at the same time as an end."

One of the strengths of the deontological position is its emphasis on the moral significance of the individual. While we sympathize with that emphasis and accept the moral centrality of the person, we feel that most deontological positions (especially that of Kant) are so extreme in their emphasis that community becomes a nonexistent moral category. The individual is so exalted that it becomes impossible for there to be any moral significance in the other. To the authors this simply does not accord with experience. Our experiences with friendship, marriage, and community living indicate that these realities are central in the moral development and moral life of the individual. As we shall make clear, society is for us the means by which the individual is educated to right reason and trained to social roles. Any position that does not give a large place to this fundamental moral relationship between the individual and society is inadequate.

As in our criticism of utilitarianism, we find that deontologism relies on an assumption that moral dilemmas can be made clear and, consequently, that we can reason ourselves out of the problem. This escape is accomplished through the use of a formal criterion that in large measure denies the role of consequences in our moral thought. The suggestion is that by looking to the formal properties of an action, we can escape the limitations of our knowledge of the consequences of that action. We suggest that this clarity is misleading, because it is attained at the cost of denying the role of social experience in understanding the dilemmas.

Virtue Ethics

The third class of ethical theory may be labeled *virtue ethics*. Virtue ethics is, unfortunately, a somewhat confusing term, since it is used as a label for two different approaches to ethics. What we call virtue ethics *narrowly defined* states that "a virtue [is] a dispositional trait of character that is considered praiseworthy in general and in a particular role." In this narrowly defined approach, "a virtue ethics [is] a systematic formulation of the traits of character that make human behavior praiseworthy or blameworthy" (Shelp, 1985, p.330).

As presented here, virtue ethics narrowly defined does not go far enough in setting up a framework for decision making about the rightness or wrongness of individual activities. Thus, while we would agree that health care professionals should be compassionate, truthful, and unselfish, these emotional dispositions do not guarantee correct decisions in treatment since more than good will is involved. Such decisions must appeal to the knowledge and the reasoning ability of the professional and rest on a specific relationship with the client. We turn then to virtue ethics broadly construed.

Virtue ethics *more broadly defined* involves not only the virtues, but the integration of the virtues with what has been variously called practical wisdom or right reason. This practical wisdom is the ability to choose patterns of actions made desirable and revealed as desirable by reasoning that has been informed not only by habits of emotional experience or virtues (Baillie, 1988) but by consideration of the widest possible range of factors with consequences for the individual human being situated in society. Reasoned consideration of this wide range of factors and the emotional dispositions are both influenced by cultural traditions about the common understanding of the good and so need to be tempered by both logic and a healthy skepticism about those traditions. Practical wisdom then requires as a foundation the development of virtues, that is dispositions, concerned with both the emotions and the intellect.

Practical reason involves not only the application of principles but the study and evaluation of all proximate and remote consequences for the individual. To act properly in a given set of circumstances involves knowing how one's actions might affect those circumstances, the societies of which one is a member, all of the agents involved, and ultimately oneself. Thus, practical reason attends carefully to the consequentialist, but not the utilitarian, point of view. In our view, everything is judged in terms of its ultimate as well as immediate effects on the total development of the individual person living in a community. As we shall see in our treatment of the dignity of the human person, mere pleasure and pain are not, as with the utilitarians, intrinsic goods.

We also wish to stress the fact that ours is not an individualistic position, for what harms other persons ultimately harms the agent. One's own dignity means very little if other persons do not have a similar value. As we shall see, in discussing the common good, the basic reason for limiting one's own freedom is the preservation of the dignity of others. This preservation of the dignity of others is not merely a question of one-on-one relationships but of harms to society, which ultimately result in harms to individual dignity. For this reason, social effects, that is, effects on the various communities of which the individual is a member, are extremely important even though they are not the central moral issue. What destroys such social goods as the family, communication, clean water and fresh air, or the health care delivery system are ultimately if not immediately and directly of great consequence for the individual.

The effects in question are not simply material effects, such as the loss of a leg or of property or even of life itself, but of such intangible but extremely important aspects of the person as human dignity and freedom of choice as well as freedom from unnecessary restrictions. While it is not always easy to specify everything that is demanded by human dignity, the authors, like American culture itself, see attacks on the freedom of choice and freedom from unnecessary restrictions as attacks on human dignity and so as prima facie, or presumptively, evil. That is to say, they are seen intuitively to be wrong, unless the opposite is clearly established.

At various points in the book we will return to the question of what is included in the concept of the dignity of the human person. For example, the implications of freedom of choice as part of human dignity will be developed in Chapter Two on the principle of autonomy. Throughout the book, we will be concerned with showing how a balance may be attained between the needs of the individual and those of society. The good of both must be maintained.

This broader definition of virtue ethics includes a consideration of the emotional dispositions and cultural factors that influence dispositions as well as the development of the reason, so that it is capable of balanced consideration of the consequences for the individual person in society. This holistic approach pivots on practical wisdom as *the primary virtue* for ethical decision making. The present work might then be called a virtue ethics in this broader sense. To avoid confusion, however, we shall call it the approach of practical wisdom.

Having located our theory relative to broad categories of ethical theory, we now wish to stress some of the key notions that underlie our positions.

The Dignity of the Individual

At the heart of this book is the assertion that the individual person is the central value in terms of whose dignity all consequences are to be judged. This dignity resides not merely in the capacity for pleasure nor in the ability to make free choices but in the capacity for warm human interaction, friendship, family relations, and for the most broadly based social life as well as for union with the whole of reality. While these capacities are not likely to be completely fulfilled, they are, nevertheless, at the core of the dignity of the human person.

The individual person is not an abstraction that can be labeled simply as "an autonomous being" or "a bearer of rights," but is a concrete individual whose life involves shared life in a particular community and sharing in some specific set of habitual social roles in that community. Thus, individual and society are not opposed concepts. They can be understood only in terms of one another. Individuals are not simply individuals; they are also fathers, daughters, nurses, teachers, and wage earners. All of these roles that entangle the individual in the lives of others and in the life of the community specify consequences which must be considered. Indeed, part of the challenge of the ethical life is the need to balance the demands of the basic dignity of the individual with the consequences of his roles and the needs of the community. The achievement of this balance, as we have already said, requires that practical wisdom be the primary virtue of the ethical life. The "person" only exists by living in society, surrounded by other people from whom and with whom it learns what it means to be a "person" at all. It is also in and through society that the person learns of the consequences of action for the individual, for other persons, and for the group itself. The society and the culture, after all, are the repositories of great knowledge based on long experience. Thus, while for us the person is the intrinsic good and so the primary focus of evaluation, that evaluation takes place in and through the community. Indeed, society may be seen as the lens through which the individual sees and evaluates the world.

It is important to note that, due to the interdependence of the individual and society, the concept of the dignity of man is not static. History has affected the concept as it has revealed further dimensions of humankind and given deeper insights into what that dignity demands for the full flowering of the person. Only in the past century did American society recognize the full evils of slavery and child labor. In our own generation, we have seen progress as our society came to consider sexism, racism, ageism, and the like as affronts to human dignity. The recognition of these evils has not removed all of them but has begun the process of reform. Unfortunately, society can forget the consequences of such insults to human dignity. Unfortunately, too, as resources become scarcer, societies are tempted to downgrade the dignity of the sick, elderly, poor, and powerless. Sometimes this is due to selfishness and shortsightedness. Sometimes it is a regrettable manifestation of the tragic in human life. We will return to the tragic dimension shortly.

For these reasons, it is difficult to define precisely what is included in the concept of "the dignity of the individual." At various points in this book, we will return to this question. For example, the implications of freedom of choice as part of human dignity will be developed in Chapter Two on the principle of autonomy. The demands of human dignity are crucial in the consideration of the distribution of health care, abortion, death and dying, as well as in the rationing of organs and the use of new modes of reproduction. Each of these problems, which will be treated in subsequent chapters, will reveal other aspects of human dignity.

The Role of Society

Society plays a necessary ethical role in that it is impossible for an isolated individual to meet the full requirements of practical wisdom for most if not all decisions. After all, it is unlikely that there would be any developed practical wisdom without society. This is due not only to the fundamental opacity and ambiguity of ethical issues, but to the limits of individual experience with regard to consequences as well as the individual's dependence on society for language and education. The society, on the other hand, though not free of opacity and ambiguity, makes possible the education and training of the individual and brings to the education the wealth of experience and knowledge it has amassed. It also brings society's particular perspective on this experience and knowledge.

Before proceeding, a few words need to be said about the words "ambiguity" and "opacity," which we have just used. The "ambiguity" of which we speak refers to situations where the clarity of the facts do not dictate the decision to be made. Thus, nothing in nature tells us whether we should drive on the right or left side of the road, though it does tell us we must do one or the other if we are to avoid disaster. Society can remove the ambiguity by law or custom. Where there are potentially dangerous ambiguities about the relationships between key individuals and institutions, society by custom or law defines the roles and relationships. In short, in the ambiguous situation, problems can be resolved by choice, especially social choices. This social removal of ambiguous roles is particularly important in applied ethics.

"Opacity" refers to situations where our knowledge is so limited and the situation so structured that we cannot arrive at an answer even with a social choice. In such situations, no matter what choices we make, serious moral questions remain unresolved. Society may attempt to treat the situation as merely ambiguous and attempt to clarify it by a decision, but the problem remains, since a mere decision does not solve it. We shall see examples of this with regard to the moral status of the fetus and the distribution of health care. The opacity of some situations is part of the tragic dimension.

Although society cannot eradicate opacity, it provides a knowledge base and a social decision-making mechanism. Among other things, this decision-making mechanism removes many problems of ambiguity. The customs and traditions of society encapsulate vast amounts of practical knowledge which influence the individual. This involves, in part, the formation of habits through the influence of role models, peer pressure, and family life. Whether we like it or not, we are all formed by social customs. These range from major principles, like the claim that we are innocent until proven guilty, to minor issues, such as the proper way to thank a host for dinner. None of us ever escapes this influence of our society, nor could we if we wanted to. What we have from social experience and cultural transmission of knowledge is extremely valuable. For example, because of the development of science and of the educational system, the average high school student in the United States knows much more about the nature of the physical world than his counterpart in Athens in 399 B.C. Or, to give a more general example, we may not be able to give a theoretical defense for democracy, but we tend to defend it on the basis of our social experience and so believe we benefit from both democracy and our defense of it.[1]

None of this is to say that society is always correct or should be accepted uncritically. Even our own society once approved slavery, the oppression of women, and the disregard of the handicapped. What we are saying is that society has an important role in evaluating and even creating consequences as well as in forming our perspective on the world and our character. In the tragic dimension, we face problems for which there is no satisfactory solution.

Society, and Moral and Legal Rights

Most Americans are acquainted with the discussion of social ethics through the language of rights. For example, the Constitution speaks of the right to life, liberty, and the pursuit of happiness. Some times, particularly in popular or rhetorical discussion, the term "right" is no more than a means of expressing a set of ideals or goals for human social development. For example, the United Nations Universal Declaration of Human Rights (1948) is best understood as an expression of hopes, rather than realities. We will not make use of this sense of "rights."

There is, however, a second use of the term "right" that plays an important role in the discussion of ethics in contemporary society. In this sense a "right" is a moral or legal claim that an individual may assert against someone else. Thus, there are two types of rights, moral rights, in which the claim is based on moral principles, and legal rights, in which the claim is based on law. Any such claim imposes an obligation on another person. For example, if you have signed a contract for a service, then you have a legal and moral right to have that service performed by the person with whom you signed the contract. Conversely, that person has a legal and moral obligation to perform that service for you. Or, if you promised your friend to meet her at four this afternoon, then she has a moral right to expect you to be there, and you have an obligation to show up.

Rights are accepted when they have been justified or made valid by an appeal to the proper set of principles. For example, a legal right may be asserted when the appropriate legislation has been made law, or when a judicial decision confirms an interpretation of law. Clearly, legal rights appear, change, develop, or disappear according to developments in a society's code of law.

Moral rights are very different. They exist as part of a moral perspective, or a set of moral principles, and as such they can be understood in as many ways as there are diverse moral positions. For example, a utilitarian will understand rights to be generated within the experience of a society as a statement of what the society finds most basic in the treatment of the individual. A deontologist would understand a right to be a moral claim which in a sense pre-exists the society, that is, the individual gets his rights from a source other than, and more important than, society. For example, a right may be a consequence of God's creation, or it may be another way of expressing the autonomy of the person.

In this book, we will speak of rights in both the legal and the moral sense. When speaking of legal right, we will of course be referring to legal rights granted by American law. When we speak of moral rights, we will speak of rights to things which are demanded by the dignity of the individual inside a particular community. To put it another way, we see rights as claims to things which are necessary to protect and advance the particular individual in that basic dignity.

We admit, however, that rights in their specific as opposed to their general form are structured by the society in which the individual exists. Thus, though there may be a general moral right to food, the right to a specific food will depend on the resources of the community and even on its culinary customs. This point will have particular importance when we discuss the general right to health care in Chapter Four.

Public or Common Good

We have insisted that practical wisdom considers the direct impact of actions not only on the individual person but on society. Our reason is simple: The good of society is one of the chief means to the protection and growth of the individual. Without the public good or common good all other goods would be difficult to attain.

The common good is understood to be the collection of goods which, having been produced by the broadest and most inclusive form of social cooperation, belong to society as a whole, as opposed to belonging to the individuals. In modern times much of this cooperation is managed by the government, but key parts of the common good such as the language and the culture are the result of even more widespread cooperation. We note, however, that when we say that the common good belongs to the society, we do not mean it belongs to the government. Society owns the language, one of the most important of the goods in the common good. The language is *not* the possession of either the government or any individuals or group of individuals. Indeed, when a government acts as if it does own the language, we are almost certainly dealing with tyranny of the worst sort.

The particular goods that form part of the common good are not written down in some easy to find handbook. Over time, the list has grown from such things as the judicial system and the economic infrastructure (roads, canals, etc.) to include the educational system, the welfare system, as well as police and fire protection. Today we are debating as to whether the health care system (or nonsystem according to some) is or should be part of the common good. This last question cannot be answered *a priori* since it depends on the social evaluation of the entire system. In short, it depends on the values of society and the resources available. We shall return to this in Chapter Four.

Each particular part of the common good is justified only in so far as it contributes directly or indirectly to the good of each and every individual in society. In other words, the common good is not some great god to whom all is to be sacrificed. It is a means to the perfection of all individuals in the society. A public sewer system, for example, directly serves not only those who are hooked up but, by preventing the spread of disease, it serves everyone in the society. The public educational system serves the students directly, but serves everyone by preparing people capable of carrying on the essential functions of society.

Ultimately, the public good exists for the good of individual persons rather than the other way around. For grave reasons, minor goods of the individual can be subordinated to the public good. Thus, most of us pay taxes to support large parts of the common good. But our very personhood does not belong to the society, and it would be unjust for society to demand that we sacrifice our life or our sanity for the common good. In short, the common good cannot justify destroying the individual human person, which is the central value and so the justification of the existence of society and the common good.

In the chapters that follow we will often consider conflicts between individual and public goods and the conditions under which one is subordinated to another.

Moral Ambiguity, Opacity, and the Limits of Practical Wisdom

All of the previous considerations point up the complexity of life as we must live it. This lived complexity gives rise to a moral complexity which often involves us in moral opacity and ambiguity. Indeed, it is in our acceptance of moral opacity and ambiguity that this book differs from other approaches to ethics. While recognizing the value of certain aspects of both deontologism and utilitarianism, we nevertheless see ourselves as offering an importantly different perspective. These other ethical positions assume that some clear and unequivocal ethical principle or ethical consequence is not only possible, but is the source of any acceptable ethical evaluation. These positions suggest that if clarity is not possible, ethics is not possible. As is clear from our discussion, our ethics presuppose no such clarity. Ethical reasoning cannot always be assumed to start from clear and distinct principles. The starting principles are often so general and vague that they can give little practical guidance. First principles such as "do good and avoid evil" may be valid but are of little value in decision making. While we strive to develop secondary principles that are more applicable, we are adding to the primary principle material that may not be absolutely certain. We are often dealing with short-term probabilities while remaining ignorant of the long-term consequences. Thus, as we shall see in Chapters Two and Three, the medical form of the principles of autonomy and beneficence incorporate social judgments that remove ambiguity by embracing the specifications of American society. We run the danger, then, of going from the overly general to the overly specific.

When applying the secondary principles we are often acting in areas where there is not only ambiguity but opacity. As we shall see, for example, in the chapter on abortion, no skill, technique, insight, or decision is likely to provide a clear unequivocal determination of when the conceptus is to be considered a person. Unfortunately, it is not possible to derive from reason alone an indisputable answer to the issue. Instead, we must look for an ethical resolution to the dilemma in the full scope of relevant material—intellectual, personal, and social. The search never removes the opacity. Sometimes the search suggests practical compromises, but these do not remove the moral anguish in making decisions about something fundamentally unclear.

When the matter is truly opaque, society must resort to law in order to preserve the social order or the value of the individual person. In such cases, law is a practical determination, not the truth. No matter how useful, such laws do not remove the opacity and do not resolve the underlying moral problem. As we shall insist in our treatment of abortion, the opacity remains and the tragic dimension of life hits us with full force.

Occasionally, we are tempted to believe that our practical compromises are true solutions. This temptation springs from an uncritical acceptance of our implicit knowledge. Our beliefs about the nature of the world and the ultimate meaning of life influence all our judgments. This occurs whether these beliefs are philosophically or theologically founded, or even unfounded. An implicit belief in divine providence or in modern science affects our evaluation of a medical problem. Similarly, the assumption that the fetus is a person or that the authority of a particular church is supreme will also have major effects.

In addition, implicit knowledge about underlying truths as well as implicit knowledge of appropriate circumstances and of the means of applying that principle to the circumstances are always there, although not always consciously. For example, the competence and rationality of patients can generally be assumed, but in many settings a conscious evaluation needs to be made. Assumptions taken over from the culture may never have been examined critically. For example, many assume that modern health care is scientific and that the doctor knows best, when in fact, as we shall see in many sections of this book, some practices have little scientific justification. As a result, when an individual thinks she knows clearly and unambiguously what is right in a situation, especially an opaque situation, she might be wrong due to implicit unexamined assumptions about action. This, too, may be part of the tragedy of human life.

Emotions and the Ethical Life

The emotions influence our ethical judgments both for better and for worse. Without "fellow feeling" we would not be so ready to acknowledge that others have the same value as we do. Love urges us to go beyond the minimum in helping others. Yet, without compassion, we might help others as if we were dealing with blocks of wood to be moved around in line without expertise. Arrogance might lead us to paternalism and to domineering behavior, even as we pretend to help others. Hatred and envy and resentment can distort our perception of reality and decision making. We are fully aware of this and shall return to it from time to time in the course of the book. We only regret that both the limitations of time and ethical theory make a full treatment impossible.

The Tragic in Human Life

Both the chance of being wrong despite the best intentions and the need to make morally wrenching decisions in the face of incomplete information or with inadequate resources bring us face to face with the tragic in human life. While humankind may believe that, granted good will, there is always a solution to every problem, there are unsolvable problems. While ethicians sometimes write as if their principles can resolve every conflict in an intellectually and emotionally satisfying manner, this is not the case. Even if ambiguity were to be removed, we would still find ourselves in situations that are opaque and where, no matter what we do, there are disastrous consequences for individuals or society. When a health care professional performs triage, that is, rations care at the scene of an accident, some are helped and some neglected. This is the damned-if-you-do, damned-if-you-don't situation. This is the essence of the human tragedy. We will face it in this book, but we do not pretend to have the wisdom, practical or otherwise, to overcome it.

APPLIED ETHICS

When the principles of ethics are applied to a situation, more than principles are required. Because the application of principles is to be made in a particular society with its particular role definitions, customs, and laws, these must be taken into consideration. As we shall see shortly, the changing definitions of the roles of physicians and nurses are a particular source of difficulty in American medical ethics.

Ultimately, the consequences for the individual must be considered, since the consequences vary in particular social situations and change over time as technique is improved. The factual study of consequences is a necessity. In the case of rule consequentialists, that factual information is concerned with the generalizable effects of an activity and with the probable effects of the activity in the particular case. Thus, while everyone agrees that it is wrong to kill innocent persons, before we can pass ethical judgment in a concrete situation, we need to know whether or not this person is innocent and whether or not this particular activity will kill. Whether pornographic material causes violence is a question that must be answered before one can condemn pornography on that ground. In medicine we shall have to look at the effects of medical treatment not only on the body, but on the spirit, lifestyle, and pocketbook of the patient, as well as its effects on society. In short, applied ethics looks to the concrete and the practical and thus demands more than theory.

In medical ethics the consequences change as technique and conditions change. One hundred and fifty years ago, before blood typing and matching, blood transfusions were almost universally fatal and so generally unethical as well. Ten years ago, the risks were small and blood transfusions generally posed no ethical problem. Today, with the spread of AIDS, there are again ethical problems with the system that supplies blood for transfusions. Sometimes our knowledge of the consequences and alternative treatments change, with the result that both the medical and ethical status of a treatment must be reevaluated. We shall see further examples of this with regard to radical mastectomy, tonsillectomies, and medical circumcision.

In the real world, we need a mutually acceptable way of deciding on the consequences and evaluating them. For example, in determining the effects of lead poisoning on children, we have certain canons of scientific procedure that, when followed, will answer (to the best of our ability) this question. Or, in determining who is innocent and who is guilty in these particular circumstances, we have the court system and the legal code. In short, applied ethics looks to the concrete and the practical, and in so doing it involves socially developed institutions and socially accepted techniques that aid the individual in evaluating moral issues.

For these reasons, when we present material regarding problems that are very much rooted in ambiguous circumstances, such as the appointment of a guardian for incompetent patients, or the definition of death, we will rely on court decisions, laws, and even statements by professional associations for what is at least a reasonable starting point for arriving at explicit content for an ethical decision. Sometimes the law even dictates what the decision should be. This is because these sources represent the thinking of interested parties who have a collective experience greater than that of any individual. These institutions are the schemas, the socially developed, that is, traditional, means by which a particular society applies for itself and its members ethical principles to specific circumstances. This is not to say we agree with, or even ought to agree with, each of these decisions and statements. The value of the individual provides us with the perspective from which critical evaluations of these procedures and decisions may be generated. Indeed, it is the task of the individual to develop these critical evaluations as his experience suggests the need for critical considerations. In the pages that follow we will be exercising this critical function to suggest ways in which law and custom might be made to better defend and promote the dignity of the individual in the health care context. At the same time, the collective experience of the society as a whole and of significant professional groups is a precious resource.

PROFESSIONAL ETHICS

Professional ethics are a special type of applied ethics. There are, moreover, different views about the nature of professional ethics. First, a set of rules might be called professional ethics because it is articulated by the members of a profession or, secondly, because it is concerned with the ethical conduct of the profession.[2] The first type of professional ethics, that is the professionally articulated ethics, is found in codes of ethics promulgated by the professional group. Occasionally, they are also found in authoritative rulings of the professional association. We will refer to such codes and rulings throughout the book, since they often indicate careful thought based on long experience with the problem. Unfortunately, some of these codes are a mixture of what may be called rules of etiquette and of professional courtesy as well as of rules about matters of deep ethical concern. Indeed, at times, the professional articulated codes have been self-serving rather than truly ethical or at odds with more general social values. Recently, for example, the government has declared the traditional professional ethical prohibition of advertising as being illegal and against the public good. An uncritical acceptance of every provision of the professional codes is not, then, wise.

The idea of the professionally articulated ethic lingers on since some professionals claim that only they know enough to judge the ethics of their own group. This claim disregards the fact that their clients or patients and society as a whole are affected, so that others have a right to participate in formulating and imposing the professional ethic. As a matter of fact, the society and the clients are part of the force that forms the role of ethics of a particular profession and so have a great influence on its ethics. If nothing else, society decides formally, through licensing laws and even court decisions, what the profession will and will not be allowed to do. Less formally, social movements, such as the patient's rights movement, change expectations and so relationships such that the ethics changes with them even before they are enacted into law. If society expects health care professionals to stop and treat people who have been involved in accidents, this will become part of the obligations of the professional role even before it is incorporated into the law. The development of the doctrine of informed consent, which will be treated in the next chapter, is a prime example of how expectation and law have changed the roles of physician and patient, thus radically influencing health care ethics.

The importance of the role definition for professional ethics is crucial. It determines what duties are specific to the members of the profession and which rights will be granted by society. The role definition, indeed, constitutes much of the health care contract of which we will speak later in this chapter.

The socially accepted purpose of the profession in its turn has a preponderant influence on the definition of the professor's role as well as on the specification of rights and duties. A profession like law is set up and approved for the promotion of justice according to the constitution and laws of a specific society. In the society of the United States with its adversarial system of justice, the lawyer has a duty to represent the interests of his clients in order to ensure a fair trial even though that might result in some perpetrators of crimes going free. Similarly, health care providers will have specific obligations that depend on what is approved as the purpose of the profession within the culture.

The Purpose of Medicine and the Health Care System

While everyone may assume that they know the purpose of medicine, nursing, physical therapy, and health care in general, a little reflection reveals that there are problems that have ethical implications. First, let us look at the medical profession, then at nursing, since they are the two largest professional groups in health care.

Is the overarching purpose of the health care professions the prevention of death or the alleviation of suffering (May, 1983)? If it is the alleviation of suffering, does this embrace not only a cure of the cause of the suffering, but also the comforting and care of the sufferer who cannot or will not be cured? Or is health care, in the context of a specific illness, only the attempt to optimize the patient's chance for a happy and productive life as defined by the patient (Robin, 1984)?

If the purpose of health care is the prevention of death, then physicians are professionally correct when they keep people alive even though in a vegetative state. If the purpose is the relief of suffering by either cure or care, the physician who uses "heroic measures" with a person in a permanent vegetative state is cruel and unprofessional. If the purpose is to optimize the patient's chances for a happy and productive life as defined by the patient, then treatment that dooms the patient to an unproductive life is perhaps unethical even though the physician and society thinks that the unproductive life is good.

Pellegrino (1979b) holds that the end (purpose) of medicine formally considered is a "right and good healing action taken in the interests of a particular patient." Kass (1983) also emphasizes healing as the primary purpose, though elsewhere (1975) he has suggested that the pursuit of health is the primary purpose of medicine, with the prevention of death and the alleviation of suffering secondary to that pursuit. Positions that put healing at the center provide a way of judging when to stop treatment because death is imminent or because healing is no longer possible. At that point the alleviation of pain becomes primary as the only humane and ethical possibility that remains.

It is impossible to define the purpose of either medicine or health care in general so that it can be engraved in stone. In the first place, the purpose changes as the condition of the patient changes. In the second place, the purpose changes as the agreement between the patient and the health care provider changes. Medicine and health care have several purposes, and all need to be considered in line with the condition and wishes of the patient.

The idea that medicine has as one of its purposes the pursuit of health (Kass, 1983) recognizes that the physician is also concerned with preventing as well as healing disease and that the individual physician seeks to maintain health at an optimum level for the particular patient. This can also have great social implications for the physician, who is then placed in an advocacy role regarding questions of public health.

It should be noted that the profession as a whole should have as its purpose the prevention of disease and the maintenance of the health of the whole population. The fact that such tasks are often relegated only to public health officials, sanitary engineers, and the Centers for Disease Control does not mean that the social dimension is not part of the purpose of the health care professions.

The authors will assume that in most encounters the primary purpose of medicine is the healing of particular patients. When healing is not possible, the alleviation of suffering by ethical means becomes primary. When healing is not necessary, the prevention of disease and the maintenance of health are the proper focus. The prevention of death and the prolongation of life may be the result of all of the activities designed to achieve the above purpose but are not goals in and of themselves without further consideration. As we shall see in Chapter Six on death and dying, the value of life and the prolongation of life can become problematic.

We have oversimplified the issues here since key words such as health and disease and associated terms such as cure, restore, and maintain are all ambiguous. In Chapter Four when we discuss the distribution of health care, the nature of disease and health becomes an important issue and we will deal with it there. We shall also return to the problem in Chapter Six when we examine, however briefly, the obligation to evaluate health care.

Statistical Lives and Identified Lives

In the above definition of the primary purpose of medicine, we stated that in most encounters the primary purpose of medicine is to heal the particular patient. This is because the particular patient has been identified to the physician or health care specialist, and as a consequence the patient implicitly asserts a right to treatment against the physician. When the patient with the identified relationship asks for treatment, the worth of that individual as a human being requires the physician to act unless there are clear and compelling prohibitions. In this case, we have the moral claim of an identified life.

In the absence of such identified lives, however, the health care specialist, as noted above, has obligations to the general health and welfare of her patients and the society at large. As a member of a health care system, the specialist has responsibilities for the prevention of disease and the maintenance of health that can be discussed in terms of statistical lives. Public health programs save statistical lives by disease prevention. The people who do not get sick are never identified, but their health is just as real a product of the system as their illness would have been. This obligation is an obligation of the entire profession as a collectivity and not merely the obligation of particular practitioners.

THE HEALTH CARE PROFESSIONS

Membership in a profession or the adoption of the role of the practitioner of a profession brings with it obligations specific to that profession and role. In this chapter, we will seek to establish the nature of some of the key professions involved in health care and to specify the roles they play.

It should be noted that the roles defined are not uniformly delineated in all societies. Indeed, the roles change over time even in a given society. This should surprise no one, for the role assigned to the health care worker is influenced by the values of a given society as well as by the goals and aspirations of the profession. Soviet medicine, or socialist medicine, is more committed to the service of the collectivity rather than merely to the good of the individual. Medicine in the United States has always focused on the well-being of the individual rather than on the social good. American medicine, moreover, was in the Hippocratic tradition, which paternalistically saw the physician in charge of everything. Indeed, it is only in the 1980 version of The American Medical Society's *Principles of Medical Ethics* that there is a mention of patient's rights and societal obligations (Veatch, 1981a, p. 25). The patient's rights movement, with its insistence on liberty and equality in line with the Western liberal political tradition, has had much to do with this change. The changes are still going on, with the result that at present there are competing versions of the role of the physician. Parallel changes are occurring in the profession of nursing, as it seeks to define and obtain social acceptance of new and expanded roles for nurses. Here, too, there are competing models and so conflicts with what is ethical and what is not.

Models for Medicine

Veatch (1972) proposed four models for ethical medicine: (1) the engineering model; (2) the priestly model; (3) the collegial model; and (4) the contractual model. We add to this (5) the covenant model, proposed by Veatch in a later work (1981a) and developed by May (1983).

The *engineering model* makes the physician an applied scientist, if not a technician. Like the scientist, the technician, or the engineer, the physician in this model tends to be interested in the facts, not in values. In this model, the health care professional is liable to speak of treating a disease rather than taking care of a patient. Indeed, the ill person can disappear under the pile of supposedly objective test results.

While the experience of Nazi physicians acting as so-called scientists and technicians should have cured us of the temptation to follow this model, it has been encountered in some physicians who want to disregard the whole psychic and cultural dimension of illness in the interests of a truly scientific approach. All of us have seen this technical approach at its worst when health care professionals talk about the disease in front of the patient as if the patient were not there and were not suffering. It may even be that the increase in malpractice suits has been in part motivated by the impersonal treatment received from technicians who ignore the person behind the role of the patient.

Pellegrino (1979b) notes that the later versions of the American Medical Association code emphasize scientific competence and avoid the language of human commitment except as might appear in a formal legal contract. He even goes so far as to say that the code is tending in the direction of a craftsman's ethics. In short, the engineering model is still alive and well.

The ethical implications of such a model should be obvious. Such a model creates a temptation to act as if you were treating a disease rather than a person. The technical goal to be accomplished is liable to become the important thing no matter what the psychic and social costs to the patient. At times the effort to keep people alive in permanent vegetative states appears to be the rule with just such an emphasis on the technical possibilities.

Carlton's (1978) study of the socialization of young physicians has as its subtitle *The Primacy of Clinical Judgment over Moral Choice*. It showed that there is a narrowing of the physician's decision-making process, so that there are key human factors left out. In particular, the religious and value preferences tend to be neglected in favor of more technical considerations. Thus, there are at least elements of the engineering model in the training of physicians.

The *priestly model* is based on the fallacy of generalized expertise. That is to say, it assumes that since the physician is an expert in medicine, he or she is also an expert about life in general. The physician assumes a moral dominance over the patient. This leads to physicians who make pronouncements such as "that is a risk you should not take," or "your family should be your first consideration." The main principle of this model is the traditional one of "Benefit the patient and do no harm." Unfortunately, because the priestly physician treats the patient as a child, the traditional principle often neglects other principles, which command the physician to respect the freedom of the patient, to protect the patient's dignity, and to contribute to the good of society.

The ethical implications of this model will be seen constantly throughout the first part of this book as we discuss the conflict between the obligation to do good and the obligation to respect the autonomy of the patient.

The *collegial model* sees the physician and the patient as colleagues cooperating in pursuing the common goal, which may be the preservation of health, the curing of illness, or the easing of the pain of the dying, depending on the situation. Such a model demands confidence and trust from both parties in the relationship and calls for long continued conversation between the two so they are sure of the goal and are in agreement about the means.

Veatch is skeptical about this model being practical at this time, since ethnic, class, economic, and value differences between patient and physician make it hard to communicate, let alone arrive at a true relationship of equality implied in the idea of colleagueship. We would add to this the fact that a relationship with specialists is so brief that there is no time to establish the trust that is a key to the collegial model. At the same time, the relationship in this model can and does exist between many patients and their family physician.

The *contractual model* sees the relationship between the health care provider and the patient as a business relationship governed by a contract or a free agreement entered into for consideration, that is, for specified goods that are exchanged. In this model, contract law supplemented by particular health care laws would substitute for ethics. In a purely contractual relationship each encounter between provider and patient would in theory start out with negotiations about the conditions of sale and the warrantees expressed and implied. While there are some virtues in clarifying expectations, most providers and most patients want the relationship to be more than contractual in this sense. Indeed, with Pellegrino and Thomasma (1981), we insist that there are obligations that arise from roots deeper than the contract. As we insist throughout this work, ultimately it is the dignity of the individual human being that is the primary ethical consideration.

If the relationship were only contractual, it would place clear but minimal obligations on both the health care provider and the patient (May, 1983). These obligations would be specified by what is stated in the contract and the current legal interpretation of the language used. Beyond the contract, the health care provider would be under no obligation to the patient.

While there is certainly a strong contractual side to the role of the health care provider, there is something more. Membership in one of the healing professions has in the past entailed the profession of an ideal, and dedication to a noble task, that is not merely the result of a contract with individual patients. This fact, among others, has led May (1983) to develop a covenant model. Though inspired by the religious idea of the covenant between God and his chosen people, covenants do exist aside from a religious context.

The *covenant model* attempts to recognize those elements of the health care relationship that go beyond mere contract. In the covenant model, the dedication to an ideal and the privileges granted by society impose obligations on the physician and nurse quite aside from a contract. This becomes clear in emergencies when the health care provider must help even in the absence of a contract. The covenant also supposes a permanent relationship, or at least one open ended with regard to its duration. This aspect can be illustrated by the fact that a physician may not terminate a relationship at will, but must provide for the continuing care of a patient. The covenant relationship is also seen in the tradition that the physician or nurse had to provide at least some care on the basis of patient need, independent of ability to pay or of merit.

In ordinary dealings, the covenant relationship between provider and patient does not necessarily involve all the legalities of a formal contract, but does involve an agreement or understanding about the role of each participant. The physician, having made an effort to discover the values of the patient, respects those values, and if he cannot agree to act in accord with those values does not enter into any contract or further agreement. Once an agreement about these values and the goals of the relationship has been set, the patient agrees to follow the advice of the physician about the myriad details of the treatment.

Though there is a basis for a covenant relationship between physician and patient, in the United States today the relationship has a strong contractual aspect, which modifies and even dominates the idea of covenant. As we shall see in the coming chapters, the contractual elements demand that the physician and patient enter into more detailed agreements than the covenant relationship would demand. For example, the patient does not by the fact that she goes to a physician agree to follow the advice of the physician. All aspects of treatment except for the most trivial remain a subject for discussion and informed consent. In any event, the operative model often depends upon the exact nature and history of the relationship between physician and patient, as found in the contrasting relationships many have with their family physician as opposed to that with a surgeon or anesthesiologist. In short, it may depend upon the *practice role* as well as on the underlying idea of what a physician is. A surgeon who seldom maintains a continuing relationship with a patient is in a different practice role than a family doctor. Specialists and consultants have different practice roles, which make a difference in the relationship with the patient and so with what must be specifically worked out in the contract.

The contract model can be modified by some of the elements of the covenant relationship so that it does not involve all the legalities of a formal contract. The modified version centers on an agreement or understanding about the role of each participant and is reinforced by a contract, since it is not founded exclusively on mutual trust. The physician, having made an effort to discover the values of the patient, respects those values and if he cannot agree to act in accord with those values does not enter into the contract. Once there is agreement about these values, the goals of the relationship are set, a treatment is agreed on, and the patient agrees to follow the advice of the physician about the myriad details of treatment. In a covenant relationship, not as many details need to be worked out.

The contractual model as we have modified it here provides for a sharing of decision making and for cooperation in the therapeutic process. It is not necessarily based on complete trust, though such trust is desirable, but on agreement about the goals of the relationship and about the treatment in general. It respects the conscience of the physician and the rights of the patient. The importance of this will be apparent in Chapter Two on autonomy and in Chapter Three on benevolence and nonmaleficence.

This seems close to what many people want and, while not perfect as a model, appears to be a realistic step in the right direction. Its realism ultimately depends on the particular patient/provider relationship involved. When the patient and the physician have developed a clearly personal relationship in which each knows the other's values and they share a mutual trust, the collegial or the covenant model is certainly ideal. This should be the case with the family or primary care physician. In many settings where the patient meets the physician only once or twice for a very particular purpose, the contractual relationship would seem to be more suitable. This occurs in consultations with a specialist or in the transient relationship with a surgeon. The operative model, then, is dictated by the actual relationship.

The Family Physician and Others

Actually, what people are looking for and society needs may be the family physician. The American Academy of Family Physicians (Smith and Churchill, 1986, p. 17) has a definition of the family physician and primary care which deserves careful study. The family physician is educated and trained to develop and to bring in practice unique attitudes and skills which qualify her to provide continuing, comprehensive health maintenance and medical care to the entire family regardless of sex, age, or type of problem, be it biological, behavioral, or social. The physician serves as the patient's or family's advocate in all health-related matters, including the appropriate use of consultants and community resources.

In the first place, the family physician is dedicated to health maintenance as well as medical care. She is not dedicated to the simple prolongation of life. Equally important, because the relationship is to be continuing and comprehensive, it is possible and desirable for the family physician to develop a truly personal relationship with the patient in such a way that a collaborative and even collegial relationship develops. Longlasting relationships reduce the need for specific contractual provisions. This may not be possible for other specialties where the relationship is intermittent, often superficial, and confined to the area of specialization. While the definition may go too far in alleging competence in behavioral and social areas, it does recognize the holistic nature of the patient and the necessity of being attentive to these factors. In view of this, the family doctor has a role that is closer to the collegial model (though the temptation is to be paternalistic). Other specialists may also develop a collegial relationship, but it is more likely that they will be involved in a contractual relationship.

Emerging Models and Roles

While we still speak of a physician/patient relationship as being a personal and professional relationship, the rise of the physician as businessman and the hospital as business has created a new model with profound consequences for both health care and health care ethics. Health care providers are increasingly scrambling for customers, employing marketing strategies and attempting to increase their profits. While this may not have immediately changed the public image of doctors and hospitals, it does change the system. As Robin (1984) remarks, the new economic orientation plus the increase in the number of physicians creates a tendency to do more for each patient in order to keep up income. As we shall see in later chapters, it also creates a temptation to supply services because patients want them, even though the services are not therapeutic. That, we believe, can turn the physician into a tradesman or retailer.

We may also expect to see the bureaucratic employee model emerge. As the surplus of physicians becomes a reality and the for-profit sector of health care grows larger and larger, more and more physicians join nurses and physical therapists in the ranks of employees (Starr, 1982). This shift can be expected to produce changes in the roles of physicians. They too will face the problems of the bureaucratic model that nursing has had to cope with. In particular, they will enjoy less autonomy in the practice of medicine. They will, for example, find themselves under pressure to increase income and decrease costs (Mechanic, 1986). There will undoubtedly be more regulation of the pace and routines of work (Starr, 1982, p. 446). Most important of all, physicians may find themselves used as replaceable units in a service delivery system that allows less time for the personal relationship with the patient and so more of a temptation to act on the basis of the engineering model. One thing seems certain, employees in a bureaucracy will be under pressure to produce profits, and the health care provider will find himself caught between the ethic which says that the patient comes first and an "ethic" which replaces the patient with the bottom line of the annual report. At the very least there will be tension between the traditional advocacy of the particular patient and the duty to allocate resources in the interests of society and all patients.

Although this book operates on the basis of a more idealistic role for the physician, nurse, and health care institution, the reality of the marketplace and of changing American values will need to be taken into consideration. This will be particularly true when we consider the principle of justice and the problem of health care distribution in Chapter Four.

Different models, it is argued, fit different circumstances (Christie and Hofmaster, 1985, p. 20). This is particularly true with the patient who abdicates all responsibility and becomes completely passive when ill. At the very least we are dealing with a sort of contract in cases like this. We say a sort of contract since the patient has agreed to let the physician handle everything for a fee. Such passivity may cast doubts on the ability of the patient to enter into a contract. As does Hull (1985), we argue that such contracts should not be encouraged since the patient, as far as possible, has an obligation to be active in both decision making and in treatment.

On the other hand, when the patient is highly educated and independent, he or she may seek a more collegial model. In addition, in the case of primary care physicians or family practitioners, no matter what role they find themselves in, it should always have an advocacy dimension, since patients rely on their primary care physician to coordinate other health care providers and institutions in order to fulfill the purpose of the relationship (Smith and Churchill, 1986). Even this obvious obligation is not without its challengers. Post (1979) argues that in some medical centers the expanded house staffs have made the role of the physician of record superfluous. He goes on to explain how the family physician is moved out of the picture. This poses great ethical problems since the patient almost certainly does not know of this (MacIntyre, 1979; Orsher, 1979). At this point, we merely want to point up another problem in the area of role definitions and the obligations that flow from them.

Nursing Models

Nursing is an independent profession and has in concert with the government and the public developed its own roles and the obligations that flow from them. Indeed, nursing is striving to expand its roles, although it meets opposition from some other health care professionals. Nursing roles are in transition. During this transition, the problems inherent in the various nursing model roles are important not only in themselves, but because they indicate some of the problems that may arise for physicians when their independence is curtailed by their status as employees.

Smith (1980) proposed three models of nursing: the nurse as surrogate mother, the nurse as technician, and the nurse as contracted health care worker. Murphy and Howard's (1983) models are more useful in our present situation. They propose the bureaucratic model, the physician advocate model, and the patient advocate models.

The bureaucratic model expects the nurse to focus on the details of institutional coordination. In this model the nurse's responsibility to individual patients is limited and team work is emphasized. In this model the physician is the authority figure, and the nurse not only has obligations to the physician but may not go against the physician. Rapport among the team members takes precedence over responsibility to the patient's needs. Loyalty to authority is a prime virtue. Murphy notes that in this system the patient is supposed to be passive and make it easy for the professionals to do their job.

This first model, which ends up making the organization more important than the patient, is very common in practice, but it also constitutes a denial that nurses are professionals and loses sight of the purpose of health care. It leads to disrespect for patients. Although this disrespect is often covered over with a paternalism, it is still disrespect.

In the physician advocate model, the nurse is an extension of the physician, the physician's hand. The nurse is there to build up the physician and to inspire confidence in him. While this may, on the surface, make for a harmonious relationship, like the bureaucratic model, it makes the nurse less than a professional and leaves the patient without the nurse as a patient advocate who will put the interests of the patient first.

It should be noted that it was only in 1973 that the International Council of Nurses dropped from their code for nurses a provision that "The nurse is under an obligation to carry out the physician's orders intelligently and loyally." The American Medical Association's Judicial Council (AMA) went much further in April 1984, when it decreed that a nurse's disregard of a physician's order in emergencies should not be looked on as a breakdown in professional relationships. For all that, many still act as if the physician advocate model was in command.

The patient advocate model takes the nurse to be an independent though interdependent professional, and so with an ethic that cannot be dictated by others. The nurse must make her own decisions even though they are made in the context of the health care team. Ultimately, in this model, the nurse is to provide the best possible care for the patient even if that means going against the physician and the administration. The nurse's primary obligation is to the patient. This model rejects the charismatic authority of the physician as leader of the health care team. Indeed, proponents of this model argue that since the nurse has more contact with the patient, the nurse should be the leader of the team.

The nurse, like the physician, can have many practice roles inside a given model of nursing (Quinn and Smith, 1987). A nurse's practice role may be as staff nurse in a hospital, but it may also be that of a clinical specialist, community health practitioner, nurse midwife, or nurse anesthetist. Indeed, the practice roles of nurses keep increasing in number even as existing practice roles expand their scope. All of these factors will affect the relationship to the patient, the physician, and the various health agencies with which the nurse is associated.

These models and roles indicate that there can be ethical problems within health care based on a failure to agree about the roles to be played by physicians and nurses as well as other health care professionals. They also indicate that in nursing, as in medicine, changes are occurring. The same may be said of all other health care specialists who operate in the American system. Physical therapists, respiratory therapists, medical social workers, occupational therapists, and medical technicians all have roles to play, and those often changing roles have ethical implications.

The Patient's Role

Everything said thus far should indicate that we do not see the patient's role as the "sick role" (Ducanis and Golin, 1979). The sick role calls for the patient to be more or less passive and subordinate to the physician because there is a built-in institutional superiority. We believe that the role of the patient should be a more active one that respects equality of persons. All too often, health care providers succeed in forcing patients into the "sick role," but this does not mean it is right or even that it is good health care. We will, in fact, go on to argue that the patient should take the opportunity to evaluate the physician prior to any illness, and that the patient's choice of a physician is one of her key acts of autonomy.

In line with what has been said, we see the role of the patient or the patient's surrogate as that of a partner in health care or at least that of a contractor who gets to specify key conditions of the relationship. The exceptions that occur in emergencies are discussed in the next chapter.

Special Practice Roles and Special Relationships

All of the previous discussion of roles assumes that the relationship between health care professional and patient is a helping one. That is, we assumed that the health care professional is committed to acting in the interests of the patient. Normally, that is the case so that the assumption is very reasonable. We must, however, attend to those instances in which the professional is legitimately committed to the interests of a third party and so subordinates the interest of the patient to that third party. This subordination is even ethical so long as the patient has been properly informed and understands the relationship and the resulting subordination.

The commitment to third-party interests occurs in the case of company physicians, nurses, and physical and occupational therapists. The company physician who examines prospective employees is screening out people who are either unsuitable for a given job or who might raise a company's health insurance premiums because they belong to a high risk group. He is not committed to treat or even inform the prospective employee of the results of the examination. Similarly, a company nurse who treats an employee is not always bound by the usual confidentiality (Chapter Five) but must report the case to the employer for the protection of the employer. There is a special role and so special ethics in these cases.

Ethical Diversity and Health Care

The previous pages discuss the roles and goals of health care professionals in terms of the culture of the United States. It should be obvious, however, that other societies can and do define the roles and goals in different ways. The differences are not only a result of differences in philosophy and religious belief, but of the history of the professions in a particular culture. A belief in fate, for example, makes some cultures less liable to approve of aggressive intervention to save life. Some cultures are more insistent on equal treatment than others. The position of the family in general and health care in particular also varies and affects the ethics of familial relations. Veatch (1981a) gives excellent illustrations of all of this in his chapter, "Medical Ethical Theories Outside the Anglo-American West." These differences, of course, work their way out into important differences in practice. In Israel, for example, the decisions about caring for newborns is influenced both by a religious tradition that stresses the sanctity of life, by memories of the Holocaust, and by concerns about the population (Eidelman, 1986). In the United States, the tendency is to treat any baby who is potentially viable and continue until it is almost certain that it will die, while the British are more likely to start treatment and then stop it as soon as it appears there is extensive brain damage (Rhoden, 1986). While the culture should not be decisive, it is a factor that must be considered.

The diversity in cultural differences in health care ethics should make us particularly sensitive to the fact that the United States, as a pluralistic society in rapid change, presents particular problems. The discussion of ethics is always difficult in a pluralistic society which permits a wide diversity of opinion on every conceivable subject. The difficulties on the theoretical level are heightened when the society is debating the roles of professionals and the obligations that flow from those roles.

Because there is no complete agreement in America about the purpose of the health care professions and the role definitions of the various professions, health care ethics are often in turmoil. At the very least they are in transition as new roles emerge and society places new restrictions on and grants new privileges to health care providers. The authors have taken a stand on what the roles ought to be at the present time. This has been done to give some coherence to the treatment of health care ethics, but with an awareness that the debate is ongoing.

SUMMARY

The present book follows the approach of practical wisdom in which the individual person situated in a concrete community is the intrinsic good. All actions are judged to be good or evil in terms of their consequences for the individual person in that society. The practical wisdom of such an approach demands that all dimensions, individual and social, be considered in assessing consequences. Particular attention must be paid to impact on the persons and on society as a whole.

Although we follow a practical wisdom, rule consequentialist approach in which the rules are formed by consideration of the general consequences of various activities, we are conscience that changing circumstances change the consequences and so the rules. We are even willing to admit exceptions when the evidence in an individual case shows that the general consequences are not present and will not be increased by the exception.

Professional ethics and health care ethics in particular involve a specification of obligations in terms of the purpose of the profession as well as the general and particular practice role of a given health professional. The purpose and role are the result of agreement between the profession, patients, and society as a whole. The society part in this definition is influenced by philosophy, religion, history, and, in short, the entire culture of the society. In the United States, a pluralistic society in rapid change, the cultural factors are not always harmoniously integrated, so that there are many disputed areas in health care ethics.

NOTES

[1]It is useful to note that common sense and practical wisdom are not the same. "Common sense," or what people are accustomed to, rests largely on the comfort produced by existing practices rather than on critical thinking. Existing practices tend to be firmly ingrained because they have been developed over time and consequently are comfortable, both emotionally and intellectually. These practices are the basis of what might be called common sense, because most people in the society are accustomed to the set of practices and have their expectations and presumptions established by it. Practical wisdom has a much broader scope, requiring that "all things be considered and considered critically." Practical wisdom tries not to take things for granted but to examine them from all sides since every event is like a pebble thrown in a pond with tiny waves moving outward from the center. Even so, practical wisdom is not infallible, as we shall see when we examine the American health care delivery system.

[2]It is difficult to define a profession. It should be clear, however, that we are not talking of a professional as one who works for pay as opposed to an amateur or one who works out of love of the activity. A profession, however, does seem to involve the following elements: first, a dedication to a way of life; second, one which involves activities important to the functioning of society; third, one which puts service to society ahead of, or at least equal to personal gain. Traditionally, a profession also controlled entrance into its membership and set educational requirements. In addition, professions were supposed to have and enforce ethi-

cal codes on their membership. Perhaps there are no professions if all of these requirements must be fulfilled. More likely, however, there are various stages of professionalization. See Garrett (1963) pp. 159-162 on the idea of stages of professionalization and Baumrin and Freedman (1983) for various ideas on professions.

Chapter Two
PRINCIPLES OF AUTONOMY AND INFORMED CONSENT

GENERAL FORMULATION

The dignity of the person commands us to *respect individual persons*. In practice, respect for the dignity of the individual involves not only leaving people alone to make their own choices, but also recognizing that no individual has the right to touch another without consent. This means that *one human being, precisely as human, does not have authority and should not have power over another human being*. This means that individuals shall not coerce others or limit their activities or impose their will on others. Even society and its instrument, the government, must respect the freedom and privacy of individuals and can interfere only when it is necessary to protect others or for very serious and overriding social concerns.

We stress that since this respect for freedom and privacy is ultimately rooted in the dignity of each individual person, the principle of autonomy in this book also calls for respecting even those persons who are not at a given moment capable of free choice. In short, persons do not lose their dignity because they are unconscious or in a coma or out of contact with reality. Even the nonautonomous person is to be respected since persons are valuable in and of themselves and not because they are useful to society, or beautiful, or the right sex or color, or perfectly healthy, or have a high IQ. This is what we mean when we say that individual persons are intrinsically good, that is, good in and of themselves and not because the person is useful or has certain accidental qualities. The individual person, then, is not to be used as a thing or treated as if he or she were inferior.

Even society may limit human freedom for only the most serious and overriding social concerns, that is, for the protection of the dignity of other persons or for the continued existence of the society as the chief means to the protection of the individual. For example, the government would be correct in limiting our right to burn brush when there is a high danger of forest fires. Similarly, the society limits our freedom to spend our money as we please when it taxes us to pay for defense and necessary public services. Aside from that sort of limit or interference, the right of the individual to freedom from interference is, in the United States, protected by the Constitution and by strict rules about the procedures and rules which control any governmental limitation of freedom. Whether or not the government has a right to interfere to protect individuals from themselves is disputed. More will be said about this later in this chapter under the heading of paternalism and in Chapter Six on death and dying.

This respect for persons in general and their freedom in particular has consequences for all the professions. A little reflection will reveal the fact that neither lawyers, clergymen, teachers, doctors, or nurses have a right to interfere with individuals or force their opinions on them, or even to act on a person's behalf without permission. A physician, a nurse, or a nutritionist does not have the right to force treatment on a patient or to enforce good health habits on others. Nor do teachers have a right to drag anyone they please into class and attempt to teach them. Specialized knowledge, even a license to practice, does not authorize professionals to control any aspect of another's life or to limit the freedom of others. Society authorizes interference by professionals only rarely and generally only under court control. This is based not merely on respect for the free choice of competent people who are our moral equals, but on the idea that individuals do not automatically have authority over those who lack the capacity for free choice. This, then, brings us to the formulation of the medical version of the principle of autonomy or, more accurately, the principle of patient autonomy.

PATIENT AUTONOMY: INFORMED CONSENT

The health care formulation of the principle of autonomy can be expressed as follows: *You shall not treat a patient without the informed consent of the patient or his or her lawful surrogate, except in narrowly defined emergencies.* The principle clarifies the meaning of respect for the person and his or her freedom in the context of health care. It not only seeks to prevent medical tyranny and to preserve freedom, but also to encourage rational decision making by the patient, who in the last analysis must live with the consequences of medical treatment or the lack of it. In law this principle is connected with both the right of privacy (right to noninterference) and with the law on assault and battery, which forbids not only unwanted touches but even the expectation of an unwanted touch. In law, as in ethics, *informed consent* is a crucial concept in medical practice.

Informed Consent

The concept of informed consent is not only complicated and easily misunderstood, but relatively recent in American medical ethics. Indeed, many older health care professionals find it strange, since their tradition called not for informing the patient, but for concealing things from the patient. They did not seek to gain the consent of patients, but control of them. Hippocrates (after whom the Hippocratic Oath is named) would find the concept of informed consent particularly strange, for he felt that most things should be concealed from patients while caring for them and that, in particular, nothing was to be told the patients about their present or future condition.

The great Greek physician obviously did not believe that he needed the patient's consent. Those who use the priestly model of the physician discussed in the previous chapter will still tend to view the relationship to the patient in this paternalistic way. Those who follow the collegial model and see the patient as a full partner in the healing process understand that informed consent is not only an ethical necessity, but a necessary component of health care. Within the contract model, the informed consent is the act by which the contract is specified.

No matter what the health care professional's attitude, the law in the United States will insist on informed consent, especially if there are any invasive procedures such as those involved in surgery or treatments with considerable risks involved. In short, to disregard informed consent in the United States of America is to risk lawsuits. The law in other countries is different, but in the United States, at least since the 1960s, the law has tended to say that the role of health care professional requires respect for the freedom of the patient and, in particular, that this respect demands informed consent.

The Key Concepts

For informed consent by the patient or, when appropriate, by a lawful surrogate, the following conditions must be present: (1) The patient or appropriate surrogate must be competent or have decision-making capacity, that is, be capable of understanding the consequences of the consent and be free from coercion and undue influence that would substantially diminish freedom. (2) The health care professional, within the demands of their particular role, must have provided the necessary information and made sure that it was understood. In general, if any one of these conditions is not present, there is no patient informed consent and so no authorization of treatment. At times, the permission of a court is required before the patient can be treated. It must be stressed that the health care professional does not have a right to treat the patient who is incompetent because she is unconscious or drunk or severely retarded. Authorization based on informed consent is required. If there is no authorization, this generally means that the health care professional cannot proceed. The exceptions will be discussed after the conditions given above have been explained more fully.

Competence and Understanding

By competence we mean the ability to perform a certain task. In the context of health care ethics, we mean by competence the ability to make choices based on an understanding of the *relevant consequences* of that choice on oneself and others. The ability to understand the relevant is to be judged by common sense rather than a technical or professional standard. According to the common sense standard, the patient must be able to understand such things as the fact that he will die or get sicker without treatment, or that the treatment will be painful and mean being out of action for a number of weeks. The competent patient is not to be judged by his educational level, nor does the competent patient have to understand everything about the condition or the treatments proposed. Often even a highly trained specialist does not understand everything about a disease or a treatment. Indeed, the physician may not fully understand how a common drug like aspirin works. In any event, the *exact how* of the treatment is not always in itself ethically important, *whereas the consequences are crucial*. We are, then, speaking of substantial common sense and not complete medical or scientific understanding. More will be said of this below when we discuss what must be revealed to the patient.

The competent patient does have to understand the consequences of her decision to accept or reject a particular treatment. In particular, the patient should understand that she is authorizing or refusing to authorize treatment (Faden and Beauchamp, 1986). The effect of the treatment on the patient's health, life, lifestyle, religious beliefs, values, family, friends, and society are all factors that bear on the ethical decision to accept or reject treatment. So the patient must be capable of understanding consequences in these relevant areas.[1]

The fact that the patient makes a decision contrary to that recommended by the health care professional, or even contrary to the general norms of society, does not prove that he is incompetent because of a lack of understanding. The patient may prefer to suffer the pain from the disease rather than the pain from the treatment. The patient may prefer to die rather than put the family through a long agony that leaves them penniless as well as emotionally drained. This is an important point, since health care providers, like all human beings, must resist the temptation to impose their values on others. Worse yet, the health care provider may forget that medical values, and even the value of health and life, are not the only valid values in ethical decision making. Neither medical school nor doctoral programs in nursing certifies a person as wise enough to make decisions for other human beings regarding the relative value of such consequences.

Most of this is neatly summarized in the following statement from a publication of the American Hospital Association (1985, p.9):

Decision making capacity is the patient's ability to make choices that reflect an understanding and appreciation of the nature and consequences of one's actions and of alternative actions, and to evaluate them in relation to person's preferences and priorities. A patient's decision contrary to a physician's recommendation does not in itself indicate incapacity.

Classifying the Incompetent

There are no handy labels that can be used to classify those who are incompetent to understand the consequences of their decisions. Each case is to be judged individually. Many children will be found to be competent from an ethical point of view even though they may not be legally competent. Someone below the age of 18 is not legally competent in most areas, but she can well be ethically competent to judge the consequences. People who have been legally declared incompetent to manage their financial affairs or who have been involuntarily committed to a mental institution might still be ethically competent to make a decision about accepting treatment. Many people who have been classified as "retarded" are quite capable of understanding that they will be in pain if they refuse treatment or in pain if they accept treatment. Even people who have been declared legally incompetent to administer their financial affairs or who have been involuntarily committed to mental institutions can still understand the consequences of their health care decisions. Health care professionals cannot ethically treat such persons against their will unless the courts have appointed a guardian specifically for decisions about treatment. The permission of a parent may protect the health care provider legally in these cases, but when the child is judged competent, the health care professional still has the ethical problem and the need for informed consent. We shall say more about this problem when we discuss surrogates.

Unconscious people are temporarily incompetent. People under the influence of alcohol or drugs may, to a greater or lesser extent, be temporarily incompetent. Some few patients have so permanently lost contact with reality that they may be incapable of understanding any ordinary consequences of their actions. In general, however, the assumption is that adults are competent unless there is clear evidence to the contrary. The publication of the American Hospital Association (1985, p.10) puts it very clearly:

> In the absence of indicators to the contrary, hospitals and health care professionals should assume that the adult patient has adequate decision making capacity.

There are, of course, cases in which the person is incompetent or temporarily incompetent. Residents of long term care facilities who are often labeled "pleasantly confused" are probably incompetent, though they may have lucid moments or days in which their ability to assent or dissent must be respected. On the whole, however, the "pleasantly confused" need a surrogate to consent for them. When there are none of the usual surrogates, a guardian needs to be appointed. A surrogate or a guardian alone may suffice for informed consent, but not for the broader tasks of protecting these patients. We shall return to the problem of advocacy and protection of patients in the next chapter.

Competency and Freedom

Competence requires not only the ability to understand the consequences of one's decisions, but freedom from coercion and such undue influence that would substantially diminish the freedom of the patient. There is not only a question of coercion, undue manipulation, or ordinary persuasion (Fadden and Beauchamp, 1986, p.337), but also of natural reactions to illness and normal circumstances of health care. High fevers and some drugs can leave anyone temporarily incapable of understanding anything.

Coercion may be seen in the use of force or of drugs equivalent to force. These will invalidate any consent. More often, however, the problem is not one of force but of undue influence. Physicians who threaten patients with the withholding of treatment in the future, unless the patient consents here and now, are guilty not only of blackmail but of invalidating the consent obtained. Although such cases exist, they are not the common source of undue influence. Family pressures may constitute undue influence and substantially reduce freedom. The sick person is often dependent on his family and so susceptible to their pressure that he cannot envisage bucking the relatives. This pressure is particularly great on children who are completely dependent on their parents.

Not only outside pressures but normal and natural factors can strongly affect our freedom. All the strong feelings that accompany a serious illness or a stay in the hospital will also have their impact. The exaggerated fears of the timid and the magical hopes of the desperate both distort understanding and affect competence. In addition, the influence of the unconscious and the individual's personal history also affect the decision-making process. These factors do not, however, take away the ability to understand the consequences of one's actions or constitute undue influence or coercion.

It is obvious that no one is ever completely free. The question the health care professional must answer is whether any of these influences, external or natural, substantially diminish the person's freedom so that there is inadequate capacity for a valid consent.

There is, of course, no easy answer to that question. The evidence of competence or incompetence should be obtained by reflective conversations between physician and patient in which the physician is aware of her own biases as well as the those of the patient (Katz, 1984, p.133). In short, the physician and all health care providers are obliged to spend time getting to know the patient and in ascertaining the state of the patient's mind and understanding. We would with Katz stress that "short of substantial evidence of incompetence, choices deserve to be honored."

The Information in Informed Consent

In this context, it should be noted that we are dealing with the need for an explicit consent. The mere fact that a patient seeks the assistance of a health care professional or enters a hospital does not constitute even implicit consent in all cases. In minor matters, however, implicit consent may be present and suffice for the purpose of informed consent. Thus, a patient who goes voluntarily to a hospital grants implicit consent for a temperature and blood pressure reading. Since nothing is at stake, this is sufficient. The patient by the mere fact of entering the hospital does not give implicit consent for intrusive procedures such as the taking of blood or the administration of an enema, let alone for an operation. When any real danger or an invasive procedure is involved, the patient needs to know what is being proposed and what the consequences might be. An explicit consent should then be given. In any event, it should be kept firmly in mind that even implicit consent can be revoked. The patient has the right to refuse to have his blood pressure taken, even though he has already submitted to the procedure a dozen times.

If the patient is to make a mature free choice with an understanding of the consequences, the health care professional and the physician in particular must provide information about those consequences. The type and extent of the information to be given depends on the criteria for disclosure. There are four conflicting rules or criteria for the disclosure of information to the patient: (a) The patient preference rule; (b) the professional custom rule, (c) the prudent person rule, and (d) the subjective substantial disclosure rule.

The *patient preference rule* dictates that the health care professional tell the patient what the patient wants to know. This rule does not make much sense. Some patients will want a lot more information than they need and can end up wasting time. Others will want no information and so avoid their own responsibility for decisions affecting their health and life. More often than not patients will not even express a desire for information. Many patients do not know that they have a right and duty to ask for information. No matter what the cause of a patient refusing information or at least not demanding it, patients will end up with inadequate data for a decision. In short, such a rule does not promote autonomy and so is not truly respectful of the patient.

VanDeVeer (1986) defends the idea that the competent patient can delegate the physician to make medical choices about specific forms of treatment under one condition: it is clear that the patient has merely delegated his right to make informed choices *about the manner of treatment and not about whether or not he will be treated in the first place.* The authors feel that, in general, this absolves the patient from too much responsibility. It makes sense, however, when the patient has a personal relationship with a health care provider who fully understands the values and desires of the patient. If such a relation exists, the physician *may* know enough to act in accord with the values of the patient. In addition, in such a relationship, the patient *may* also have enough experience with the health care professional that there are specific and individual grounds for trust in this person. These conditions, of course, are not to be assumed but to be established.

The *professional custom rule,* also called the professional community standard, says that the health care professional shall tell the patient what is normally or customarily told patients in similar situations. For a long time this was the operative rule. It is still the rule used by many physicians. There are two major objections to this rule.

First, it leaves the health care professional free to abrogate the rights of the patient by suppressing very relevant information. Such suppression can be the worst sort of manipulation, even though it is intended for the good of the patient. Indeed, in some cases it was customary to suppress information that might cause the patient to refuse treatment. One study (Rosoff, 1981, p.326) notes that as many as 50 percent of the patients would have refused treatment if the potential complications had been revealed to them. As we shall see when we discuss the so-called therapeutic privilege, that motive for suppressing information is neither ethical nor legal. Secondly, research indicates (Rosoff, 1981, pp. 313–457) that the professional custom is a myth. In other words, there is no such thing as a professional standard. In practice, then, the rule means the physician is using her own bias or ignorance as the standard.

The *prudent person rule,* also called the reasonable patient standard, rests on the assumption that the physician's disclosure to the patient should be measured by the patient's need for information material to the decision to refuse or accept treatment. Thus the rule would have the health care professional provide the information that a prudent, reasonable person would want before making a decision about treatment or the refusal of treatment. In practice, this is generally understood to include the first six items below (Rosoff, 1981, p. 318). We have added a seventh, since a reasonable person will want to consider those factors as well.

1. The diagnosis.
2. The nature and purpose of the proposed treatment.
3. The known risks and consequences of the proposed treatment, excluding those eventualities that are too remote and improbable to bear significantly on the decision process of a reasonable person or are too well known to require statement.
4. The benefits to be expected from the proposed treatment, with an assessment of the likelihood that the benefits can be realized.
5. All alternative treatments that might reasonably be used. All the information mentioned in three and four above is to be given about the alternatives as well.
6. The prognosis if no treatment is given.
7. All costs, including the amount and duration of the pain generally involved; the potential impact on lifestyle and ability to resume work, as well as the economic costs of both the treatment and the aftercare. The patient should also be told if insurance will cover the bills.

The *subjective substantial disclosure rule* (Faden and Beauchamp, 1986) calls for the health care professional to describe to the patient everything that would be material or important to the particular patient and not merely to a fictional reasonable and prudent person as he makes the decision. A factor would be material or important if it could change the decision of that particular patient. This rule brings in the subjective and objective factors important to the individual patient and not merely those important to a hypothetical objective prudent person. The application of this rule demands that the health care professional really get to know the patient and ascertain what is important to him. This in turn calls for real dialogue between patient and professional or between surrogate and professional.

We favor a combination of the prudent person and substantial disclosure rules since together they best assure that the particular patient will have the information needed for a sound decision from the patient's point of view. Thus, the patient should be informed of all the things a prudent person would want to know, plus the things that are of importance to this particular patient.

In this context it should be pointed out that the consent forms used in many hospitals do not provide the information required by any of these principles. They are too close to blank checks to have any moral or ethical value. In the authors' opinion, they do not suffice as ethical authorization of treatment even though the law may give them some weight.

Making the Information Understandable

Since the purpose of the information is to enable the patient or the surrogate to make choices based on an understanding of the consequences, there is an obligation to present the information in such a way that the patient or surrogate understands the consequences. In short, the obligation to obtain informed consent before proceeding involves an *obligation to actually communicate and not merely an obligation to spout facts*. A recital of all the technical details and the use of technical language may not only fail to increase comprehension, but may actually destroy understanding. The mere fact that a patient has signed a consent form saying she has been told the fact does not mean that informed consent has been obtained. To be content with a mere recitation of the facts and the signing of a form makes a mockery of the patient. Even when the law accepts such forms as proof of informed consent, ethics demands that the health care professional make sure the patient understands the consequences in terms of the things that are important to the patient. If there is no understanding, there is no agreement and so no authorization to proceed.

Difficulties with Informing the Patient

We have already spoken of the obstacles to effective communication with the patient. At this point, it is necessary to mention a very real professional problem that occurs both because of the nature of medical knowledge and the emotional blocks of health care professionals.

While medicine speaks of itself as being scientific, the knowledge in the field is anything but certain (Bursztajn et al., 1981; Duncan and Weston-Smith, 1984). To a very large extent, the health care professional knows only the general probabilities for classes of patients. When it comes time to apply those probabilities to individual patients, the probabilities lose much of their predictive value. That is to say that the odds that a cure will result or that a certain side effect will occur are largely unknown in the case of a particular patient.

There may be difficulty in deciding how much of the health care professional's uncertainty should be shared with the patient (Gorovitz, 1982). This is an emotional problem for the physician, the nurse, the physical therapist, or any member of the health care team, since sharing uncertainty may take away some of the professional mystique as well as upset the patient who may want assurance. Though too much uncertainty can paralyze the ability to act, the refusal to face uncertainty and ignorance has sometimes led to irresponsible treatments (Katz, 1984). In other cases certainty is purely subjective, a result of the physician's personal preference rather than of scientific research. It can be argued that sharing the uncertainty can ultimately build trust and that in any event the failure to share uncertainty is inimical to shared decision making between physician and patient. Informed consent calls for just that sort of sharing. Ethically, then, the difficulties of sharing uncertainty must be faced by the health care professional.

Is Informed Consent Possible?

All the difficulties and distinctions made thus far can call into question the very possibility of informed consent. If we add to this that the health care professional is often an authority figure with power and the patient a more or less powerless individual under great stress, the question of the possibility becomes more serious. Before attempting to answer the question of the possibility of informed consent, let us first clarify the point at issue.

Informed consent does not demand full freedom of choice. Indeed, few human acts are ever fully free, and certainly no human acts are made without the influence of many factors. Second, though impartial presentation of the facts and perfect understanding of the consequences is the ideal, this ideal is seldom reached. People under stress, both patients and health care professionals, operate at less than optimum rationality. It follows, then, that a perfectly informed consent is impossible.

If one assumes that perfectly informed consent is perfectly rational, that is, objectively and unemotionally derived from certain premises in the manner of geometry, then a perfect informed consent is not desirable. Ethics is concerned with good and evil. Of necessity, then, it is bound up with love, fear, hate, ideals, ambitions, and so with the emotions. In such situations, the ethical health care professional will be trying to persuade the patient even as he provides information as honestly as possible. The concern and convictions of the health care provider are important and need not be suppressed, only controlled. On the other hand, the fears and ideals of the patient need to be respected since they are connected with the patient's values and history and are not merely annoying obstacles to communication.

Therapeutic Privilege

Physicians have long claimed, and the law has often recognized, an exception called the therapeutic privilege (Rosovsky, 1984, pp. 98–102). *Therapeutic privilege*

is the privilege of withholding information from the patient when the physician believes the disclosure will have an adverse effect on the patient's condition or health.
Even those who justify the privilege limit it by placing three conditions on its use. First, the actual use of the privilege must not be based on generalities but on the actual circumstances of a particular patient. That is, it must be used on a case-by-case basis. Second, the physician must have a founded belief based on an intimate knowledge of the person that the full disclosure will have a *significantly adverse effect* on the patient. The mere fact that the patient will be disturbed by bad news is not a sufficient justification for the use of the privilege. Third, reasonable discretion must be used in the manner and extent of the disclosure. The physician may not be justified in concealing all the information. For example, though a physician might argue that even the word "cancer" would seriously harm the patient and justify concealing the diagnosis, this would not justify concealing the fact that the treatment was extremely painful. The same general principles apply to all health care professionals, though it is not clear that the law will protect them.

According to Rosovsky (1984, p.101), the privilege cannot be legally used in a case where the reason for withholding the information is the belief that the patient will refuse treatment if told the whole story. In short, the privilege does not justify denying a person the ability to choose just because one suspects the patient might choose differently than the physician. Rosovsky also notes that the privilege is not a justification of the misrepresentation of significant facts or fraud or willful misrepresentation. It is one thing to withhold information, another to deceive the patient. There will be additional discussion of the problem of deception in Chapter Six on confidentiality and truthfulness.

While the therapeutic privilege may sound reasonable enough at first glance, there are two serious problems with it. In the first place, research fails to find cases where the disclosure of information has a significant adverse effect on the patient's condition or health. In the second place, it is a denial of patient autonomy.

Exceptions in Emergencies

The obligation to obtain informed consent before proceeding to treat a patient included an emergency exception in its very statement. For there to be an emergency justifying treatment without informed consent, three conditions must be present (Rosoff, 1981, p.14).

1. The patient must be incapable of giving consent and no lawful surrogate is available to give the consent.
2. There is danger to *life or danger of a serious impairment of health.*
3. *Immediate* treatment is necessary to avert those dangers.

The authors believe that from an ethical perspective the first condition should be modified to include the words "and the wishes of the patient are not known." If the wishes of the patient are known, if there is a living will or a clear directive beforehand, the fact of incompetence does not destroy the wishes of the patient. Both the surrogate and the health care professional should follow those known wishes, since one is not dealing with a narrowly defined emergency.

While the authors' clear support of advanced directives is not universally accepted, we base our support on two basic ideas. First, health care professionals need informed consent in order to lay hands on the patient. This consent is not to be presumed when the patient has given advanced directives to the contrary. Second, the authors' basic stand on the relation of the individual and society demands the principle enunciated by the New Jersey Supreme Court in the *Jobes*[2] and related cases. This principle stressed the general primacy of the right to self determination over the state's countervailing interests. Exceptions to that general rule should be determined by the legislature or the courts since only the society is competent to decide when its interests are preeminent.

A careful look at these conditions will indicate that most visits to a hospital emergency room do not involve the sort of emergency that justifies treating without a consent. There are many so-called emergencies where treatment can be delayed (without danger to life or a risk of serious impairment of health) until the person regains consciousness or until a surrogate can be reached.

This narrowly defined emergency exception is justified on the ground that consent can be safely assumed in such cases where a reasonable person who accepted the ordinary community view of things would consent if properly informed. This is a reasonable assumption and is probably verifiable in the vast majority of emergencies in this narrowly defined sense. Thus, no one raises serious questions about the use of the exception. The question of whether similar assumptions hold when the person is of doubtful competence and in a nonemergency situation requires separate consideration.

Exceptions in Nonemergencies

In line with what has already been said, the following statements can be made. If the person is competent and refuses treatment, there should be no treatment in either emergencies or nonemergencies. If the patient is doubtfully competent and refuses treatment in a nonemergency, the benefit of the doubt goes to the patient, unless the health care provider seeks and obtains a court order. Problems arise, however, with clearly incompetent persons in nonemergency situations.

We must at the very start recognize that there is a temptation to justify treatment of the incompetent patient, because any decent human being, especially one dedicated to the healing arts, finds it difficult to stand by and let another suffer when something could be done. The emotions seem to dictate that the principle of benevolence—"do good" (see Chapter Three)—should take precedence over the principle of autonomy and the necessity for informed consent. The traditional medical ethics based on the priestly model certainly gave benevolence the first place over autonomy. That this is the correct answer is not clear either legally or ethically. Some law courts have held that a physician can treat without consent not only when there is serious danger to life or health, but when it is necessary to relieve great pain and suffering (Rosoff, 1981, p.16), but that appears to be the exception today. Indeed, Rosovsky (1984, p.90) simply states that "when patients are incapacitated but do not require life or health saving treatment, practitioners cannot proceed." Legally, then, the health care provider generally proceeds at his or her own risk when they treat incompetent or doubtfully competent persons in nonemergency situations.

Ethically, it remains questionable that the mere fact that it is possible to do some good *authorizes* a person to treat a incompetent or doubtfully competent person when no surrogate is present to give or refuse a consent. At this point, basic attitudes towards life and one's neighbor enter into the picture. On the one side are those who believe that they are their brothers' keepers and see the possible good as justifying intervention. On the other side are those who, like the authors, hold that we are *not* our brothers' keepers and so permit no additional exceptions to the need for informed consent.

The position of the authors can be stated very simply. As a rule, one individual does not have authority over another. If the health care professional feels she must act in nonemergencies when (a) competency is nonexistent or doubtful or (b) there is no advanced directive such as a living will (see Chapter Six for living wills), the legal system should be used to get a guardian who can give a consent. In short, the freedom of individuals should have the protection of due process and the law even in health care settings.

When In Doubt There Are Courts

In the discussion above it is assumed that there were no surrogates available to give or refuse consent for the incompetent or doubtfully competent person. In serious nonemergencies it is always possible to seek the help of the courts which can, on brief investigation, appoint a guardian *ad litem,* that is, a guardian for this specific instance. That court-appointed guardian is, then, the lawful surrogate who can give or refuse treatment in line with the best interests of the patient or the rational choice principle. This procedure can also be used when the health care provider thinks that the surrogates are not acting in the best interests of the patient. In any event such recourse to the courts protects the health care providers from lawsuits even as it keeps them from assuming unjustified authority over patients.

The courts are not the ideal way to make decisions, for the intrusion of the legal system into patient care can be cumbersome, expensive, and insensitive. But in the absence of patient competency, proper surrogates, or clear legislative directions, societal protection of rights through the courts is both necessary and appropriate. Even The American Hospital Association (1985, p.13) suggests that the courts should be consulted in the following five cases:

1. The incapacity is great and likely to be prolonged and there is no obvious surrogate.
2. The capacity of the patient is questionable and the decision to be made is significant.
3. The views of the surrogate are strongly at variance with the medical judgment or the patient's known views.

4. The choice of the individual to serve as surrogate is controversial and all efforts to resolve the matter at the hospital level have failed.

5. Family members radically disagree about the course of action in the case of a patient who lacks adequate decision-making capacity.

While no one wants the courts to practice medicine, it is clear that the suggestions given by the American Hospital Association recognize that human rights and not merely health care are involved. The courts are rightfully concerned with human rights.

The Consent of Children and Adolescents

There is not enough time in an introductory text to treat all the problems involved in the ethics of consent of children and adolescents. Interested parties should consult Morrissey et al. (1986). His treatment of the law in this area also raises the key ethical questions. It is important to recognize that the ability of the child or adolescent to consent depends on both actual and legal status and the need of the patient, that is, the seriousness and nature of the health problem. Moreover, since society does not appear to have a uniform outlook on the matter, no easy solution is possible. The law, whether in statutes or court decisions, gives social specification of rights and obligations. Unfortunately, in the case of the health care for children, the law is a blend of older theories, which gave preference to the rights of parents, and later theories, which gave first place to the child's welfare and more recently to the rights of the child.

The Role of Institutional Ethics Committees

In some cases, Institutional Ethics Committees (IECs) are now consulted in cases where surrogates are involved. Institutional Ethics Committees are multidisciplinary groups of health care professionals, frequently with community representatives set up in health care institutions to educate about biomedical ethics, to help in policy development and to act as consultants in difficult cases (Gibson and Kushner, 1986). The consultation function is controversial since in some cases it has led to the committee making decisions or unduly influencing decisions that are more properly the province of the patient, the surrogate, or the individual health care professional (Siegler, 1986). In addition, although the legal status of these committees is not at all clear (Wolf, 1986), some writers (Lo, 1987) feel that the courts will respect committee recommendations.

The 1986 New York State Task Force on Life and Law proposes using the ethics committee rather than the courts in resolving conflicts and dilemmas about patient care. This would make the committee into a mediator. While this sounds admirable, the following cautions seem in order (Lo, 1987). First, since the goals of the committee are not always clear, some committees dominated by health care professionals might end up confirming prognoses, providing emotional support for health care professionals or reducing legal liability rather than protecting the rights of patients. Second, many committees limit participation by patients and families so that the most important actors in the ethical drama are left out. Indeed, many committees have no nurses on them, even though nurses are the profession most in contact with patients and their families. If, in addition, the committee is loaded with physicians, the mediations and recommendations may reflect the value of the medical profession rather than the values of the patients. Finally, the tendency of some committees to operate in secrecy, to omit recommendations and reasoning in the medical record, as well as refusing to permit review of their recommendations, casts doubt on the integrity of some committees.

The Hasting Center *Guidelines* (1987) contain a valuable section on ethics committees. In its treatment of review of ongoing cases (prospective review), the *Guidelines* stress points that, as a matter of policy and sound ethics, should be made clear to patients and surrogates. Among other questions that demand clear answers are the following:

1. Is consultation of the committee optional?
2. Are recommendations merely advisory?
3. Must the patient or surrogate consent to a committee review?
4. Does the committee consider only ethical problems?
5. What constitutes a quorum of the committee?
6. Do recommendations require a consensus?
7. Will a written record be kept in the patient's record?

Every one of those questions demands serious thought since it involves an ethical issue. Since we do not have easy answers to the questions, it should be clear why the ethics of the Institutional Ethics Committee are still being debated. Only experience and time will allow us to form a final judgment about their utility and the ethicality of particular features of the committees.

Despite the problems, the authors would like to insist on three points. First, from an ethical point of view it seems clear that the IEC is not a surrogate and so is not authorized to make decisions for incompetent patients or their surrogates. Only the law can give such authorization. Second, even though the IEC is not a surrogate, when consulting on ongoing cases, the Ethics Committee can and should act primarily as a guardian of patient's rights. Third, the functions of the committee should be clearly and publicly announced and its recommendations and decisions open to review.

PATERNALISM: WEAK AND STRONG

The conflict between respect for autonomy and the desire to help the patient brings us to the problem of paternalism. The word paternalism is derived from the Latin word *pater*, meaning "father." In its dictionary meaning it refers to a ruling or controlling of others in a way that suggests a father's relationship with his children. In the context of health care ethics, paternalism involves acting without consent, or even overriding a person's wishes, wants or actions, in order to benefit the patient or at least to prevent harm to the patient. There are two elements here: first, the absence of consent or even the overriding of consent, and second, the beneficent motive (the welfare of the patient).

It is not paternalism when the health care provider acts to prevent the patient from causing serious injury to others. This is a delegated exercise of the police power of the state and is authorized by law. There is also no question of paternalism if the health care professional overrules the patient for the convenience or profit of the provider. The nurse who in a desire to finish her charting gives a painful treatment before a narcotic has taken effect is not being paternalistic. Such cases constitute pure tyranny. Nor is there any paternalism if the health care professional refuses to go along with the patient's wishes because these wishes are against the conscience or professional standards of the provider. In this case, the professional is acting for the sake of his own conscience and not specifically for the welfare of the patient. In any event, the health care professional is not the mere servant of the patient.

Paternalism exists, however, when the health care worker intervenes to prevent patients from harming themselves in some serious way. This paternalism is authorized by law in the case of those attempting suicide. Whether it is ethical depends not only on the factors discussed in this chapter but on deeper issues of life and death, which will be discussed in Chapter Six on death and dying.

It is useful to distinguish between strong (also called extended) paternalism, which attempts to overrule or override *the wishes of a competent person,* and weak (or limited and restricted) paternalism, in which consent is missing or the health care provider overrules or overrides the wishes of an incompetent or a doubtfully competent patient. Weak paternalism is sometimes called cooperative paternalism when one of its purposes is to restore the person's competence so that the patient may give informed consent.

Strong paternalism involves the usurpation, that is, the coercive seizure, of the patient's right to make decisions. As noted at the beginning of this chapter, even the government does not have the right to overrule its citizens except when necessary to protect the rights of others or when there is an overriding state interest.

In practice, many governments, even the United States, practice paternalism. Strong paternalism on the part of the government is justified only for the promotion of substantial state interests and the protection of the rights of others.

The government more frequently engages in weak paternalism, although the justice of this is debatable. The law does recognize the right of parents over their children on the assumption that the children are not fully competent, although the extent of even the parent's right to be paternalistic is debated (Aiken and LaFollette, 1980). Also, most states authorize involuntary commitment to a mental institution of a mentally ill person whose actions are dangerous to himself (Beis, 1984, pp.114-135). If we make the judgment that mental illness is an indication of doubt about competency to give informed consent, this is a form of weak rather than strong paternalism.

Even so, this weak paternalism is surrounded by all sorts of legal protections including the right to counsel.

The government, however, *has not authorized health care providers to use strong paternalism* and appears to authorize weak paternalism in only a limited number of cases.

From an ethical point of view, writers generally reject the right of health care providers to use strong paternalism. Quite aside from the fundamental issue of authority over others, there is a basic question of the competence of an individual to decide what is best for another person and, in particular, for a competent adult. The competence to make such decisions would require both a knowledge of the other person's values and of all the factors influencing their lives. Health care providers and patients do not necessarily share the same values. The health care professional, for example, may believe that life is precious no matter what. That patient may believe that life without the ability to move about is meaningless. Health care professionals certainly do not have the right to enforce value judgments on the patient on the grounds that "doctor knows best." Finally, it would be a rare health care professional who knew all the factors influencing the life of a patient. In short, the professionals lack the competence to decide what is best for another and so have no right to use strong paternalism.

Sometimes those who justify strong paternalism in health care act as if there were only one correct decision in every case. It is well to remind ourselves that there is often more than one good decision possible, especially when we are operating not in a world of certainty but in one where probabilities are often all we have to go on. Most of all we must stress the fact that decisions about health, life, and death are not merely medical decisions but involve the good of society and the good of third parties, as well as the values of the patient. While the health care provider is competent to give advice about the medical aspects and even give the medical odds, the patient has the right and obligation to make the decision and to place his bets.

While it appears impossible to justify strong paternalism in the health care setting, the problem of weak paternalism remains. As we noted above in the discussion of exceptions in nonemergency situations, the courts have sometimes allowed treatment without informed consent to relieve serious pain or suffering. To the extent that this treatment will remove doubts about the competency of the person and allow informed consent, we tend to think it is justified. Here the treatment is directly in the service of autonomy.

Another example of weak paternalism may be found in the use of restraints. In the hospital setting the temporary use of restraints is often justified on the grounds that the patient is confused, disoriented, and so liable to injure herself. Hospitals recognize the dangers of this policy and typically surround the use of restraints with various safeguards, such as periodic visits to the patient, approval of supervisors or the physician if the restraints are to be used over a long period of time, and a written justification of their use. Granted all the proper institutional safeguards, restraints may be justified by weak paternalism.

The problem of paternalism is even more complicated in the mental health setting. The American Psychiatric Association urges that law permit at least a short period of involuntary confinement and treatment if *all four of the following conditions are present*. First, there must be evidence that the person's mental illness is treatable and the treatment is available. Second, the person must be obviously so mentally ill that he is incompetent to make medical decisions. Third, there must be clear evidence of mental deterioration such as delusions or hallucinations. Fourth, the person must obviously be suffering.

While the authors are not completely at ease with this approach, it is a genuine example of weak paternalism and would appear ethically justified as long as there are time limits put on the involuntary hospitalization. Although we admit that there are cases where weak paternalism is justified, we insist that there is *no general authorization* for even weak paternalism.[3] Each case needs to be studied carefully, and the exceptions should be made with regret.

The principle of autonomy and its relationship to paternalism cannot be fully understood until we have studied the principle of benevolence. We note that the struggle between paternalists and those who put autonomy in the first place is a struggle about whether benevolence or autonomy is primary. This will appear more clearly after the consideration of benevolence in the following chapter.[4]

Surrogates

The previous section made it quite clear that surrogates are important in health care ethics. Surrogates or substitutes are people who are authorized by law or custom to make decisions when the patient is incompetent or doubtfully competent. There is, however, no handy list of surrogates that can be relied on with certitude. Ordinarily, parents are considered surrogates for their minor children, spouses for one another, adult children for parents, when parents are lacking, grandparents for grandchildren, and, when sons and daughters are lacking, adult grandchildren for grandparents, not to mention brothers and sisters as well as uncles and aunts. In our society, the surrogates pretty well follow the kinship lines *on the assumption* that these relatives are liable to know the values if not the desires of the patient and can at least be trusted to act in the best interests of the patient.

Assumptions, however, yield to the facts. In many cases health care providers will find themselves caught in a cross fire between two or more potential surrogates. The father of the child may consent to treatment while the mother refuses. The wife may say yes while the brothers and sisters of the patient shout no. Equally difficult is the situation where the provider suspects a conflict between the interests of the patient and the interests of the surrogate. For example, the surrogate may want the patient to die in order to make life simpler even though the patient could still have a reasonable life if treated. As noted in the previous section, the health care professional may know that what the patient desired when competent is at odds with the decision of the surrogate. The patient may have expressed a desire to have life-saving measures omitted when he becomes terminal, while the spouse may want heroic if futile measures continued.

In all of these cases the health care professional must proceed with caution and be ready to seek court intervention when the desire of the patient or the patient's apparent best interests are being neglected. In short, surrogates do not and should not always have the last word.

Who Shall Inform the Patient or the Surrogate?

Most writers on medical ethics assume that the physician has the obligation to inform the patient or surrogate. There is no doubt that the physician has the primary and principal obligation to inform. Other health care providers, especially those who, like nurses and physical therapists, are legally independent practitioners, also have obligations in this area. Finally, hospitals and other health care institutions would appear to have at least supervisory responsibility to make sure that their employees have informed the patient when it is their duty to do so (Annas, 1981).

One of the roots of the obligation of informed consent is the legal idea that an unwanted touch is a battery. As a result, everyone who touches the patient needs the patient's informed consent (Graber, 1985). While it may be assumed that the signature on a consent form gives consent or that the physician has gotten such consent for treatment, nurses, physical therapists, medical technicians, and respiratory therapists will encounter cases where this is obviously not true. When the patient asks what is going on, what drug is being administered, or why she is being given an enema (a procedure that invades the body, if only in a minor way), the question should be answered *within the limits of the expertise of the particular health care provider.* That is to say that the provider should not go beyond their own professional competence. If the patient does not even know that they are being prepared for an operation (and these cases do occur), supervisors should be informed and more formal procedures instituted and formal, detailed written proof of informed consent obtained.

The report of the American Hospital's Committee on Biomedical Ethics (American Hospital Association, 1985, p.8) notes the following obligations of the hospital with regard to informed consent:

1. To ensure that informed consent has been obtained for diagnostic and therapeutic procedures performed in the hospital.
2. To develop educational programs that teach effective ways of getting ethically and legally acceptable informed consent.
3. To make certain that patients are aware of their right to consent or reject proposed procedures and treatments.

The AHA report also suggests that hospitals may wish to have materials available that can be understood by patients or to have arrangements with libraries for obtaining such materials. Such suggestions are in line with the spirit as well as the letter of the law in the area of autonomy. Indeed, they indicate a sensitivity to the need for a provider-patient cooperation that not only respects patients but improves health care in general.

The Right to Refuse Treatment

The principle of patient autonomy clearly implies that the patient or the surrogate has a right to refuse treatment. The right does not depend on whether or not the refusal makes good sense to someone else, but only on the competence of the patient. Mental patients have the right to refuse treatment, though the exact scope of the right is sometimes blurred (Ennis, 1978, p.132; Beis, 1984, p.153). Even in a psychiatric facility, the right to refuse treatment remains unless specifically ordered by a court.

The American Hospital Association's Bill of Patient's Rights summarizes this right rather neatly.

4. The patient has the right to refuse treatment to the extent permitted by law and to be informed of the medical consequences of his actions.

This right to refuse, however, does not imply that the patient is ethical in refusing treatment in any and all cases. While the health care provider is not ethical in forcing treatment on the patient or, with rare exceptions, in treating without informed consent, the patient, like the health care professional, must respect the principles of beneficence and nonmaleficence, which will be discussed in the next chapter.

Problem Areas

As already indicated, the principle of autonomy poses special problems in psychiatric facilities. The same is especially true of nursing homes (Uhlmann et al., 1987). Since nursing homes have an ever-increasing number of residents, the ethical problems will only increase rather than decrease. Many of the residents of these homes are threatened by dementia, physical frailty, and prejudices against the elderly. It is estimated that as many as 50 percent of the residents are intellectually impaired. In many cases it is hard to find out what the resident values or wishes, while the usual surrogates such as spouses and relatives may not be easily available.

In the face of these problems, nursing home administrators and health care professionals should take at least the following steps to protect autonomy. First, before or shortly after admission, the resident or, if incompetent, his or her surrogate, should be informed of various decisions that may have to be made in the future. They should then be asked for a written directive, if not a living will or a durable power of attorney, which will specify their wishes in important medical decisions. It is understood that these directives are subject to change. (We will return to the living will and durable power of attorney in Chapter Six.) Second, a surrogate should be appointed by the resident if competent or by a court. All of this should be attached in writing to the medical record.

A fuller development of these ideas, along with a sample form and policy which present both principles and applications, may be found in Uhlmann et al. (1987).[5]

SUMMARY

The principle of autonomy demands that a health care provider not treat a patient without the informed consent of the patient or the patient's surrogate except in narrowly defined emergencies. In order to follow this principle, the health care provider must decide if the patient is competent to understand the consequences of the consent to or refusal of treatment and is free enough to give consent. To help the competent patient or the surrogate in making a decision, the health care professional and, in particular, the physician must give the diagnosis, prognosis with and without treatment, and reasonable alternative treatments as well as inform the patient of the economic, psychic, and social costs of the treatment. In addition to the emergency exception, there are cases where weak paternalistic intervention can probably be justified. In cases of doubt, a court order should be sought. These obligations created by the principle of autonomy often seem in conflict with the principle of beneficence, which will be treated in the following chapter.

Special procedures are needed to protect autonomy in places such as psychiatric facilities and nursing homes.

CASES FOR ANALYSIS

NOTE: Although actual events and sometimes the public record supplied the raw materials for these cases, they have been edited so as to illustrate ethical problems rather than as actual detailed reports. In most cases we have changed names. We have retained actual names only when the case is so famous as to require that identification.

Since some of the events described took place many years ago, the state of health care reflected is not up to date in all cases. The ethical problems are real for all that.

1. Mrs. G. has an aneurysm in the brain, which if untreated by surgery will lead to blindness and probably to death. The surgery recommended leads to death in 75 percent of the cases. Of those who survive the operation, nearly 75 percent are crippled. Mrs. G. has three small children. Her husband has a modest job and his health insurance will cover the operation, but not the expenses that will result if she is crippled.

When informed of all this, Mrs. G is in great turmoil for a week or so until she makes her decision. She refuses treatment because she did not like the odds. There was, after all, only one chance out of 16 for a real recovery. In addition, she could not see exposing her family to the risk of having a cripple on their hands. Six months later Mrs. G. was informed that her case had been misdiagnosed.

2.   Zenobia, aged 80, lives alone about 50 miles from a town with medical care. About a year ago cancer of the colon was discovered. The physician who diagnosed the condition wanted to use chemotherapy, which he estimated had a 50 percent chance of bringing about a remission of several years in a woman her age. Zenobia refused treatment because the treatment was painful, expensive, and involved trips to another town 100 miles distant. Aside from the cancer, Zenobia had excellent health for a woman of her age.

Now Zenobia has been put in the hospital for pneumonia. She was delirious when a neighbor brought her in. There are no children or relatives. She will die of cancer in a few weeks.

3.   Mary, using self-examination, detects a lump in her breast and goes to Dr. Zippo, her long-time gynecologist, for a full examination. After palpation of the breast, but without further examination or tests, Dr. Zippo tells Mary that the lump is probably malignant and says that a radical mastectomy is necessary. He does not tell her that a radical mastectomy involves removal of the breast, the underlying muscle, and the nodes in the arm pit. He fears she would refuse the operation if she knew this. He does not tell her about advances in the treatment of breast cancer since he does not believe in them. Mary, a normally timid person and very respectful of authority, is very afraid and agrees to the surgery.

4.   Mrs. Ursula Stack, a 75-year-old housewife, became aware of breathlessness and was easily fatigued. She was known to have had a heart murmur for two years. She consented to come to a research hospital for cardiac catheterization, which confirmed the presence of severe, calcific aortic stenosis with secondary congestive heart failure.

Because of the unfavorable prospect for survival with this lesion without surgical intervention, the recommendation at the combined cardiac medical-surgical conference was for operation. The physician explained the situation to Mr. and Mrs. Stack and recommended aortic valve replacement. It was noted that the risk of surgery was not well known for her age group, that early mortality was usually around 10 percent, with 80 percent good functional results after three years. Her lack of other obvious disease made her a relatively "good" candidate for a successful surgical outcome despite her age.

Mrs. Stack appeared to understand the discussion and recommendation but requested deferral of the decision and *showed signs of denial of the problem*. She had no other medical problems, her husband was in good health, and their marriage appeared to be a happy one. They were financially secure and enjoyed a full set of social and recreational activities. She returned on three subsequent occasions for simple, supportive attention. The physician decided not to employ psychiatric assistance or other measures to reduce her denial and began to use conversation in such a way as to reduce her anxiety associated with the decision she appeared to have made.

5. John, 17 years old, was seriously injured while jumping from a train on which he had been hitching a ride. Taken to a nearby hospital, he was given emergency treatment by Dr. Lycanthropus, who judged that the boy's right arm would have to be amputated below the elbow because it had been *crushed beyond repair.* Two other physicians were consulted and agreed that the amputation should be done immediately in order to protect John's life.

John was unconscious as a result of an anesthetic administered to allow the suturing of a head wound which was bleeding profusely. Attempts to contact the boy's parents in a neighboring town were unsuccessful. Dr. Lycanthropus amputated.

6. Mary, age 11, was left in the temporary custody of her two sisters, Jane, age 18, and Margie, age 21. Margie, a registered nurse, took Mary to the physician because of a persistent sore throat. The physician recommended a tonsillectomy-adenoidectomy. Margie agreed and Mary was admitted for the procedure. The child, Mary, died in the course of being anesthetized for the operation.

7. Matilda died in childbirth because there was a four-hour delay in performing a Caesarean. The delay resulted from the fact that Matilda refused to consent to the procedure since she desired to have a normal delivery. Matilda was fully competent at the time of her refusal and understood the physician when, in the presence of witnesses, he informed her that he could no longer be responsible.

8. Jerry, age 11, was hospitalized and diagnosed as having schizophrenia. His parents were told that he should be given an antipsychotic medication which would clear up his thoughts. Having been told that only this medication would help, the parents gave consent without any additional information. Jerry was given Prolixin. After he was on the drug for two months he started to develop strange movements. All of a sudden his arm would jerk straight up over his head or his foot and leg would jerk from time to time. These movements were uncontrollable. This was diagnosed as tardive dyskenesia (TD). These are side effects suffered by most who use the drug for a long time. In 1 or 2 percent of the cases the side effects will severely incapacitate the patient. Some experts argue that there is virtually no danger if the antipsychotics are used for only a short time.

9. Mary, confined to a wheelchair, has no living relatives and no friends. She is a very lonely 19-year-old. She seems to have no interests in life except taking care of her long red hair and reading True Confessions. She has been diagnosed as having small cell cancer of the lung. This cancer sometimes responds very well to chemotherapy. If it does not respond to the treatment almost at once, it is fatal and the patient dies within months. The treatments leave you very weak for a long time and cause you to lose your hair. The physician tells her of the diagnosis and prognosis without treatment but tells her nothing about the side effects lest she refuse treatment.

NOTES

[1]Some writers make the conditions for competence so strict that, if applied, most people would be judged incompetent most of the time. Thus, Joel Feinberg (1975) wrote that, for a fully voluntary assumption of risk, there must be calmness and deliberation, an absence of distractions and disturbing emotions, and no misunderstanding or neurotic compulsions. If there are drugs or alcohol involved, there would in this view be less than perfect voluntary decisions. While we might agree with Feinberg in theory, in practice, perfectly voluntary decisions are not required. This would be true especially in the medical sphere, where there is nearly always some emotion disturbing a person's philosophic calm.

[2]The Jobes case may be found in *Bio Law,* 1987, pp. 571–80.

[3]In the context of paternalism in general, VanDeVeer (1986) has developed a principle of hypothetical individualized consent, which would permit and justify interference with a competent or doubtfully competent patient if the following conditions are met. First, the health care provider knows the values of the individual in question so that the interference would promote the values of the particular patient. Second, in view of the first condition, the provider knows that the patient would validly consent if (a) he were aware of the relevant circumstances or (b) the patient's normal capacities were not substantially impaired. Third, the interference would involve no wrong to the provider or third parties.

Especially in a medical context, the first condition assumes that there is a truly personal relationship such that the values of the patient are well known and not merely assumed. In the health care setting, the first part of the second condition must also assume that there is not sufficient time to inform the patient of the relevant circumstances. The assumption of substantial impairment, of course, makes this and the theory of weak paternalism very similar.

[4]One of the better explanations of the conflict between benevolence and autonomy is found in Engelhardt (1986). For other views see Beauchamp and McCullough (1984) and Culver and Gert (1982).

[5]While the authors praise the Uhlmann article, they disagree with his idea that the institutional ethics committee is a suitable surrogate. As noted earlier in this chapter, ethics committees are for education and advice, not for decision making. We are also concerned with, though not completely opposed to, the idea that the physician may be appointed as surrogate. Actually, a nurse who knows the patient better would be a more suitable health care professional surrogate in most cases. In the last analysis, a non-health care professional is more liable to have the comprehensive view that the patient should have. We will discuss the patient's comprehensive view in Chapter Three.

Chapter Three
PRINCIPLES
OF BENEFICENCE
AND NONMALEFICENCE

INTRODUCTION

In its most general form, the principle of beneficence says no more than: "Do good." Similarly, the principle of nonmaleficence tells us to: "Avoid evil." Unfortunately, those formulations are so general as to be useless. This becomes painfully clear when we realize that we cannot do all good or avoid all evil. Those impossibilities will show us why we need more specific formulations to help us sort out the possibilities and to make ethical choices.

The Impossibility of Doing All Good

The impossibility of doing all good arises both from the nature of time and space as well as from our own limitations and the limits of the instruments available to us. There is just so much time in a day. Indeed, there never seems to be enough time to do all that we want to do or plan to do. The limits of time limit us no matter how efficient we become. Space, too, hems us in. We cannot directly and immediately do good to those who are far away. Indeed, because we can only be in one place at one time, most of the people in the world are beyond our direct touch and so cannot be helped personally.

Our own limited talents also limit our ability to do good. Not everyone has the brains to be an atomic physicist or a designer of supercomputers. Some have better health than others, some greater strength, others better coordination. The relative strength of intellect, body, and coordination thus put limits on what a person can do. It should be noted, however, that even those who have enough intelligence to master any given task do not have a enough time to master them all. The person who is both physician and lawyer is rare, the person who is physician, lawyer, electrical engineer, mechanical engineer, nuclear physicist, biophysicist, anthropologist, chemist, paleontologist, carpenter, plumber, bricklayer, and agronomist seems as real as a winged horse. Even if such a person did exist, time and space would still limit the good she could do.

Finally, our ability to do good is limited by the state of the art in a given area as well as by the availability of state of the art tools. The lack of immunosuppressant drugs held back transplant surgery, since without those drugs the patient's body rejected the new tissue. Today, immunosuppressant drugs exist, but their availability is still limited by their high cost. Without them even the finest surgeon is limited in what he can do for the patient who needs a new kidney.

Our obligation to do good is also limited by our obligation to avoid evil. In other words, the principle of nonmaleficence limits the principle of beneficence. The sight of a child drowning in a raging stream filled with floating ice urges one to attempt a rescue. One is stopped by the realization that there is serious risk to one's own life and the fact that one would probably not be able to save the child in any event. The evil involved is a price to be paid for attempting a rescue. While we might praise the rescuer as a hero, we would not say she had a duty to jump in. Indeed, we call such people heroes because they do *not* have a duty, but do more than could be normally demanded.

Clearly, more specific formulations of the principle of beneficence are needed to help us in deciding what should be done. It should be clear, too, that doing good and avoiding evil will not simply be a question of principles but of practical wisdom weighing the relevant aspects of the factual and social situation as well as the concrete meaning of human dignity in a particular time and place.

The Impossibility of Avoiding All Evil

Nearly everything we do has some undesirable side effect or at least the risk of some evil. When you cross the street you run the risk of being hit by a car. When you take aspirin you risk stomach problems or possibly Reye's syndrome. When you undergo major surgery, you risk your life. Life is inherently risky. If we tried to avoid all harm and risk of harm there would be time for nothing else. Indeed, if we tried to avoid all risks by staying in bed, we would risk bed sores, deterioration of our muscles, and stationary pneumonia. There is no escape from all risk and so no escape from all evil.

Quite aside from the inherent riskiness of human life, we must also face the fact that because life is social we are involved in actual evils to a greater or lesser extent. We are members of a society that, despite considerable progress, still oppresses minorities and women. Many work for companies that are destroying the environment. Some teach in schools where at least some professors are grossly unfair to students. A few are employed in hospitals that tolerate incompetent physicians or nurses. By continuing to cooperate with groups that cause or permit evil, we are to some extent tainted by evil. Yet we cannot avoid all of this evil. If we go off as hermits, we have cut ourselves off from the benefits of social life and increase the risk to our lives and even our sanity. Worse yet, our flight from evil often leaves the villains in charge and the victims in worse shape than before. There is no easy way out. We need, then, specifications of the principle of nonmaleficence which will enable us to make at least rough judgments of what evils we have to avoid.

SPECIFICATIONS OF BENEFICENCE

As we noted in the first chapter, the individual person is the intrinsic good and all other things are to be judged by their consequences for the individual. In practice, some things are *necessary* for the dignity of the human person. Other things, such as gourmet foods or designer clothes, are merely useful. These merely useful goods, not necessary for human dignity, may, under certain conditions, be subordinated to the good of other persons and of society.

The things necessary for the person to remain human and maintain dignity are at the top of the list of goods to be done. Ordinarily, the list of necessary goods contains nourishment, including both food and water, shelter and clothing, as well as memberships in social groups necessary for the psychological growth of the person. Many people would also include health care, as defined by their society, as a necessary good. We say that these things are ordinarily necessary for the person to remain a human being since in medical ethics we will come across cases in which even the provision of food or the continuance of medical care may be destroying human dignity and maintaining a "vegetable" rather than a human being (see Chapter Six).

Often, however, it is not merely a matter of deciding which goods are necessary and which are merely useful for ourselves, but of situations in which the effort to better or to preserve ourselves may conflict with the good of other human persons. In these cases our betterment is often subordinate to their survival. At times, the obligation to respect others may limit the obligations to attain even these basic, necessary goods. At very least, humans are generally free to sacrifice even basic goods for themselves in order to preserve basic goods for others. Thus, a person may forgo medical care to keep from impoverishing the family and depriving them of basic goods.

As we have already seen in Chapter Two on autonomy, even the health care provider's right to help is limited by the respect due to the freedom of the patient and by the need for an informed consent from the patient or a lawful surrogate. As we have already pointed out, there is a tension here between respecting freedom and securing what a health care professional may consider the best interests of the patient (Engelhardt, 1985).

The societies we belong to are among the most necessary of goods. We are dependent on society for nearly any conceivable good and so are obliged to be members of various societies and to participate in and contribute to those societies, as well as observing the rules of those societies. The necessary goods of these societies place obligations on us. In line with the demands of practical wisdom, these social obligations must be considered in making our decisions as to which goods must be done. This assumes, of course, that the society is just and does not seek to subordinate the individual totally to the group.

In practice, most of the goods we have to do are specified by social agreement, whether through law or custom as well as through relationship, roles, or agreements. These specifications result from the acts of both societies and individuals. As a result, there may be considerable variation between societies and individuals. Thus, although all societies have common general obligations, there is a great deal of variation in specification between societies. All societies must demand contributions from their members, but they exact different contributions such as taxes or personal service, depending on history and form of government in a particular society. Again, though all people need to have an income, they vary greatly in the way they choose to acquire that income. Some hire themselves out and acquire one set of obligations; others enter into individual contractual relations with a series of customers and so have different duties. The marriage contract, for example, sets up a relationship and specifies a set of obligations that exclude certain other relationships. The relationship of father and mother to their children creates specific obligations which have priority over other obligations. The roles of health care providers have similar effects.

In the health care professions, law, custom, relationship, and contract are particularly important. As we saw in Chapter One, the specific role of the provider determines the relationship to the patient. The professional, moreover, professes to do certain things implied in the purpose of the profession. These are the general goods that he is obliged to provide. The contract between professional and patient further specifies the particular good to be done in this case. Note that the physician or nurse cannot profess to do more than their particular education and skill permit, nor can they do more than the patient agrees to.

A health care provider is not a sage capable of solving all problems, and so should not attempt to even if the patient were to let him. These two limits or specifications (the one by talent, the other by agreement) are to be kept in mind at all times in health care ethics.

All of these general and specific obligations in beneficence are also limited by the obligation to avoid evil. Before giving even more precise specifications for beneficence in health care, it is necessary to consider at least some general rules about the obligation to avoid evil, since we cannot avoid all evil.

SPECIFICATIONS OF NONMALEFICENCE

Because most people realize that it is impossible to avoid all evil, ethicists have devised various general rules to help in deciding what evils can be tolerated. Perhaps the most famous is the principle of double effect developed by deontological natural law thinkers.[1] The deontological notion that some acts are good or evil independent of their consequences is quite prominent in the formulation. The *principle of double effect* provides that a person may perform an act which has or risks evil effects if all four of the following conditions are verified:

1. The action must be good or morally indifferent in itself.
2. The agent must intend only the good effect and not the evil effect.
3. The evil effect cannot be a means to the good effect.
4. There must be a proportionality between the good and the evil effects.

In line with the practical wisdom approach, which considers all relevant factors and looks to the consequences of acts, this book uses a simpler formulation, which may be called the *principle of proportionality*. This provides that:

> Provided the action does not go directly against the dignity of the individual person (the intrinsic good) there must be a proportionate good to justify permitting of risking an evil consequence.

The proportionality contained in both principles is to be judged by considering the following four factors:

1. Whether or not there are alternative ways of attaining the intended good with no evil or less evil consequences.
2. The level of good intended and the level of the evil risked or permitted.
3. The certitude or probability of the good or evil intended, permitted, or risked.
4. The causal influence of the agent.

Alternatives

If there are alternative ways of attaining the good with less evil or less risk of evil, common sense dictates that the alternative be chosen. To put it another way, *the good is to be done with the smallest amount of evil possible.* In medical practice this would mean not using a drug with harmful side effects if it were possible to treat the condition with diet or exercise. The possibilities, of course, would depend on both the self-discipline of the patient as well as the effectiveness of the diet and exercise.

It should be recalled from Chapter Two that the health care professional has the obligation to inform the patient of the alternatives and the relative benefits and risks involved. The patient has the obligation to consider these, weighing proportionality.

The Level of Good and Evil

Everyone recognizes that not all goods and evils are equal. Losing a few hairs from one's head is generally considered very minor compared to losing an eye. Saving a human life is, for most of us, more important than keeping a pet well fed. At base, we recognize that some things are *merely useful* for the life of the human person, while others are *necessary* for human life and dignity. There is, of course, much room for discussion as to what goods fall into which class as well as to which is more or less useful or more or less necessary. It is generally accepted that in the United States a formal education is necessary in order to earn an income, but there is no agreement about which level of education is necessary. People can agree that vitamin A is necessary and still disagree about the best way of getting vitamin A into the system. For all that, there is considerable agreement that certain things are seriously evil and others very minor.

The loss of life, or of the freedom of choice, or even of movement is considered a great evil; the loss of a favorite sweater or a small sum of money at cards is not. In short, what threatens basic human rights and dignity or what threatens life or physical integrity in a major way is considered serious. In practice, the hope of a serious good is needed to justify even risking such evils.

Certitude or Probability of the Good or Evil

Some serious evils are remote, that is, the risk of them is so small that in practice we treat the evil as not serious. While you risk your life just about every time you cross a busy street, the risk is so small that you feel no moral uneasiness about crossing as long as you are careful. If the odds are very small that an operation will save my life and very high that it will leave me crippled, the life saving aspect becomes a lesser good and the risk of being crippled assumes more serious proportions. In practice, then, proportionality involves very complicated if not always precise balancing of the levels of goods and evils with the probability or certainty of those same goods and evils.

Certitude, Probability, and the Wedge Principle

In arguing about the certitude and probability of consequences, particularly evil consequences, ethical thinkers often invoke, implicitly if not explicitly, the wedge or camel's nose principle. The wedge analogy assumes that if you put the tip of a wedge in a crack and strike, you will split the log apart and destroy everything. The camel's nose analogy imagines that if you let the camel get its nose under the tent, that the rest of the beast will soon follow. In a general sense both expressions operate on the underlying idea that in defending a given position even a small concession will destroy that position.

There are two forms of the wedge principle. The first or logical form is concerned with logical consistency and not necessarily with the actual effects. Assuming that ethical principles should be universal and cover all individual situations, exceptions are seen as the logical wedge which will undermine the principle. Thus, some religious thinkers argue that if you say contraception is ethical, you must also accept homosexual activity as ethical. They say this is logically consistent since both involve unnatural acts. The argument has no force, of course, with those who see no evil consequences in either contraception or homosexuality. Similarly, deontologists will argue that if you permit any justified lies, you logically undermine the whole prohibition of lying. This version of the wedge principle does not say that you will increase lying, but only that you logically undermine the principle.

The empirical form of the wedge principle does not worry about logical consistency, but about the actual consequences of the act or the exception to the rule. Will the exception increase lying and so threaten social interaction? Will the practice of contraception lead to an increase in abortions? Will sparing the rod spoil the child? These are questions of fact that must be answered by experience or careful studies. Often, however, the careful studies are lacking and we are given general impressions or so-called common sense answers to what are questions of fact. This is an invalid use of the empirical wedge principle, since evidence and not opinion is needed.

It is not always easy to discover the consequences of such things as pornography, violence on television, or the effects of Caesarian sections or circumcision. Because answers are often hard to come by, decency demands that one investigate carefully before invoking the empirical wedge principle and then tossing around prohibitions on the basis of what you guess might happen. Here, again, all the rules on proportionality come back in as the good and the evil consequences are calculated. Even though there may be harmful consequences from an action, there may be even more harmful effects from trying to suppress it. Prohibition, which aimed at suppressing alcoholism, not only failed but contributed to the beginnings of organized crime. Suppressing pornography, for example, might do great harm to freedom of speech and so not be justified. The justification, however, is a question of fact and not a matter of mere opinion.

The Causal Influence of the Agent

Most effects are the result of many causes such that a particular agent is seldom the sole cause of the consequences. Lung cancer, for example, may have been triggered not only by smoking, but by conditions in the work place and in the general environment as well as by hereditary factors. The smokers and the polluters are responsible for the lung cancer to the extent that they caused it. They are not solely responsible since hereditary factors also play a role.

In some cases the action of a particular agent may be a very minor contributor to the evil. For example, the cleaning staff in a hospital that is overcharging patients helps keep the place going, but hardly makes any great contribution to the evil. The accountants, on the other hand, are more deeply involved. The board of directors is directly and largely responsible for the overcharging.

While there is no excuse for the board since it has the controlling causal influence, the cleaning staff needs no more good than their need of a job to justify their continued employment. The accountants, having tried to change the situation, can tolerate the involvement if they feel that they can prevent other serious evils by continuing to work for that particular hospital.

In this context, it should be stressed that in many cases, there is no causal influence and no possibility for a given person to change the situation. In these cases there may be no obligation to avoid or remove the evil simply because it is impossible to do so. We shall discuss this in Chapter Eleven on self-policing and the problem of "whistle blowing."

Preliminary Summary

The detailed consideration of the principle of proportionality brings us to a reformulation of the principle: "Avoid evil." The principle of nonmaleficence now reads: "Avoid evil and evil consequences unless you have a proportionate reason for risking or permitting them."

This reformulation of the principle of nonmaleficence calls for a more precise working of the principle: "Do good." The reformulation of the principle of beneficence now reads: "Do good unless the consequences of doing good produce a disproportionate evil."

In practice, the good to be done depends on the seriousness of the matter and on the whole network of social roles and contractual obligations that define the particular good that this individual should do. It is time, then, to return to the statements of beneficence and nonmaleficence specific to those involved in health care.

THE PATIENT'S OBLIGATION

We start with the patient's obligation, since the patient is the center of health care and the reason for its existence. Equally important is the fact that the patient must make health care decisions in a context that includes obligations to family, society, and the values of things other than health and mere biological existence. As we noted at the end of the last chapter, the fact that a patient has a legal right to refuse treatment does not mean that there is also an ethical right to do so.

What is the patient's ethical obligation with regard to preventing disease and maintaining and restoring her health? In view of the fact that health is only one among many goods and the obligation to take care of health only one of many obligations, many medical ethicists have given the following summary statement: "*Individuals are obliged to use ordinary but not extraordinary means of preserving and restoring their health.*"[2]

The explanations of ordinary and extraordinary make it clear that this is really only a form of proportionality. "Ordinary," for example, does not mean common, usual, or everyday. Rather it means *that which, all things considered, produces more good than harm.* "Extraordinary" does not mean unusual, rare, or exotic, but *such as will, all things considered, produce more evil than good.* For example, the use of Valium, a minor tranquilizer, would be extraordinary in a patient whose adverse reaction to the drug is rage. On the other hand, the implantation of an artificial heart might be an ordinary means if that is the only way a person can prolong life long enough to put it in order.

The ordinary/extraordinary terminology may be confusing and so it is better to word the principle as a special case of proportionality. The patient's formulation of the principle of benevolence in health matters, then, reads as follows: "*Take care of your health so long as, all things considered, this does not produce more harm than good.*" The phrase "all things considered" is important since it not only distinguishes the patient's obligation from that of the health care professional but also from that of the surrogate. As we shall see a little later, both the professional and the surrogate do not have to consider all things.

The phrase "all things considered" also stresses the need to balance out all the obligations of the patient. The phrase includes not only the impacts on the self, but on the family and society; not only the pain, cost, and health benefits, but the meaning of life and the quality of life as the patient sees it. Health care that barely keeps a patient alive while its costs reduce the family to fiscal poverty and emotional exhaustion is not necessarily a good thing. Indeed, the patient can reasonably judge it an evil to be avoided. Similarly, treatment such as a blood transfusion that conflicted with a religious obligation, would not be a good let alone an obligatory good. On the other hand, neglecting exercise, proper sleep, and nutrition is nearly always wrong because such basic self care procedures hardly conflict with other obligations.

In this context, it should be emphasized that the health care provider cannot make these decisions, if only because the professional does not know all things much less all things that are pertinent to the decision of the patient. Above all, the health care provider is not competent to judge the meaning and value of life for other people. Certainly, the health care professional is never in the position where she is qualified to say that the quality of life of the patient makes him unworthy of life or unworthy relative to other persons. The proper nature of health care professionals' judgment of quality of life will be treated later in this chapter.

THE HEALTH CARE PROVIDER'S OBLIGATION

While the health care professional is not competent to make a judgment of proportionality *all things considered,* he has a professional role and is competent in a given area. This area is the area in which the health care professional must judge the proportionality of consequences. In the case of physicians we call the specific formulation of beneficence *the medical indications principle.* For nurses it would be *the nursing indications principle,* and so on for each of the professions involved. Here we will develop only the medical indications principle for physicians.[3]

The medical indications principle states that, *granted informed consent, the physician should do what is medically indicated such that, from a medical point of view, more good than evil will result.* To put it another way, the medical benefits are to outweigh the medical burdens on the patient. The following example, taken from Ramsey (1978, p.182), illustrates the principle in action.

There are two groups of babies with *spina bifida.* The first group will die within a few days or weeks. The second group will live for months or years or more even if untreated. This second group of babies, who are not dying, is further divided into group A and group B. The babies in group A have such a wide wound on the back that it is not suitable for an operation. An operation might not heal and might leave the wound infected and the final condition of the baby worse than the first. Group B contains babies who were seen to kick at birth and so have some muscle power. In this case an operation stands a good chance of reducing the handicap and improving the child's chances in life without making things worse.

Treatment is not indicated for group one since they will be dead in a short time and there is nothing to be accomplished by the operation. In this case the surgeon should not urge the operation. In the case of group A, the operation is not medically indicated because the specifics make the child unsuitable for an operation, indeed, create a risk of making the child more handicapped. Treatment is medically indicated for group B since more medical good than harm should be accomplished. The surgeon should propose the operation and even make a strong case for it.

In order to see the significance of the principle more clearly, it will help to alter the case by supposing that in group B there is one child who is severely retarded. Is the operation for *spina bifida* still medically indicated for that child who is not dying and who has an operable condition? The answer is yes. There is *more medical good than harm* to be gained by operating, so the operation is medically indicated. Medically, the benefits of the surgery are greater than the burdens resulting from it. The fact of severe retardation is not a *medical* counterindication no matter how one feels about retardation. A judgment about the value of life of retarded people should not enter in here because that is not a medical question. It is a profound personal or philosophic question to which there is no easy answer. We shall return to the quality of life problem in Chapter Six when we discuss the value of life to the person who possesses that life.

Let us look at yet a third case in which a severely retarded neonate is dying from a pneumonia. The child's life can be saved with antibiotics. Is treatment of the pneumonia medically indicated even though saving the life will leave the family and society with a severely retarded child on its hands? Does the fact of severe mental retardation change the medical indications? The answer is no. The treatment of the pneumonia is medically indicated since medically it will produce more harm than good. The treatment is medically indicated unless the patient is dying of some other untreatable disease or unless the treatment will cause more harm than good from a medical point of view. The fact that the child will never lead a full life as defined by the physician or by society is not a medical counterindication. Rather, it is once again the sort of quality of life decision that goes beyond the consideration of medical benefits and burdens and so beyond the scope of medicine and beyond the competence of the physician.

The impact of the decision on the family and the society is also not a medical question, though it would be part of the patient's consideration of benefits and burdens. Perhaps, as we shall see, it may at times be a part of the surrogate's decision. Indeed, an attempt to make such factors part of the medical indications approach would detract from the central idea that the health care professional, except in industrial, military, and some judicial settings, is to seek the good of the patient and not the good of other parties involved.

The so-called Baby Doe rule,[4] though it is still debatable, is an example of one attempt to apply the medical indications principle and speaks to these situations rather clearly (Murray, 1985). Two points should be noted in the following quotations. First, the rule speaks of life threatening situations and not merely of patients in a terminal condition. Second, nutrition and hydration are considered part of treatment.

The Department of Health and Human Services rule (1985b, no. 4) condemns the *withholding of medically indicated treatment* where "withholding" is defined as follows:

> the failure to respond to the infants life threatening conditions by providing treatment (including appropriate nutrition, hydration, and medication) which, in the treating physician's (or physicians') reasonable medical judgment will be most likely to be effective in *ameliorating all such conditions.* (italics added)

Three exceptions to the condemnation are listed, though appropriate nutrition, hydration, and medication must be provided even in these cases.

1. The infant is chronically and irreversibly comatose;
2. The provision of such treatment would merely prolong dying, not be effective in ameliorating or correcting all of the infant's life threatening conditions, or otherwise be futile in terms of the survival of the infant; or
3. The provision of such treatment would be virtually futile in terms of the survival of the infant and the treatment itself under such circumstances would be inhumane.

The requirement that appropriate nutrition, hydration, and medication be provided even in these three cases is questionable (Lynn and Childress, 1983). Nutrition, hydration, and mediation may only prolong the dying process. Further, though we may have strong emotions about something as everyday as eating and drinking, nutrition and hydration in hospital settings are often painful and uncomfortable medical procedures rather than simple everyday acts. Nasogastric and gastric tubes need medical justification and are not to be taken as ordinary methods of feeding and hydrating. (This point is more fully developed in Chapter Six on death and dying.) Here and now we want to stress that keeping the patient alive at all costs is not automatically medically indicated.

THE SURROGATE'S OBLIGATIONS

The obligation of the surrogate in giving or withholding consent depends on whether the wishes of a once competent patient are known or can be deduced, or whether the person has never been competent, or where the wishes are unknown. If the wishes of a once competent patient are known either orally or in written form or can be easily deduced from a person's actions and values, the surrogate should decide in accord with the wishes of the patient. This is sometimes called the substituted judgment principle. To overrule those wishes would be a violation of the person's autonomy.

When the person has never been competent or has been competent but never manifested his wishes, two principles have been proposed for the surrogate: the best interests principle and the rational choice principle. The best interests principle requires that the surrogate act in the best interests of the patient, *disregarding the interests of others*, including the interests of the family, society, and those of the surrogate. The best interests principle thus demands that the good of the patient and nothing else be considered.

The rational choice principle commands that the surrogate choose what the patient would have chosen if competent and had considered all available relevant information and the interests of relevant others. The rational choice principle goes beyond the narrowly defined interests of the patient. It recognizes that patients are obliged to and generally do consider the interests of at least some others in making their decisions. The rational choice principle would allow the surrogate to judge that even a very painful treatment should be given since many people depend on the patient for moral support. The principle might also justify refusing the treatment on the grounds that the treatment would impoverish the patient's family and leave the patient a cripple.

Each of these principles entails problems. The best interests principle asks the surrogate to do what is nearly impossible—judge what is best for another. Further, it does not face the fact that the interests of the patient and the interest of the surrogate may be in conflict. Not all surrogates can surmount their own interests.

The rational choice principle assumes that we could know what the patient would have chosen if competent and if she had considered every relevant factor. That is a very "iffy" assumption. We doubt that anyone except God can know what a person would have done in those circumstances. Among other things we generally do not know what relative value the patient would have given to the interests of others. In practice, the rational choice principle probably leads to the surrogate choosing what, all things considered, the surrogate deems best. The difficulty of the task is illustrated by in the following cases.

1. A wife faces the prospect of a husband who will be a vegetable forever or a cripple requiring constant care at home if the treatment works. If the treatment does not work, he will be dead within a year.
2. A son who wants his inheritance as soon as possible must decide if his father should be given care that will prolong life for years, even though the father will not know where or who he is most of the time.
3. A mother is faced with the decision whether or not to treat a seriously deformed and profoundly retarded child who will never recognize her and be little more than a large animal in the house for many years to come.

In all of these cases the motives are mixed and the choice agonizing. While we will all condemn the son for letting the father die in order to get his inheritance sooner, we also recognize that both the father in the first case and the mother in the third have legitimate interests and concerns. The best interest principle, which asks them to disregard those concerns, seems to ask something unreasonable if not impossible. The rational choice principle, on the other hand, is reasonable but creates a fear that we will open up a Pandora's box of evils. The wedge principle reappears. We are left asking if the rational choice principle will as a matter of fact lead to surrogates violating not autonomy but the patient's right to treatment or even to life.

The introduction of ethics committees may provide more advice to health care workers and even to surrogates, but it does not solve the problems of surrogate decision making since the committees do not, barring a legal delegation, have legal authority to make the decisions. Ethically, the ethics committee might perhaps supplant the surrogates only temporarily and if there were evidence that the surrogates were not following one of the approved principles of surrogate decision making. Even in these cases, however, a court order should be sought as soon as possible. In any event, we need more experience with the ethics committees, their composition, and values before taking any definitive stand about them.

All of these problems point to an underlying problem in pluralistic societies that lack a community consensus about what is right or wrong. Such societies end up substituting laws which set down the minimums, only to find that the minimums do not solve our problems. When the pluralistic society becomes increasingly infected with distrust, not only of professionals but of government, law seems to lead to malpractice suits and increasing demands for lay review and control of health care decisions. In the absence of a community consensus and its accompanying trust, everyone in health care must feel isolated and very alone when faced with the difficult problems involving incompetent patients.

The Quality of Life Problem

Health care providers, in using an "indications principle" appropriate to the particular profession, can and legitimately do make judgments about the benefits and burdens of medical, nursing, or respiratory care or its omission. The quality of life judgment has a different status when there is judgment about the value and meaning of life itself. An "indications principle" forbids health care professionals to make quality of life decisions about the relative worth of persons or their lives as beyond their competence. Thus, a nurse may ethically judge that a given nursing intervention will leave the patient worse off. Nursing science, however, does not permit a judgment that a treatment should be omitted because this particular life is no longer worth living. This is particularly true in a pluralistic society in which there is no social consensus about such questions. In Chapter Six on death and dying, we will have to face the related question of whether or not a given life is a human life.

Unfortunately, in a world of scarce resources, there will come a time when society and its instrument, the government, must make at least minimum decisions which indirectly judge what life and health are worth in monetary terms. At least society will have to decide how much it will pay to preserve life or provide health care. The increasing cost of health care will ultimately force the society to make a judgment to limit the good that a health care professional can do because it will limit the reimbursement they will receive for it. This will be discussed in Chapter Four on justice in the distribution of health care. Here we will stress some of the value issues other than justice.

At the very beginning of Chapter Two, we stressed that the individual person is the intrinsic good and not good merely because he is useful to society or to others. In short, persons are valuable because they are human and not because they produce something. We must, however, ask what makes biological life valuable to the person. Mere vegetable or animal existence is surely not valuable to the person without qualification. That question will be considered in Chapter Six on death and dying. We must also face the question of whether human life that has a potential for personhood has value. We will look at that question in Chapter Seven on abortion. All of these problems are painful, precisely because we do not have a community consensus about values. At the same time, they are crucial problems since they concern what have always been considered to be basic values.

Professional Power and Benevolence

Writers on health care ethics (e.g., Kass, 1983; Pellegrino and Thomasma, 1981) emphasize the ethical obligations that arise from the unequal power relationship between the patient and the health care professional. There is need for concern about this inequality in practice. There is some evidence that all relationships between health care professionals and their patients involve some problems of power and territory (Rosenthal et al., 1980). This would not be the case in a perfect world, where both the principle of autonomy and the principle of beneficence were perfectly observed and where the compassion of the caregiver overcame all annoyances from the patient. In the real world, and on a day–to–day basis, the temptation to use power for one's own convenience and comfort is real and almost constantly present. We include a few examples of the abuse of power to illustrate the type of ethical problem that is generally not discussed. Once described, the following common abuses of power need no commentary.

1. To maximize income, the physician schedules three patients for the same time. If they all show up, two of them have to wait and so waste their time for the convenience of the physician. As the day goes on, the waits become longer and longer and have been known to add up to three or four hours. Most patients are too intimidated to complain, let alone to bill the physician for their lost time.
2. The nurse, knowing that the orthopedic surgeon likes to move fast, uses hot water in preparing the casting compound since that speeds up the setting time. She disregards the fact that it also makes the cast very hot and uncomfortable, especially for children with tender skin.
3. The patient is told to take all of her clothes off, put on a paper gown, and wait for the physician in a cold examination room. Two hours later the doctor shows up and makes no excuse, let alone a legitimate one, for the inconvenience.

4. A small town physician tells patients that he will never treat them again, not even in an emergency, if he ever hears that they went to the new doctor in town.
5. The patient in room five does not wash himself when told to do so. The nurse punishes him by waiting 20 minutes to answer the patient's call bell.
6. The supervisor puts a family member out of the patient's room because the relative makes the nurse nervous when taking a pulse and a temperature.

Medical Indications and Unnecessary Surgery

Studies indicate that there is considerable unnecessary surgery, that is, surgery that is not medically indicated at all or not indicated because there are less radical alternatives. Some studies in the early 1980s estimated that as much as 36 percent of all cataract surgery, 36 percent of knee surgery, 43 percent of hemorrhoidectomies, 31 percent of gall bladder surgery, 29 percent of prostate surgery, and 28 percent of hernia repair surgery is unnecessary (*Perspectives,* 1985). The fact that second opinions significantly reduce surgery indicates that some "unnecessary surgery" may be due to a difference of opinion among surgeons. At the very least, this indicates that medical indications are not precise but as much a matter of opinion as of scientific research. More disturbing is the fact the second opinions indicate that many surgeons are too quick to take up the knife before less drastic measures have been tried. The Wennberg variations, which tie the number and type of surgeries to the number and type of surgeons in an area, give some credibility to this interpretation. The most disturbing interpretation of all would hold that some surgeons merely cut with or without medical indications. Such conduct would involve exposing the patient to unnecessary risk, defrauding the insurance company, and wasting health care resources. Fortunately, this seems to be rare.

The Health Care Provider as Patient Advocate

Chapter One spoke favorably of the nurse as patient advocate model. In the light of the principle of beneficence as expressed in terms of medical indications or nursing indications and all parallel professional indications, we want to argue that every health care professional has an obligation to be a patient advocate in the area of their expertise. This advocacy does not authorize the health care provider to overrule patients or lawful surrogates, but does, when everything else has been attempted, authorize or even oblige them to seek court protection for the patient whom they suspect is being abused or made the victim of a conflict of interest.

Chapter Eleven will deal with self-policing and whistle-blowing as part of the advocated role. Here, we would like to stress the problems of patients who are particularly vulnerable and so in need of protection not only *by* health care professionals but *from* health care professionals. Problems in this area will grow as the population ages and long-term care, whether in the home or long-term care facilities such as nursing homes, becomes more common.

Nursing homes often have a large number of patients who, if not confused, are weak and physically vulnerable. At times the nursing home patient may have been made confused or incompetent for the convenience of the staff. Overmedication or "snowing" of patients has been documented on several occasions (Cushing, 1984). The fact that tranquilizers such as Thorazine and Mellaril account for as much as 20 percent of the drugs prescribed in nursing homes gives rise to questions about induced incompetence.

The consent of such patients and the consent of surrogates can easily be overridden. They can be punished for failure to bow to the whims of the staff. The punishments can be as severe and obvious as the use of physical abuse or as hard to detect as withdrawal of attention and concern for the patient. While there are federal and state regulations governing long-term care and even periodic visits from state inspectors, these do not provide 24-hour-a-day protection. Registered nurses, licensed practical nurses, aides, and administrators who are on the spot have the obligation to protect the patient and to provide, as far as possible, conditions that foster not only the health, but the dignity of the patient. This is an enormous challenge. The budgets are often low and the staffing may sometimes be inadequate both in terms of numbers and training. Often there are only a handful of professionals to oversee a host of aides. The truly ethical health care professional, then, may find himself involved in a continuous and even losing battle for the proper care of the patient. At this point, the obligation to be a patient advocate can change to the obligation to support the political advocacy of the professional organizations which have the power to influence the allocation process (discussed in the next chapter).

Beneficence and the Right to Refuse Patients

Except in emergencies, health care professionals and health care agencies do not have to accept every patient who presents herself for treatment. Americans, however, are shocked when they hear stories of the "dumping" of indigent patients or even of patients who lack adequate health insurance. Yet as far back as 1982, it was estimated that about one million families a year were refused health care for financial reasons. In some cases, as many as 90 percent of the cases transferred to public facilities from emergency departments at other hospitals made the trip because they lacked adequate medical coverage.

All of us are shocked when we read such newspaper stories, since physicians, nurses, and health care institutions profess to care for the sick. At the same time, it is clear that these professionals and institutions cannot treat everyone who comes along and can treat only a limited number without payment.

The institutional problem and the problem of social justice involved in these situations will be treated in the next chapter. Here we will treat the basic principles covering the obligation of the health care professional practicing in a noninstitutional setting.

Traditionally, health care professionals, except in emergency situations, have had the right to select or reject patients who came for care. This was based on the idea that the professional/patient relationship was a very personal one and so not something that could be forced on either the health care professional or the patient. The profession of healing powers was not an offer to serve all who come.

In more recent times, we have begun to see that the power to reject and accept patients can be abused. If the rejection or acceptance is not based on factors relevant to the professional/patient relationship, we have an unfair discrimination, which is a rejection of the dignity of the patient. Our ideas of fairness no longer approve of an unqualified right to reject patients. At the same time, no one would say that the health care professional must treat all who present themselves for care.

There are, of course, legitimate reasons to reject a patient. In the first place, the physician may lack the skills to treat that particular patient. In the second place, she may lack the time because her practice is already over subscribed.

Can a health care provider ethically reject a patient because of inability to pay or to pay what the physician requests? The answer is both yes and no.

The health care professional who never does charity work is certainly not practicing the profession of healing as much as engaging in a business. In our opinion, he is unworthy of the name of health care professional. During most of American history, charitable service was so much a mark of the life of the physician that the vast majority of them had very low incomes (Starr, 1982). At the same time, the health care professional has a right to earn a good living and so must have some discretion as to how many nonpaying clients should be accepted. While the physician's role calls for charitable work, it does not call for becoming a charitable institution. We note that nurses in many parts of the country are still so underpaid that much of their work must be considered a charitable contribution to the sick and poor. We are left, however, with a problem of justice in the microallocation of health care, which will be treated in the next chapter.

While ethically the physician has wide latitude in selecting patients, there is less freedom in dropping a patient. Both legally (Annas, 1981; Cowdrey, 1984) and ethically, a physician is guilty of abandonment if in a nonemergency situation she does not continue treating a patient and so expose him to danger. There are, of course, good reasons for terminating the relationship. Termination of treatment requires that the physician provide for continuity of care by handing the patient over to another qualified professional.

The appearance of AIDS has raised old questions about the right of health care professionals to refuse treatment to a patient because of danger to themselves. Two points need to be considered in answering the question. First, all the rules of proportionality apply. Second, because the professional professes to serve society and the sick, the risks of harm must outweigh that professional obligation as well as the other goods involved. In short, it takes more than normal risk to excuse health care professionals because of danger to themselves.

In the case of AIDS, all current research indicates that the risk of a health care professional being infected by a patient is very small, *if proper procedures are followed.* There is no danger if the health care professional with open cuts or breaks in exposed skin avoids working with the AIDS patient until the cuts and cracks are healed. There can, then, be temporary ethical excuses for not working with AIDS patients. On the other hand, a refusal based on a dislike of homosexuals or drug users appears contrary to the whole spirit of the health care profession.

SUMMARY

It is impossible to do all good or to avoid all evil. It is necessary, then, to have principles that specify which good is to be done and which evils are to be avoided. In practice this specification involves a judgment of proportionality between the good intended and the evils risked. In health care there are different specifications for the patient, the patient's surrogates, and the health care professionals. In the case of health care professionals, the further specifications arise from the nature of the profession in question. The medical indications principle is a prime example of the principle of proportionality and the professional obligation joined in one principle. Quality of life judgments are not within the expertise of the health care professional.

A patient should not be turned away except for relevant reasons, nor should the relationship be broken even for relevant reasons without providing for continuity of care.

CASES FOR ANALYSIS

1. Joseph and Edmund Campion were born as Siamese twins, joined below the waist and sharing the lower part of their digestive tract and three legs. There were internal abnormalities as well. At birth, there were respiratory problems and they were in such critical condition that they were not expected to live more than a few days.

The father, a professional, and their mother requested that there be no treatment and no feeding. A nurse wrote on the chart, "do not feed in accordance with parent's wishes." This was countersigned by the physician in charge. Some of the nurses disregarded this order and fed the babies. The twins did not die in a few days as expected. After intervention by the Children and Family Service, who got court-ordered custody of the twins, they were fed. Four months in the neonatal intensive care unit was reported to have cost $166,000.

Tests indicated that the twins would not survive a surgical removal. When returned to the family they needed constant care.

2. Joseph Saikewicz—age 77 IQ 10 mental age two years and eight months—has been institutionalized for 40 years. Joseph can communicate only with gestures and grunts. He is unaware of danger. He becomes disoriented when removed from familiar surroundings. He has no living relatives.

His health had been generally good until he was diagnosed as having acute myeloblastic monocytic leukemia, which is inevitably fatal. In approximately 30 to 50 percent of these cases chemotherapy can bring about a temporary remission which usually lasts between two and thirteen months. Results are poorer for patients over

60. The chemotherapy often has serious side effects including anemia and infections.

In April, 1976, the Probate Court appointed a guardian *ad litem* with authority to make the necessary decision.

3.   Angela Merici is an extremely beautiful woman in the eyes of everyone but herself. Angela is convinced that she has a big nose that detracts from her appearance. Despite the assurances of friends and family, she persists in this belief. Angela goes to a plastic surgeon to remedy her condition. The surgeon points out that there is no need for the surgery and lists all the inconveniences and the expense of the work. Angela persists in her demands. Finally, the surgeon flatly refuses to meddle with the nose. Angela then goes to a second plastic surgeon, who believes that the psychological effects of the surgery justify the risks and the expense. The second surgeon performs the operation, modifying the nose so little that friends hardly notice the results. Angela goes around seeking compliments on her new appearance and is devastated when no one notices the "new" Angela.

4.   Mr. Capricioso has just moved to Center City and seeks a new family physician. During his first visit he asks the physician to give him a prescription for Valium, a tranquilizer, and to continue with the B_{12} shots that his former physician had given him every month. Nothing in the medical history or the examination indicates a need for either tranquilizers or B_{12} shots. The physician informs Capricioso of this and refuses to go along with either request.

5.   Mrs. Selbstmord, age 55, has chronic asthma. She keeps two cats to whom she is very attached, even though she is very allergic to cat fur, smokes a pack of cigarettes a day, and insists on getting emotionally involved in all family squabbles. Her family physician, Dr. Babadillo, has lectured her constantly on the fact that all three factors are complicating her asthma. He is reluctant to prescribe most asthma medicine because of the side effects, but most of all because a change in Selbstmord's lifestyle will do more good than any medication. After a year of unsuccessful patient education, he refuses to treat her any further unless she does her part and changes her lifestyle.

6.   Miss Regina Maris, never married, age 27, is a very successful young business woman. At the time of her annual check-up, she requests a sterilization by tubal ligation. When questioned about her motives, she merely replies, "I'm not taking any chances." She rejects suggestions for other methods of contraception. When the physician suggests that she may want children in the future, she rejects the idea vehemently. Even after the physician points out the dangers of the procedure, she sticks to her request.

7.   Rose Timony, R.N., is a nurse practitioner and works for the Home Health Agency. Matilda Ervin, one of her patients, is suffering from a long-standing sore throat and swollen lymph glands. The physician in charge has prescribed an antibiotic. Mrs. Ervin does not respond. Because of this, Nurse Timony suspects that the infection is

viral and terminates the antibiotics when the physician, informed of the situation, refuses to do so.

8.   James, age 14, was afflicted with a harelip and cleft palate and needed a common operation that promised to improve both his appearance and his speech significantly. The boy's father, a believer in mental healing, refused to permit the operation. The physicians explained the operation to James, who expressed a desire to "try for some time longer to close the cleft palate through natural forces."

9.   Brother Fox, age 93, a member of the Society of Mary, suffered a heart attack while undergoing corrective surgery for an inguinal hernia. He sustained substantial brain damage, slipped into a coma, and was placed on a respirator in an intensive care unit. Two neurosurgeons stated that there was no reasonable possibility that he would regain consciousness.

Father Eichner, who had been Brother Fox's close friend for nearly 26 years, knew that Brother Fox would want the respirator taken away. The two of them had, in the past, discussed the Quinlan case, and Fox had stated that he wanted no extraordinary means used if he were ever to be in this situation.

10.   Mary, an unmarried mother, is admitted to the hospital in the fortieth week of her pregnancy. Her membranes had broken a number of hours before. There are numerous signs of fetal distress so that the physicians believe a Caesaran section should be performed for the sake of the child. Mary refuses. She confides to the nurse that she does not know who the father is and does not care what happens to the child. Besides, the operation would be a lot of trouble. "Why look for more trouble than you have?" is Mary's motto.

11.   Procrustia is a registered nurse at the Bona Mors nursing home. The job is within walking distance. In any event, Procrustia does not drive and there is no other job she could get to without spending hours on public transportation. She works the three-to-eleven shift so that she can care for her mother during the day when her brother is absent. Her salary and that of the brother barely cover living expenses and the medical expenses of the 85-year-old mother, who is pretty well bedridden and in need of constant care.

After four years on the job, a new company buys the nursing home. Changes start to occur. Staff is reduced dramatically. The quality of food declines and even the heat is lowered three degrees during the day. All of these changes start to have an adverse effect on the residents. First there are more upper respiratory infections. Then there is more pneumonia. Bed sores are on the increase since there is insufficient staff to turn the patients often enough. Slightly disruptive or demanding patients are now "snowed," i.e., given heavy doses of tranquilizers to keep them out of the way.

The staff feels it cannot survive under the new conditions unless they can keep the patients very quiet. Procrustia complains to the management and is put off quietly. She complains a second time and is told that she is free to quit if she does not approve. She debates calling in the state inspectors, knowing that if they close the place down she will have no job and most of the patients will have no place to go since the area nursing homes are filled to capacity. In the end she does nothing and stays quietly on the job.

12. Femur, a registered physical therapist, is in private practice. She receives numerous referrals from physicians and, despite the prohibition of the professional code of the American Physical Therapy Association, also accepts patients without physician referrals. Before accepting any patient, she first checks their insurance coverage or possession of a Medical Assistance card or their participation in Medicare. If they have none of these normal guarantees of payment, she demands prepayment before beginning therapy. With this system she has done quite well and is earning between $40,000 and $50,000 a year. When paid in cash, she does not report this to the government.

Femur went through school on loans which she is still paying back. In addition, she is the sole support of her aged parents and a younger sister, who is going to college. She is a generous contributor to her church and to the local United Way. But she refuses to do any charitable professional work. When pressed by peers she replies, "I am free to be charitable where I please, and it does not please me to give my services away."

13. Joe is 11 years old, affected with Down's syndrome, and suffers from mental retardation. He has never lived at home and has been institutionalized since birth. At the time of the case he is in a home for 19 multiply handicapped children and is attending school at a special center. He is able to write his name, has good motor and manual skills, can dress himself, is toilet trained, and can converse reasonably and take part in school and Boy Scout activities. It has been recommended that he be placed in the county's sheltered workshop following his education. This means that he can be occupied in some gainful employment.

When Joe was six, a pediatric cardiologist made a preliminary diagnosis of a ventricular septal defect (a hole between the two chambers of the heart which elevates the pulmonary artery pressure). The pediatrician recommended cardiac catheterization to define the exact nature of the problem. The parents agreed. The tests showed a condition which, if untreated, generally leads to an average life expectancy of 30 years. About 25 percent of people with this condition die suddenly; the rest deteriorate slowly. Children untreated cannot run and play. The pediatrician recommended corrective surgery with a risk of death placed at 3 to 5 percent. He noted that he did not recommend the surgery for those with lower IQs since little was to be gained.

Joe's parents refused since they do not want Joe to outlive them. They believe geriatric care in the country is terrible. Besides, they felt that Joe would be a burden on their normal children.

NOTES

[1]The principle of double effect is common among Roman Catholic moral theologians. Those interested in the complexities of it and the contemporary debate about it should see Richard A. McCormick,

How Brave a New World? Dilemmas in Bioethics, pp. 413–429. Yet more detailed work can be found listed in the index in McCormick, *Notes on Moral Theology 1965–1980.* Those interested in a more traditional use of the principle should see Benedict M. Ashley, and Kevin D. O'Rourke, *Health Care Ethics: A Theological Analysis,* pp. 194–196.

[2]This ordinary/extraordinary means principle was originally developed by Catholic moral theologians as early as the sixteenth century. It originally arose because some treatments, even common ones, were so painful that it would be unreasonable to oblige a person to undergo them. In time, the principle became more general and became a proportionality principle. See McCartney, (1980, pp. 215–224).

[3]Paul Ramsey (1978) holds that the patient and the physician are both bound by the medical indications principle. He seems unwilling to trust the patient and overly concerned with the wedge principle. We object to this approach because it once again makes the physician the judge of what should be done and does not accept the fact that decisions about health are not purely and simply medical decisions.

[4]The Baby Doe rule can be found in 45 CFR Part 1340, Federal Register, April 15, 1985, pp. 14878–901.

Chapter Four
PRINCIPLES
OF DISTRIBUTION

INTRODUCTION

In the present chapter we will attempt to establish principles for the distribution of goods and services with particular emphasis on health care. To put it another way, we are asking what principles society should follow in attempting a just or at least a reasonable distribution of the goods necessary to protect the dignity of the individual person. It must be stressed that this is largely a question of social justice, that is, the principles of justice governing society rather than the individual. This is true since ultimately only the society as a whole is in a position to effect a just or fair distribution such that the dignity of each individual is protected. We shall discuss this point in greater detail a little later on.

At the very beginning we must realize that distribution is concerned with scarce resources. By scarce resources we mean that we are dealing with situations in which the demand for a resource outstrips the supply. In the first part of this chapter we will be concerned not merely with the theory governing the distribution of health care, but with the distribution of other goods such as clothing, education, food, and shelter as well as of security and the chance to work. The distribution of all these rather basic goods, which are often in short supply, needs to be considered in terms of the overall needs and dignity of the members of society.

JUSTICE, DIGNITY, AND SCARCITY

Scarcity and Distribution

At the very start there are several ethical and practical problems which every theory of distribution must face. First, the dignity of the individual person and the demands that flow from it must be respected. Second, need is the basis for the individual's claim to any basic good. Third, any system must permit some inequalities in distribution in order to recognize unequal contributions. Fourth, any pattern of distribution will have economic and political consequences which will influence the development and even survival of the society.

First, the method of distribution devised by practical wisdom should recognize the dignity of the individual. This will mean that we must avoid paternalism and in so far as possible respect the right of the individual to make his own mistakes. While there is always a temptation to say that everyone should eat such and such or be sheltered in such a way rather than another and even to dictate how much medical care a person should consume, the fact of the matter is that people have different needs and tastes in these areas. This is a result not only of differences in biological and social needs, but also of differences in subgroup membership and individual choices. As long as individual choice, subgroup autonomy, and individual differences are valued in American society (and it is our position that on moral grounds they should be in any society), they should be respected in the distribution of the basic goods.

Second, the need of the individual person must be the basis of the claim to basic goods. While need may be difficult to define precisely in every case, the disregard of individual and unequal human needs amounts to neglecting individual human beings. The demands of human dignity are the demands of individual persons in whom that dignity resides. We shall say more about this when we discuss the theories of justice that fail.

Despite this insistence on individual need, it is clear that needs grow and so create ever increasing demands on the society. The restless human animal is forever discovering new and better ways to satisfy the need for shelter, food, education, defense, and health care. Each new invention creates a demand, if not a need, for itself. We will, then, have to distinguish between needs and desires in the actual circumstances of a given society.

Third, though distribution should be on the basis of need, society must recognize that it must reward contribution in order to motivate people to contribute to society. Every society, even communist societies, ultimately discover that they must allow for some inequalities of distribution in order to motivate people to make contributions to the society. In American society, the free market, while imperfect, is the major method for the distribution of goods and for balancing economic contribution and economic reward. In societies where there is no recognition of contribution, whether through productivity or participation, stagnation sets in and everyone is worse off.

Economic contribution is not the only form of contribution. Individuals make a variety of political and social contributions. All of these contributions should be weighed in a fair and prudent theory of distribution. For example, the Veterans Administration, with its educational benefits, home mortgages, hospitals, insurance plans, and other programs, is designed to reward those who served in the military. These benefits are intended to be rewards for service and inducements to continued service. The political and social health of a society depends directly upon continued contributions in key areas of the society.

Finally, the economic and political consequences of any system of distribution must be considered for the sake of preserving the society. The dignity of the individual can be defined and acknowledged only within society. The individual's need for society is the ground for society's right and obligation to protect itself from such problems as political unrest and economic instability. To do this, the society has certain needs, such as the power to defend itself from insurrection and invasion or the power to enforce regulations which preserve the economic system. These concerns are different from those of the individual and must be decided upon by the political authority of that society. In effect, the society is under an obligation to the individual to promote the common good.

Social Priorities

To avoid social disruption, priorities must be established on some rational basis that accords with the goals and values of the society and set in such a way that expectations are regularized as a means of preventing social unrest and achieving social goals.

These political and economic realities force us to acknowledge that costs of basic goods, including health care, must be considered when dealing with scarce resources. One cannot simply say that cost should not be considered just because it is unpleasant to consider it. Here as elsewhere the basic dilemma of guns or butter remains prominent. No society can provide everything that everyone needs, let alone what everyone wants. Just as political considerations must be acknowledged to avert the danger of revolution, economic considerations must be acknowledged to prevent destroying the economy.

There can be no general right to the best a society can offer, because in an era of scarce resources (which will most likely be our permanent condition), a society would destroy itself if it tried to provide its members with the best of every material advantage.

A sound theory of distribution, then, must provide for *priorities* and a system of allocating resources that at least *regularizes expectations* in the light of what is politically and economically possible. Appeals to such norms as equality or equality of opportunity are useless if there is not and never will be enough to go around, or if such appeals define their terms in ways alien to the society.

For these reasons we emphasize the centrality of practical wisdom in ethical decision making. As our ability to recognize and tackle social problems, including health problems, develops, as our political understanding of such issues improves, and as our economic ability to satisfy human needs changes, we will be called upon time and again to rethink our ethical decisions and commitments. Our practical wisdom must balance the shifting demands and possibilities our changing circumstances present.

THEORIES THAT FAIL

There are many theories proposed for solving the problem of distribution. Most of these theories fail because they disregard one or more of the reality factors we listed above. We will take a look at several of these approaches (justice as entitlement, as equality, as fairness, as need based, as rights based, and as utility) as examples of flawed theories, each of which nevertheless can teach us something about the nature of just distribution.

Egalitarian Justice

The egalitarian theories of justice call for equal distribution of goods in society or at least the distribution of equal opportunity. These theories appeal in one way to the fact that each individual person is intrinsically good, and so the equal of every other person.

The appeal to the fundamental equality of human beings sounds good, but it is abstract and therefore easily misleading. It overlooks the fact that human needs are not equal and, consequently, if the dignity of each person is to be protected, these needs must be satisfied in unequal ways. For example, the equal distribution of goods in a very simple-minded way would lead to everyone getting exactly the same whether they needed it or not and whether they wanted it or not. This would leave some with too much and others with not enough to protect life and their dignity. Such a disregard of the actual needs of individuals not only denies the dignity of individuals but in fact makes society pointless.

Equality of opportunity is frequently cited as the proper way of justly providing for human equality, but this also leads to arrangements which do not recognize the dignity of unique individuals. A learning-disabled child may have the same opportunity to go to school as a healthy child, but the learning disability will make it impossible for him to take advantage of that opportunity in the same way. Equal opportunity is meaningless if individuals do not have the talent and power to avail themselves of the opportunity. In short, the attempt to protect basic equality by demanding equality of distribution can end up destroying basic equality because it disregards the inequality of needs.

A further problem with these schemes of distribution is that they do not allow for the problems of scarcity. If there is not enough to go around equally and provide all with a basic decent minimum, then everyone but the healthiest or the least demanding will suffer. In the context of the scarcity of resources, the attempt to provide equality would lead to the destruction of those individuals who had great needs.

These egalitarian theories also disregard the fact of human selfishness. Like it or not some people will be motivated to produce and produce a surplus only if they are given a greater share of the goods of society. If egalitarianism destroys the reward system, which recognizes selfishness as a strong factor in human life, it can create a society in which the scarcity of resources actually increases. This leads to not just an economic problem but also a political one, as the failure of society to provide for its members becomes clear.

Justice as Entitlement

According to an entitlement theory of justice, goods ought to be distributed according to a system of contracts, and the only claims of justice are those surrounding the meaning and performance of those contracts. Unless a person has a valid and enforceable contract stating a claim to a good, such as health care, she has no claim to it. A valid contract involves an agreement between a legally competent person for consideration, that is, for something of value.

A system of entitlement is found in an economic market system such as we have in the United States. Unless you can pay for something, or have a contract for it, you have no claim to it. At its simplest, this would mean that if you could not pay for your medical care or did not have some medical insurance (a company contracted to pay for your health care), you would rightly receive no medical care at all. Since the theory of entitlement is central to a market economy, and the market strongly influences our lives, this entitlement sense of justice is often the first that comes to mind.

The entitlement theory of justice, however, offends our common moral sensibilities on some important points. The most important, for our purposes, is that it seems wrong that a person be denied certain basic social goods, such as housing or food or medical care, because, through no fault of their own, they lack some form of contractual entitlement to it. We tend to feel that the dignity of even an incompetent or an indigent person demands that they should receive at least basic food, shelter, and medical care even if they cannot pay for it. Indeed, we are shocked when we hear of people sleeping on heating grates in the winter, eating out of garbage cans, or being "dumped" at the public hospital and then dying because they were not taken to the closest hospital. We feel that people can justly claim a good on the basis of need. Because this basic good is somehow vital to their dignity and their lives in this society, they in justice should receive it. Some things are more important than the ability to pay.

Entitlement theory, by disregarding need, disregards the dignity or intrinsic value of the human person by replacing it with a contract. Fortunately, Americans have never consistently followed entitlement theory in all areas.

Justice as Fairness Theory

In theories of "justice as fairness" (principally Rawls, 1971), an attempt is made to balance the basic equality of people with the inequality of their abilities and circumstances. On the one hand, the moral equality of individuals is protected by a system of liberties designed to assure the basic political equality of all citizens. On the other hand, since inequality of abilities and needs will affect the individual's place and success in society, justice as fairness allows inequalities as long as any pattern of unequal distribution is evaluated from the perspective of its effect on the least advantaged people in the society.

These inequalities result from a "natural lottery," which distributes such factors as genetic endowment, family support, and an individual's driving ambitions. These natural endowments will affect one's economic and political success, but they are, in this theory, advantages or disadvantages that are undeserved. Consequently, a central concern of a system of distribution is to counterbalance the effects of this "natural lottery."

By emphasizing the effect of schemes of distribution on the least well off, justice as fairness accounts for our common-sense moral intuition that human dignity requires special consideration be given those disadvantaged. This leads to a concern that social institutions work to overcome the effects of this natural lottery by offsetting natural inequalities with mitigating distribution patterns.

Our objection to justice as fairness rests on two grounds. The first is that the principle of evaluating any distribution scheme by its effect on the least advantaged is dangerously vague. Whose judgment and what criteria should be used in evaluating the effect on the least advantaged? If the advantaged are to be the judge, justice as fairness puts the fox in charge of the chicken coop. So many schemes of distribution can be justified in this manner that the principle would never prevent the "haves" from exploiting the "have nots." If, on the other hand, the disadvantaged are to judge, we run the risk that there will be inadequate provision for leadership and other long-range political concerns.

The second objection is that justice as fairness ultimately denies the dignity of the individual. It is certainly the case that natural differences affect a person's success and happiness. But it is also the case that identifying how these differences affect the person can easily lead to subordinating the dignity of the individual to the convenience of the society. In other words, when a society tries to define "disadvantaged" does it serve its own interest or the interest of human dignity? As we argued in the first chapter, the dignity of the individual rests in part on her uniqueness expressed through personal choices and preferences. By understanding the society's reaction to the natural lottery as an attempt to overcome its effects, justice as fairness comes dangerously close to rejecting the differences implied by these personal choices and preferences in favor of a uniformity based on social convenience. To give society the full power to identify what qualifies as an effect of the natural lottery and also the power to correct those inequalities is to give society too much power over the choices and preferences of the individual.

In short, we consider justice as fairness to give too little weight to both the individual's autonomy and the problems of paternalism. It is valuable, however, because of its attempt to incorporate, at least initially, individual differences into the system of justice. It fails in its attempt to make society too tidy by overcoming these differences.

Utilitarian Sense of Justice

The utilitarian theory of distribution calls for realizing the greatest good for the greatest number. It involves a calculation of the consequences of an action, counting pleasures and benefits as positive factors and pains and losses as negative factors. These factors are summed up, and the state of affairs with the greatest total is the proper one. Utilitarianism is not a theory of justice or of distribution, but a theory of the public good in which justice plays a subordinate role. A just distribution in utilitarianism would involve no more than maximizing the benefits of goods and services within the society.

We often see utilitarianism at work in large bureaucratic organizations, which make rules to maximize the good of the organization. This procedure is intuitively attractive, and at times this is what society often has to settle for. But it has serious ethical limitations.

Since it deals with aggregates, utilitarianism loses the individual. In such a system, the individual has what we might call dignity only in so far as she has utility for the operation of the group. Precisely because the ethical theory in this book makes the individual person the ethical center and sees the public good as a means to the good of the individual, utilitarianism is viewed with great suspicion (note our discussion in Chapter One).

A further, and equally serious, criticism of utilitarianism is that it creates the expectation that all problems might be solved. Yet there is no reason to assume that human capabilities stretch so far. A tragic element is present in any attempt to meet health care needs in conditions of scarcity. No human system can expect to accomplish everything, to make distribution entirely just, to relieve all suffering. Utilitarianism buries this tragic reality in its attempt to view the good as an aggregate, in which aggregate suffering is simply outweighed by aggregate pleasure.

Justice and Needs

A system of justice based on need alone holds that a just system provides goods to its members simply on the basis of their demonstrated need and their inability to satisfy it on their own. The individual is the exclusive focus of this sense of justice, and the individual is understood in his uniqueness, that is, in terms of his particular problems and possibilities. For example, because an individual has allergies, he has a need for specialized medical treatment. Simply because he has this need, he is entitled to receive treatment for it. If he cannot get the treatment on his own, the individual has a claim for treatment against the larger society.

This system has an intuitive attractiveness, but there are two major difficulties. First, need is a difficult concept to identify clearly. How does one distinguish between needs and wants? We can easily see that difference between someone needing treatment for bronchial pneumonia and another wanting a face lift. Most issues are not so clearly distinguishable; for example, does an indigent person suffering from a correctable deformity, such as a clubfoot, need or "merely" want corrective surgery? Does a terminal patient need to be on a respirator for the last few days of his life? Does every teenager need braces on her teeth? These questions are intimately connected with the problem of defining health and disease, which we will consider shortly. We stress that needs are as much psychosocial as they are biological and the distinction between needs and wants is one of degree and social estimation rather than of kind.

Second, since needs tend to grow in the presence of the means to satisfy them, distribution based on need would create an impossible demand on the wealth and resources of even a "rich" society. Even prescinding from all basic goods except health care, a health care system based solely on need would overwhelm the resources of any society. When we consider all the social goods we need such as food, clothing, shelter, defense, public sanitation, transportation, and education, it becomes clear that simple need cannot be the sole criterion of fair distribution for the uncompromising reason that such distribution is impossible.

In the last analysis, need, if it can be identified clearly, should be the basis of distribution of necessary goods, yet it cannot be the only basis and, in a situation of scarcity, it cannot be satisfied completely. We will return to this when we consider the system of macroallocation.

A Rights Theory of Justice

As we have seen in Chapter One, rights theories of justice assert the right, or justified claim, of the individual person to certain goods on the grounds that they are necessary for maintaining the life and dignity of the individual. These claims are against either other individuals or the society, and they impose obligations on the other.

Social contract theorists argue that society was created to protect the individual's rights from encroachment by others. We all have, for example, a right to life which all other individuals are supposed to respect. But in the state of nature, prior to society, one could not trust others to respect the right to life, or any other right, and so the enjoyment of one's rights was uncertain. Society, in these theories, was invented to protect one's rights and to enforce the limitations and claims that rights embody. Thus, society stands behind us to ensure that others do not kill us, and we have a right to expect society to continue to do so.

Justice in a rights theory can be stated in a number of ways, depending upon how rights are interpreted. Some rights theories of justice are based on equality, others on entitlement, still others on needs. This implies the recognition that while one can easily say that justice is served when one has his rights satisfied, it is a much more complicated issue to describe what these rights are and how we know them. To put this in the language of the previous paragraph, what a rights theory of justice means depends very much upon how rights are *justified*.

PRACTICAL WISDOM AND A SENSE OF JUSTICE

It is the authors' contention that justice as distribution is accomplished through the application of practical wisdom to meet the demands of human dignity in the social circumstances of the time. Justice thus involves respecting human dignity and satisfying human needs and recognizing human contributions within the system and in ways that are characteristic of the system.

The specific definition of human dignity, and the specific demands that flow from it, will fluctuate according to a number of factors: the traditions and goals of the particular society; the available economic and social resources; the current understanding of the meaning of appropriate social ideals; the power and persuasiveness of political authority; the consensus of the society in the distribution; and the preferences of individuals.

Any account of human dignity must also take into account the weakness of human nature and the limits that that weakness places upon human accomplishments. To recognize human dignity is to accept the individual as an individual, that is, to recognize individual differences. Such a recognition cannot avoid acknowledging that people have different strengths and weaknesses. Just as our strengths allow accomplishment, our weaknesses function both to limit and to modify those accomplishments. For example, capitalism as an economic system tries to encourage people to be industrious and frugal (as socially beneficial ideals) by rewarding their selfish interests. Human weakness (self-interest) is a source of common good (the productivity hard work causes). The capitalist system may not be an ideal system (that is, it has flaws), but it might be the most practical system because it accommodates people both in their strengths and their weaknesses.

The changing nature of the demands of human dignity or at least the changing social specification of human needs means that the actual practical principles of justice can be specified only through the historical circumstances of a society. As we have stated, the dignity of a human being imposes formal constraints on what justice can be, such as the principles of autonomy and informed consent (Chapter Two), or the injunction to do good (Chapter Three). But as the very subject matter of this book suggests, these principles are in themselves abstract and useless without further specification. In medical ethics, the principle of autonomy becomes specified through the discussion of beneficence, nonmaleficence, and informed consent.

Both the identification of general principles and the specification of these principles take place in a social tradition. This tradition embodies the experiences and the explanations, the hopes and goals of both the society and its members. There is a rough form of practical wisdom at work as the community faces the tasks of surviving through changing circumstances. This practical wisdom works through the history and language of that tradition, where concepts are informed and understood in the terms of that tradition, and social consciousness exists as its derivation. For example, modern American attitudes towards civil rights are the result of American (and consequently Western) cultural history. From the original doubts of the Founding Fathers about the institution of slavery, through the Civil War, to the civil rights movement of the 1950s and 1960s, American culture has evolved an understanding involving both knowledge and emotion regarding the practical issues of civil rights. This understanding is fragmented among different factors of the society and is changing (one hopes improving) as new issues are raised, such as hiring quotas and reverse discrimination. In short, justice in practice is not the result of the application of a few simple principles, but also a question of politics and social consensus. It is a ragged sort of justice, but all we have in the face of the reality of human existence. This chapter, then, is a misnomer to the extent that there is no simple principle of just distribution.

In the complex health care system in the United States, distribution takes place on several levels so that we can expect to find several sets of specifications. The goods must be parceled out between the need for defense, fire and police protection, as well as food, shelter, air, clothing, health care, and public health measures. The distribution, moreover, must take into consideration the autonomy of the individual. Thus, the distribution should not demean the recipients by treating them like beggars or children whose preferences are to be disregarded. In short, the distribution must allow for the recipients to prefer more food over more health care, and more defense over public health measures. The specifications of the right to health care may also favor public health or preventative measures over restorative measures on the grounds that this is the most efficient use of scarce resources. Throughout, society must remain concerned with the effect of distribution on human dignity and so at least with the adequacy of basic goods available, such as food, shelter, and health care.

JUSTICE AND HEALTH CARE

At this point, we have developed some general norms of fair distribution. To summarize quickly, any fair system of distribution must respect the dignity of the individual. This respect is accomplished by responding in a culturally appropriate way both to the needs and to the contributions of that individual. The structure and content of a fair distribution is determined by the practical wisdom of the society, which in turn is informed by social goals, ideals, and traditions, and by the extent of the resources available.

In this section, we will show how these general norms regarding fair distribution can be a guide to evaluating the American system of health care delivery. This involves describing how the dignity of the individual is served by health care. Our means of evaluating this service is, as we have said, practical wisdom, the weighing and balancing of all things in the light of human dignity.

In order to facilitate the evaluation of health care, it is necessary to discuss such basic concepts as the nature of disease and health, the limits of health care, and related items. First, we shall present the psychosocial nature of health and disease since distribution aims at promoting the one and preventing and curing the other. Second, we will discuss the limits of the good we call health care: its presumptions and its potential accomplishments. Third, we will consider the problem of allocating resources between public health measures, which are largely preventative, and treatment of individuals, which is largely curative. Fourth, we shall discuss the concept of adequate care for basic needs. Finally, we shall begin the discussion of the distribution of health care as the satisfaction of basic needs.

A Definition of Health and Disease

The first step in this evaluation involves understanding the psychosocial nature of health and disease. This requires first a definition of terms and second an indication of how variations in this definition can affect what is expected from the health care system. We are not attempting here to define any particular condition, but we wish rather to show how social expectations and habits influence what we perceive to be significant. What we perceive to be significant lies at the heart of particular health conditions and so ultimately determines society's recognition of a need for health care.

Health and disease can be understood only in terms of what is perceived to be significant, because to talk of health and disease is to assume a privileged position. Biologically speaking, there is no health or disease; there are only different organisms competing for survival in the ways available to them. For example, a dog with fleas is not sick unless you care for the dog, which gives the dog a privileged position. If you are raising fleas, then the fleas have the privileged position and the dog is not sick at all. Thus, like justice, though perhaps more surprisingly, health and disease can be properly understood only in their social context.

In noting the social context of definitions of health and disease, we do not mean to deny the scientific nature of much of what contributes to health care. We simply mean that health and disease are not exclusively biological or physiological. On the contrary, health and disease are loaded with social and subjective concerns as well as objective scientific criteria. Indeed, most scientific considerations are nested within larger and controlling social and subjective issues.

These social and subjective considerations take several forms. Social conditions influence and may control the recognition of a problem and, once recognized, its degree of seriousness. In other words, people may suffer the symptoms of a disease without ever considering themselves to be ill. The point at which a collection of symptoms is admitted to be an illness varies greatly with social background (Spector, 1985; Starr, 1982). For example, some people will not admit they are ill until they cannot continue to work. Others consider themselves ill if they feel any discomfort or pain. Even the type of symptoms counted varies with social background.

Because of the influence of social concerns on the recognition of disease, we define a "disease" as *any deficit in the physical form or physiological or psychological functioning of the individual in terms of what society wants or expects from that individual or in terms of what the individual wants or expects for himself.* As defined, disease involves a reference to the desires of the society and those of the individual, and not merely to physiological functioning.

This definition of disease emphasizes the role of the society and the individual in defining disease. Certainly the biological and physiological elements are included. If a tumor causes such pain that the individual cannot get out of bed or even think, then it meets the criteria of a disease. On the other hand, an individual with arthritis may not consider himself as having a disease as long as he can function effectively. Similarly, society may consider the arthritis a disease only when it makes the individual unable to contribute anything to society. Thus, by recognizing or emphasizing (or by denying and de-emphasizing) particular physiological conditions, social and individual expectations and history influence the presence or absence of disease.

Given our definition of disease, health is easily understood as the *lack* of any deficit in the physical form of psychological functioning in terms of what the society wants or expects from that individual or in terms of what the individual wants or expects for himself. If you can do what you want or expect to do, or what society wants or expects, then you are healthy.

Disagreement in Defining Disease

The conceptions of health and disease held by individuals and society may vary widely enough to allow two people to look at the same condition and evaluate it very differently. There are health authorities who argue that the low body fat levels, the enlarged heart, and the stress on muscles and ligaments characteristic of athletes indicate an actual decrease in their health, while many argue that athletes, who "suffer" from all these conditions, represent the genuinely healthy individuals in our society. Not only is it necessary to understand the social circumstances and personal expectations of the individual in order to be able to understand their "health" or "disease," but it must be further recognized that one will bring to that analysis presuppositions, or prejudices, that will strongly influence the analysis. If the presuppositions and prejudices enlarge the scope of disease, they will create a demand for health care which makes it even more difficult to distribute scarce resources for the service of all members of the society.

Not only may there be differences between individuals in their understanding of disease, but there may be differences between the individual and society as well. As we have seen, both have different concerns, interests, and responsibilities, which may lead to conflicting evaluations. A father, caring for his desperately ill son, may not accept society's judgment that his son should not receive the organ transplant he needs. While society sees a boy too ill to be likely to survive treatment, and thus an inappropriate risk of scarce resources, the father sees only his son. Both are correct. Yet when it comes to the distribution of health care, the society's judgment will prevail when the individual cannot afford to pay for treatment or when resources are apportioned.

The tragic dimension of this conflict results from the irreconcilability of the two perspectives under the current historical and material conditions. Only so much can be done, and given differences in perspective, the judgment of what should be done will be contested. The danger to any fair system of distribution is that the power society holds be used to silence the anguish of the individual. Fair distribution, and even political stability, require a continuing dialogue between the society and the individual on what counts. To maintain this dialogue, the potentially tragic dimensions of distribution must always be acknowledged, and the society must restrain itself and hear the individual. This irreconcilability between the view and concerns of the society and those of the individual is not simple ambiguity: it is a genuine difference in interest and perspective that will remain in any system. It is only by an honest attempt to mediate both concerns that there will be growth in the understanding of what fair distribution is all about.

Health Care Has Its Own Limit

In addition to these difficulties, there is a limit intrinsic to health care based on the limits of medical and health care knowledge. The knowledge of a health care professional is the combination of science, experience, and compassion. Much importance has been placed on health care as a science, but questions have been raised recently about what it means to say that health care is based on scientific knowledge.

According to Bursztajn et al. (1981), Americans have exaggerated ideas of the power of health care and medical knowledge because they have a dubious concept of science in general and of medical knowledge in particular. Many people believe that health care is simply a matter of scientifically and certainly identifying the cause of a problem and treating it with a scientifically validated drug or procedure. They expect that this cause can be identified by a diagnostic procedure, which will give a clear and unambiguous answer. They further expect that the treatment will be equally precise and straightforward. It is as though medicine, in particular, is a kind of magic, which offers cures and restoration beyond the frustrations and limits we find in other areas of human life.

Medical advances and reports in the popular press seem to validate this attitude. The advances made during the twentieth century stem from identifying the causes of diseases such as influenza, polio, smallpox, whooping cough, and many others. Once identified, these diseases were treated with recently developed "miracle drugs" or vaccines, which drastically limited their destructive effects, leading to an increase in life expectancy and to a decrease in infant mortality.

But whatever their impact on the daily lives of people, these successes have created an impression about health care that obscures the nature of many health problems. For example, hypertension, a clinical problem which figures in many diseases, is apparently the result of several different factors: genetic history, health habits, and stress. Identifying the contribution of each of these factors, and even how they influence one another, is a much more complex problem than identifying the virus that causes smallpox. Health care for these problems must settle for diagnoses that are probable rather than certain, as the diagnosis reflects the recognition that a disease may have many interrelated causes. Indeed, some of the causes of a disease may be beyond the reach of any health care.

The limits of medical diagnosis, and of all forms of health care, need to be acknowledged if we are to have a realistic view of the extent to which they can satisfy needs and should be supported by society. Indeed, the removal of exaggerated views about the magic of modern health care can do much to mitigate the demand for health care and so decrease the costs. Such realism should result in making it possible to serve more people with fewer scarce resources. This point needs to be stressed since even the wealthy American society has arrived at a point where the cost of health care can no longer be disregarded.

By Way of Summary

In the last two sections, we have shown that health care cannot be divorced from social and individual concerns. Far from a "purely objective" and scientific pursuit, health care is very much rooted in the beliefs, expectations, and habits that form the community and the individuals within it. Values (and differences in values) are important for health care because they provide standards against which states of body and mind are judged. These values strongly influence determinations of what counts as health or disease, and their appropriate care. Ultimately, these factors have an enormous effect on the costs of health care and the availability of resources, and so on the actual distribution of health care.

Is Health Care Always Good?

The questions about the nature of medical knowledge, and its focus, lead quite naturally into a question about its purpose. It is usually assumed, as part of our "common sense," that health care is a good. It is, however, an instrumental good, that is, it is not good for its own sake, but a means that helps us attain some other good. What is this good that health care helps us attain? We have already listed three such goods, and we now look more closely at those three goods.

One possible goal of health care is to prolong life. If so, then our attitude toward medicine and its goals has its roots in our concern with, and perhaps fear of, death. Modern medicine has been developed over the last 300 years in the light of a hope that all human dysfunction can be eliminated, suggesting that death may be put off indefinitely. In other words, we expect medicine to help us avoid death. But death is clearly not a disease, at least not in the sense that it is unnatural. Every living, natural organism dies, so it is difficult to see something normal and universal as being a disease. The hope that science may forestall death is not based on death's abnormality; that hope is a social intention that overlays the scientific investigation.

This hope, based on impossible roots, can have a devastating effect on both human dignity and on a society's resources. There is now a wide variety of technical means to extend life: respirators, mechanical hearts, dialysis machines, etc. But what kind of life is maintained under such conditions? The increasing number of well-publicized cases of mercy killing indicate a growing unease with the vision of life hooked up to such devices. (We will return to this question in Chapter Six.) It is also the case that such life-prolonging efforts are tremendously expensive. For example, one-quarter of all Medicare funds are spent during the last year of a person's life, and most of that is spent during the last month (Kleiman, 1985). Much of this money is spent prolonging death and represents scarce resources that could be used to maintain and improve health.

Another possible goal of health care is to alleviate suffering. Most of us will agree that people should live their life as free as reasonably possible from pain. But what is pain or suffering? Pain is a personal or private experience, and it is very difficult to accurately comprehend the pain another individual is suffering. Also, what is the purpose of alleviating suffering? If we alleviate suffering without dealing with the cause of that suffering, we are simply masking the pain. Is it better to mask pain, or should we be left suffering so as to be forced to act to change the conditions that caused the suffering?

For example, painkillers are certainly useful and appropriate in many cases. A woman suffering from incurable cancer is aided by morphine in a way that many see as totally consistent with her dignity. But another woman, suffering from disorientation and loneliness, is kept sedated in an understaffed nursing home against all understanding of human dignity. Human beings ought not be warehoused like used machinery.

There are less dramatic examples of how the alleviation of suffering can be abused. There are drugs on the market, for example, that are highly effective in treating ulcers by stopping acid production in the stomach. In most cases, such treatment does not deal with the underlying cause of the ulcer, such as stress or excessive use of alcohol. Thus, the drug effectively masks the true problem, allowing it to continue and perhaps cause greater problems elsewhere in the body.

These issues raise again the possible difference between the individual's and the society's definition of health and disease. As we will see in Chapter Six on death and dying, there can be a wide variation of estimates of what counts as too much suffering. If health care takes on the task of alleviating suffering, it is going to have to confront that variety and be responsible for judging private emotional as well as physical conditions.

The third possible goal is "to optimize the patient's chance for a happy and productive life as defined by the patient." A problem with this suggestion is that, as we have already seen, society has a decisive role in defining health and disease. This is a role that society cannot abrogate because of its own need for survival. In the context of socially financed or socially delivered health care, the debate on the meaning of "optimum" would be endless, and probably lead to no improvement in government-sponsored health care.

The consequences of optimization for fair distribution are also quite significant. Enormous amounts of resources will be affected by even small gradients of change in the meaning of "optimum." Take as an example mental health. Should we be free of only those anxieties that prevent us from functioning at all, should we be free of all but minor anxieties, or should we be free of all anxieties? An attempt to free the members of a society of all but minor anxieties would not only be fantastically expensive but probably impossible.

We should also note a further problem in identifying the goal of health care. Not only may health care have an obvious, or generally intended, purpose, but in its instrumental capacity, health care can be used to serve several extrinsic ends. In our economic system and social system health care delivery not only takes care of patients, but it also pays the salaries and provides social status and psychic satisfaction for health care providers. Any understanding of the purpose of health care is going to be influenced by the economic, social and psychic concerns of health care providers. Such concerns are not the goal of the health care system but can easily be treated as if they were.

For the present, we will proceed as if health care is generally a good. We will, however, keep in mind those cases where it is not a good, and we will recall the potentially self-serving aspects of the role of health care providers in defining health and providing health care.

Health Care versus Public Health

Even if we assume that health care is a good, we are still faced with the problems of distributing resources between health care, health education, and public health measures. Ultimately, health care is a good because it promotes health. Professional health care is, however, not the only thing that promotes health (even if it is the only form that pays health care providers). A person's lifestyle and genetic endowment are key determinants of health. Equally important is the social health system, that is, the public health measures provided by the society. Pure air, pure water, effective garbage disposal and sewer systems, healthy working conditions, and public feeding of the poor and deprived children have done as much to improve health as all the health care in existence. Society, then, must allocate money to public health measures as well as to health care. The Environmental Protection Agency, the Occupational Health and Safety Agency, and the school lunch programs are health programs that should not be neglected in the name of health care.

In allocating resources, society must decide how much it wants to dedicate to public health and health education, which will prevent disease in the future, and how much to health care, which seeks to cure or rehabilitate here and now. It is not obvious that, in general, one should have precedence over the other. One major difficulty is that education and public health measures save statistical lives, rather than identified lives. No one ever knows that he was saved from a disease by public health measures, even if the incidence of that disease has dropped significantly. On the other hand, anyone sick who is cured by a physician or nurse fully appreciates the influence of health care on her situation. The emotional difference between the influence of public health and that of health care must be recognized in forming a policy on public health. Once again, the actual situation, the resources available, and the definitions of a given society will have to be weighed and balanced to allocate efforts in a manner consonant with human dignity.

Humane Health Care

Society will be working toward a distribution of basic health care that is adequate for the restoration and preservation of health as society defines it. This basic and adequate health care may be called humane in so far as it protects the dignity of the individual person.

When the absence of a certain type of health care leads to early death, disfigurement, or loss of functions necessary to take one's place in society, we have certainly fallen below the basic minimum of health care. In other words, the absent care is part of the basic and adequate minimum. It is basic because, in our society at our stage of ethical, scientific, and technological development, the dignity of the individual demands that we employ reliable and ordinary means to maintain a certain minimum level of treatment. This minimum requires that the individual gain relief from pain, which destroys the higher human functioning, and restores at least the minimum functioning valued by society; that she be spared a death that is the result of trivial or avoidable circumstances; that she be spared disfigurement that will make her repugnant to her society and herself; and that she be spared a loss of function that will make her unable to share the actions, burdens, and accomplishments that membership in society demands.

In this area, the society has limited freedom to specify what basic needs are and how they will be met. What limits the freedom of society in specifying these needs are the demands of human dignity and the extent of the society's resources. Both concerns are limits, for the society must not only protect its members by protecting their dignity, it must also protect itself by protecting its resources. Thus, the society must refer to considerations broader than those viewed by the individual, considerations such as the individual's contribution to society and the cost/benefit ratio of any treatment. It will not be obligated to treat a private in the Army in the same way as the president, nor will it have the obligation to provide the most expensive false teeth if a cheaper pair will do the job. Granted a superabundance of resources, society might specify a right to all these things, but we can see no general right which would call for such specifications.

In these decisions, the functioning desired by the individual cannot control the definition of adequate care, since we know that resources would not permit satisfying all those desires. The distribution, then, will undoubtedly leave some individuals sick, that is, below the level of functioning they desire. We cannot argue that a person who demands social payment for health care has a right to establish for themselves the level and type of treatment they will receive. Only the reasonable desires of the individual for health care need to be satisfied and then only if we understand that *reasonableness of the desire for restored function is dependent on the judgment of society as well as of the individual.*

In deciding difficult cases, the factor of contribution or potential contribution becomes important, even critical. When the basic needs for health care as defined above have been met, society has discretion in the use of its funds for health care or any of the other essential goods, whichever promotes the public good. Here the utilitarian principle of the greatest good for the greatest number seems justified, within the general limits of human dignity.

A presumption of these conditions is that not all needs have an equal urgency or involve the dignity of the individual in the same way. This is particularly clear in the case of health care, where treatment may be useful for well-being, but in no sense basic to human dignity. Not every cut needs to be stitched, nor every headache cured, nor every variation in blood pressure corrected. Those who wish to pay for such treatment out of their own funds have a right to do so, but they do not in the absence of a social specification have a *prima facie,* that is, a presumptive, right to direct help from the society.

Dangers of Social Power

However, as society assesses the extent of its own social needs and the limits of its obligations, there is a tendency to overlook the dignity of the individual. This is especially true when resources are scarce. The society might stop listening to the needs and expectations of the individual, in particular powerless individuals. But the dignity of the individual requires that society listen to the individuals who are potential patients. The dialogue must continue despite the conflict between social and individual definitions of disease.

Society may also diminish the dignity of the individual by labeling him "diseased" without some clear and overriding social justification. Such a process is acceptable only when, all things considered, it is necessary to protect the dignity of other members of the society. Thus, quarantining an individual might be acceptable if she has a highly communicable disease. On the other hand, such labeling is not acceptable if she does not have the proper political ideas or fails to bathe every day. Even though social concerns are legitimate factors in a decision, the needs of a society are not trump cards that simply override individual dignity.

In labeling or categorizing people for the public good, practical wisdom cannot avoid issues regarding the quality of life. These issues are beyond the scope of medical competence, as, for example, when contribution is included as a factor in awarding care. This opens up the possibility of abusing the dignity of individuals who do not fit the expectations or preferences of those making the political decisions. Thus, the practical requirement of establishing a hierarchy of health care needs raises issues that the society must treat very carefully, for they open the door for a potentially strong paternalism, or even political tyranny. At the same time, there appears to be no other even semiprincipled way of approaching the problem in a world where scarcity is a fact and the need to apportion resources is disregarded at peril to both the individual and society.

Compounding the problem is the fact that the socially accepted concept of human dignity changes over time and reflects the circumstances of society. This changing social ideal of human dignity must be continuously and critically examined. The examination must involve the entire society in dialogue with all social and political authorities. After all, the demands of dignity do place some limits on what society can impose on the individual. At the very least that dignity requires society to hear the individual in determining what human function and health care mean. This will be difficult and painful because the discussion must always face the tragic dimensions of human life. If, however, the society fails to hear the individual, it has not merely neglected but destroyed the dignity of the individual.

Summary

A just society seeks to protect the dignity of its members and to satisfy their basic needs. Ordinarily, a society accomplishes these two tasks by giving its members the opportunity of satisfying their own needs in their own way. When members cannot satisfy their own needs, the just society specifies how it will attempt to satisfy those needs directly and humanely. In short, society must decide what constitutes a minimum level of satisfaction consistent with human dignity and the resources available. In making this specification and setting this minimum, the society is limited and influenced not only by the need of members and the resources available, but also by the need to keep itself functioning. These concerns must be weighed and balanced within its own culture, values, and history. Since resources are always scarce, this direct distribution involves a judgment evaluating various sorts of basic needs and various ways of satisfying them directly. In particular, this judgment must recognize the need for rewards for those whose contributions keep society going or produce the surplus from which direct distributions can be made.

Directly provided adequate humane health care should include the care necessary for the individual to avoid premature death as measured statistically, to function in society as a productive member, and, when such functioning is no longer possible, to be free of unnecessary physical pain in life and death. Society may decide that it has the resources do to much more than this minimum. That would be a desirable situation. It is not, however, a situation necessary for every society.

There are no easy answers to the question of what is the minimum in a given society and how it is to be attained. As we have suggested, human dignity is maintained only by consistent attempts to be consciously aware of its demands.

A balanced distribution is not the result of society's efforts alone. The individual must be present in the dialogue. In health care the presence of the individual occurs through not only the political process but in decisions made in seeking and offering health care. That is, the distribution of health care is influenced not only by political and social decisions, but it is also influenced by microallocation.

MICROALLOCATION: INDIVIDUAL AND INSTITUTIONAL

Though society can control macroallocation, individuals, lay and professional, as well as institutions such as nursing homes and hospitals, are deeply involved in microallocation on a day-by-day basis. Both the patient and the health care professional are engaged in triage or at least the allocation of their time and energies. Hospitals and health care institutions are faced with rationing decisions on the basis of their resources and the ability of the patient to pay. All these groups have great impact upon what health care is offered an individual, but their influence is limited by the macroallocation of the society.

Allocation of Resources by the Patient

The patient must make decisions about the allocation of his resources among all needs, including those of the family. For example, a parent under 65 with no medical insurance and no claim to Medicaid will have to decide to take a child to the doctor or hospital while taking into consideration not only the medical condition of the child, but also the potential economic damage to the family that might be incurred by the resulting bills. Patients are already constrained by the economic and social organization of health care and make decisions on allocation in terms of a careful calculations of results and costs. There appear to be no clear ethical priorities for the decisions of the individual except that she must consider all relevant factors.

Microallocation: Triage and the Health Care Provider

The term "triage" originates in military medicine, where it means the process of sorting sick and wounded on the basis of urgency and type of problem so that they can be sent to the proper treatment facility. The triage rules for emergency surgery in war call for giving first preference to the slightly injured who can be quickly returned to battle, with second place being given to the more seriously injured who need immediate treatment. The hopelessly wounded come in the last place.

By extension triage can be used for the prioritizing of treatment in catastrophes and in emergency rooms. In a disaster, for examples, rules like the following apply. Give first preference to those who need treatment in order to survive. Give second place to those who will survive without treatment and last place to those who will not survive even with treatment. Emergency room triage may introduce additional distinctions. First place might go to those who have life-threatening conditions which, if not treated immediately, will cause serious physical injury. Emergency rooms may well put the third priority military group in this first position, even though they will not recover with treatment. Second come those who will require treatment within 30 minutes to two hours before being threatened with serious physical injury. Finally there are those who at the time of examination are not critical and do not require treatment in order to survive.

Because most triage is done in an emergency or crisis situation, it generally and correctly disregards everything but the medical indications and the good of the individual patient. While emergency room triage sometimes disregards medical indications when it treats a hopeless patient, this is a reflection of a social belief in the magic of medicine, which suggests that no one is really beyond help and that everything possible ought to be done.

It should be noted that military triage and any triage which is based not on individual need but on social concerns might be quite different. In military triage the good of the group is given precedence over the good of the individual, so that the contribution made by an individual to the group rather than the need of the individual is made the primary criterion of judgment. Jonsen et al. (1986) notes that when penicillin was scarce during World War II, it was given first to soldiers with venereal diseases rather than to the wounded. Those with VD could be returned to the battle much more quickly than the wounded. Such a subordination might be justified in crisis situations if the individual person is not destroyed in the process.

We can expect current triage practices in emergency situations to change as cost factors make society aware that we cannot afford to use resources where no good can be accomplished. Cost factors and other considerations involving a recognition of the limits of health care may erode the belief that no one is beyond help and that everything possible ought to be done. Indeed, we may even see a lowered priority assigned to those who have a life-threatening condition but little or no contribution to make to society. This is a shocking thought because it involves judging the value of human life in terms of social utility. Yet this type of judgment may become a fact of life as society is forced to give more consideration to efficiency under the constraints of scarcity.

Microallocation: The Institutional Sphere

Health care institutions are divided into for-profit groups and not-for-profit groups. The not-for-profit groups can be further subdivided into those that are run by the government and those that are controlled by voluntary associations. These, in turn, can be classified as general community hospitals or specialized facilities devoted to only one illness or even a single class of patients. Because each stands in a different relationship to society, the distributive ethics will vary.

The for-profit institutions clearly operate under an entitlement theory and, at the present stage of history, this is correct in so far as they pretend to do no more. To put it another way, inside a socially approved market economy, they are as institutions ethical, if not admirable, when they take those who can pay and reject those who cannot.

Government owned and operated general hospitals should be open to all, with priority granted to the needy on the basis of need. These hospitals are paid for out of general funds and should be for the good of all citizens, but priority is to be given to the needy on the basis of need on the assumption that those with health insurance or sufficient wealth can obtain services elsewhere. Government hospitals for specialized populations, such as those run by the Veterans Administration, should distribute within the limits of their purposes. All of this assumes that society has reached some consensus on the levels of need and how they will be satisfied.

Private, voluntary not-for-profit groups are a more complicated matter. They do not derive their funds from the general funds of society, but do have special privileges such as tax exempt status. In short, the voluntary, not-for-profit hospital is burdened with the public interest because they receive support and income from both the government and their communities. They also derive much of their income from government programs such as Medicare and from other tax exempt institutions such as Blue Cross and Blue Shield. These hospitals are, moreover, so much a part of the local community that they have special relations with and possibly obligations to that community.

Some specialized voluntary hospitals such as those in academic medical centers often give preference to "interesting cases," which are particularly important for teaching health practitioners and increasing knowledge in the field. This is allocation on the basis of potential contribution to society rather than on the basis of patient need alone.

The Economic Dimension on the Institutional Level

As we noted in Chapter Three, health care providers, whether individuals or institutions, are not charitable institutions who can supply all services free of charge. Those institutions that received federal monies for certain purposes such as construction are legally obliged to care for a certain number of the poor free of charge. This obligation, however, does not call for free treatment of all indigent patients. The needs of the indigent poor would soon overwhelm the resources of any voluntary health care institution. Economics, then, becomes a central factor in an institutional distribution policy.

Up to the present, society has permitted economic considerations to enter into microallocation of the institutional level. In order to prevent such considerations from dominating admissions decisions, the society permitted differential pricing. For example, hospitals were allowed to charge one class of patients more so that it could subsidize the care of the poor. Changes in how medical bills are paid, such as third-party payers (for example, Blue Cross and Blue Shield), have made such attempts to shift economic burdens ineffective. New mechanisms must be developed to cover those without the means to pay while meeting the needs of the institutions that offer the care.

Society is faced with the problem of the extent to which it will require health care institutions to care for the poor without recompense and to what extent the society will pay for the care of those who cannot pay. In short, we are back to the problem of macroallocation. In the long run, the problems on the institutional level cannot be solved without recourse to the societal level.

Institutional Allocation and Procedural Rules

Some advocate institutional fair allocation by the use of procedural rules which either eliminate bias or minimize its effects. Although these rules do not come to grips with the basic economic problem, they should be considered.

One set of procedural rules proposes selection by lottery or by some form of the first-come-first-served rule. Behind these rules is the belief that equality or equality of opportunity should be the governing principle in allocation decisions. We reject these procedures for the same reason that we rejected the egalitarian view. The rules disregard the difference in need and the fact that the differences must be acknowledged since they are relevant to the dignity of the individual person. If all things were equal, which they never are, then the lottery or first–come–first–served principles might be applicable. In the real world of scarce resources and unequal needs, they merely dodge the issues. Fortunately, these rules are generally not used in practice.

A better proposal is that there be some sort of due process in the allocation of resources. Thus, the allocation might be done by a committee which represented a cross-section of the community. Such a method, it is argued, should prevent any one person from having too much power and so unduly influencing the decision in favor of his or her biases. This proposal has great merit precisely because it looks to the incorporation of a community judgment. The judgment of the local community, however, may not be enough in the face of the economic problem, which seems to call for decisions on the national level. In any event, it should be recognized that committee decisions can lead to trading and back scratching as well as to balanced judgments. Thus, due process is a step forward, but not a final solution.

In the long run, only some sort of a national policy which represents the broadest possible community judgment will prove reasonably though never completely satisfactory. At every step of the way, there must be a dialogue between the society and its members about the nature and meaning of human dignity and how its demands may be met given the abilities of the society.

Chapter Five
PRINCIPLES
OF CONFIDENTIALITY
AND TRUTHFULNESS

INTRODUCTION

In medicine, as in the rest of human life, truthfulness and confidentiality exist in an often uneasy tension. On the one hand, all social cooperation depends on truthful communication. On the other hand, telling everything could lead to disaster. We do not go around telling everyone what we think of them for the simple reason that this would destroy human relationships and in some cases lead to violence. We soon learn two important and interrelated truths. First, telling the truth is not the same as telling the whole truth. Second, some truths should be kept confidential. It is difficult, however, to decide what may ethically be concealed and what must be revealed.

In Chapter Two we outlined the basic truths that a health care provider *must* provide the patient in order to get informed consent. In that context, the patient had a right to the information and so there was an obligation to communicate it to him. The context of informed consent, however, does not cover all the problems of truthfulness. In the present chapter, we will develop principles to cover cases where it is not a question of informed consent or where the physician is dealing with someone other than the patient or a lawful surrogate. For example, should a physician write on a death certificate that the patient died of AIDS? Should the physician tell the patient that he is sterile if this was discovered by accident and is not connected with the patient's visit?

In the second part of this chapter, we shall develop principles to cover the cases where the truth ought to be kept confidential, that is, concealed from parties other than the patient. Must the physician conceal from a wife the fact that her husband has herpes? Must the nurse conceal from a parent the fact that a 16 year–old daughter had an abortion? When can a physician reveal sensitive information to a nurse or another physician?

TRUTHFULNESS

The ordinary ethics of truthfulness is generally summed up in two commands. First, do not lie. Second, you must communicate with those who have a right to the truth. These commands are too simple to come to grips with the complex problems met in real life. As a matter of fact, both of these are really hypothetical commands. The first really says, "*If you communicate,* do not lie." The second says, "You must communicate, *if the other person has a right to communication.*" Neither one says that you must tell everyone everything you know or everything they want to know. The first command leaves you free not to communicate—to remain silent or to evade the question or even to tell a falsehood which, as we shall see, is not the same thing as a lie. The second command opens up the question of who has a right to communication of the truth.

Lying

There are obviously many very different approaches to the problem of lying.[1] In line with our general approach, we will judge the ethics of lying in terms of its consequences for the individual and for the social system of communication.

Traditionally, a lie was defined as speech (communicative expression) against the mind, that is, which communicated something at odds with what the speaker believed to be true. From a consequentialist point of view, it is difficult to see how such speech universally or even generally has evil consequences. For this reason, we prefer to call such speech against the mind a falsehood and to define a lie as *a falsehood in those circumstances in which the other has a reasonable expectation of the truth.*[2] When the other has a reasonable expectation of the truth, a falsehood breaks down communication and renders social cooperation extremely difficult, if not impossible. Ultimately the breakdown of social cooperation hurts every individual, including the liar. In this approach lying is wrong because of the social effects and not because the other person has a right to the truth.

The revised definition of lying appears lax until the nature and range of reasonable expectations have been examined. These expectations vary with (1) the place of communication, (2) the roles of the communicators, and (3) the nature of the truth involved. All three of these are connected with both the obligation of confidentiality, which will be discussed later, and with the right to privacy.

These three factors, which determine the reasonableness of the expectation of the truth, are in large part specifications of the obligation to minimize evil and to justify the tolerance of evil by a proportional good. All the factors studied in the treatment of proportionality in Chapter Three can be usefully reviewed at this point.

A person does not have a reasonable expectation of the truth if the communication would take place in circumstances where people could overhear information that might be damaging. For example, if someone asks a professor about the faults of a student in a public place where others can overhear, there is no reasonable expectation that she will tell the truth and so hurt the student. The expectations would be different in the privacy of an office.

The role of the two communicators also helps establish the reasonableness of the expectation of the truth. Ordinarily, the dean of the college asking a professor about a student would have a reasonable expectation of the truth. Even the dean of the college has no reasonable expectation of the truth if he asks for information that the professor obtained when counseling a student. That counseling relationship was confidential and the obligation of confidentiality changes expectations. Similarly, if a stranger walks up to me and asks for the intimate details of my sex life, he has no reasonable expectation that I will share them with him. A person sensible to cultural norms would know that strangers do not even ask such questions, let alone expect a truthful answer.

Even a very good friend would not reasonably expect a truthful answer to a question about very private matters, such as one's finances, sex life, or secret ambitions, nor about such potentially damaging information as the fact that I have a criminal record, suffer from AIDs, or formerly belonged to the Klu Klux Klan.

A physician doing a health history in her office would have a very reasonable expectation to a truthful answer to all the questions bearing on diagnosis. The role, the place, and the nature of the matter all create the expectation in that case. The patient who goes to the physician for a diagnosis also has a reasonable expectation of the truth.

Many people have unreasonable expectations of the truth. In the ideal order, these people, who are frequently prying busybodies, should be rudely told to mind their own business. In practice, the demands of social life often require that we get rid of them in less abrupt ways. When they have no reasonable expectation of the truth, I retain my right to conceal the truth and to protect both my privacy and the good of myself and others. As we shall see in the section on confidentiality, people do not ordinarily have a reasonable expectation that a health care provider will tell them the truth about anyone but themselves.

Society recognizes that you have no reasonable expectation of the truth when someone is asked to testify against himself. It is for that reason that a person on trial cannot be forced to testify. On the other hand, the society through the law does specify certain situations in which an individual has a reasonable expectation of and perhaps even a right to the truth. The law on truth in lending, fraud, and on the revelation of latent substantial defects in a product provides examples of reasonable expectations of the truth. In most situations, however, the law says that buyers have an obligation to find the truth for themselves.

It is not a lie to conceal the truth, though it may be unethical for other reasons. If I keep my mouth shut or evade the question or give an ambiguous answer or even tell an outright falsehood when I am asked many of the questions mentioned in previous paragraphs, I have not lied. Indeed, because I used those means to avoid an evil, I have, granted proportionality, done something virtuous. It would be quite different if I told a falsehood to a person who asked me the way to the nearest restroom or the price of a hotel or the name of the mayor. There is no reasonable cause for keeping those things secret, and so the other has a reasonable expectation of the truth.

Our examples thus far have covered cases where the other person asks for information. The situation is different in those circumstances where I am not asked for information but volunteer it. In these cases the other has a reasonable expectation of the truth. By volunteering the information, I announce that I intend to communicate and so create a reasonable expectation of the truth. There are exceptions to this when it is clear that I am merely fooling around, telling a tale, or am so biased that you should expect nothing from me. In general, however, volunteering information creates the reasonable expectation.

Even when I volunteer information, the other person cannot reasonably expect the whole truth unless I tell them they will get the whole story. Absent such a promise, there is no reason to think I am volunteering the whole truth. In most cases, the whole truth is not particularly useful or even a good thing. Indeed, people who attempt to give the whole truth often bore us to death with irrelevant details or scandalize us with their lack of respect for the reputation of others. There are even cases where giving the whole truth actually leads to deception, since the important truth can be concealed in a pile of irrelevant detail.

The Right to the Truth

More difficult questions arise with regard not to the reasonable expectations of truth, but with *the right* of a person to the truth. As already noted, the patient has a right to the information needed for informed consent because he needs that information to make decisions about treatment. In other cases when there is no question of treatment, the patient may have a right to truthful information because he has paid for it. That is, the person may have a right to the truth by purchase. For example, the patient who goes to a genetic counselor for information pertinent not to a treatment but to marriage has a right to the truth. In this setting, it is precisely information that he has paid for.

There is a third set of circumstances where the patient has a right to information even though there is no informed consent involved and no explicit purchase of information. The patient has a right to the information when he needs it to make important nonmedical decisions or to avoid great evils. Here, as in the case of informed consent, the need of the patient for the information gives birth to the right to the information. The principal example of this is the nonmedical need of the patient to know that he is dying. Religious thinkers stress that the dying person needs to make peace with God. There is also the need to set one's financial and personal affairs in order so that survivors may not suffer more than necessary. The personal affairs may involve no more than a goodbye but can also call for a reconciliation with enemies or estranged family members. These are not medical issues, but they are important. Even if one tries to deny the patient's strict right to know that he is dying, the concealment of this truth denies a person a chance to take care of these duties. The denial treats such important duties as trivial and in the process mocks the dignity of the person, whose needs are more than medical.

The Placebo Problem

A placebo (Latin for "I will please") is "*a preparation devoid of pharmacological effect given for psychological effect, or as a control in evaluating a medicinal believed to have pharmacological effect*" (Blakiston, 1972). In short, it is something that chemically should not have an effect. In more popular terms, it is a sugar pill. Though useful, the definition may be too narrow, since many other things, from the physician's diploma to nurse's bedside manner, can have therapeutic psychological effects. Indeed, some writers (Carlton, 1978) say that until recent times most medicines were placebos. Further, it can be argued that psychological factors such as the faith of the patient in the physician are still important placebolike factors in helping people. One way or another, placebos are still used not only for research and psychological effect but for keeping the patient satisfied and off the physician's phone. Sometimes the physician is really using a placebo without knowing it. This happens when the physician believes the treatment helps even though there is no scientific evidence for it. In view of the above, and leaving aside the use of placebos in research, we will redefine the placebo as *anything that is used to affect a therapeutic outcome or anything that does affect the outcome when the entity used is not supposed to have active biological powers.*

The ethical problem is clear. Does the use of the placebo involve unethical deception of the patient?

Before attempting to answer that question a few remarks are in order. First, even drugs with active pharmacological properties have enhanced effects when the patient believes in them. Second, the Hawthorne effect in industrial psychology shows that merely paying attention to a worker will increase productivity and cooperation. The same certainly holds true in health care. Third, placebos or at least belief in the placebo have been shown to have effect on the immune system and even to produce addiction (Brody, 1987).

All of this need not surprise us, since the effects of drugs depend not only on the pharmacological properties but on the attitude, i.e., mental set of the user and the setting in which the drug is taken. In addition, though many have a tendency to see disease in terms of biological causality, many diseases have psychological dimensions (Weiner, 1977), which, of course, can be influenced by the placebo. When we are dealing with multicausal systems in which the observer affects the observed and when we expect only probabilities rather than certainty, it is easy to make place for factors such as placebos, even though they cannot be neatly pinned down.

In view of all this, whether or not a placebo is deceptive depends on the exact way in which it is presented. If the physician says, "I am going to prescribe something that often helps in these cases and has no bad side effects," it is hard to see how he is deceiving the patient. Certainly, he is not lying. Indeed, the physician is far more likely to deceive with regard to a pharmacologically active drug if he says,"This will make you better." That is promising too much, whether said of a placebo or a test drug.

In such a presentation, the patient knows what she needs to know in order to give informed consent. No untruth is spoken and no information to which the patient has a right is suppressed.

While deception is not the ethical issue in the use of the placebo, there are other problems with placebos, such as overpricing or using them in place of accepted treatment. Overpricing can be condemned as a form of theft, and the failure to use accepted treatment when it is called for is simply malpractice.

Summary

It is wrong to tell falsehoods in those situations where there is a reasonable expectation of the truth. The expectation of the truth varies with the place of the communication, the roles of the communicators and the nature of the material to be communicated. When we volunteer information, we create a reasonable expectation of the truth but not necessarily of the whole truth. We have an obligation to communicate only when the other person has a right to the information as a result of contract, relationship, or special need. The use of the placebo is not per se wrong as long as the patient is not told a lie.

CONFIDENTIALITY

Introduction

All of these obligations must be seen not only in the context of truthfulness, but in the context of confidentiality. Indeed, it is only after we have considered confidentiality that we can tackle the difficult and often neglected questions about the health care provider's right and/or obligation to communicate with families and other third parties about the condition of the patient.

Confidentiality is concerned with keeping secrets. A secret is knowledge which a person has a right and/or obligation to conceal. In the present section we will concentrate on obligatory secrets.

The obligation to keep secrets arises from the fact that harm will follow if the particular knowledge is revealed. There are three types of obligatory secrets, which are distinguished by the type of harmful consequences that result from revelation. These are the natural secret, the promised secret, and the professional secret.

The *natural secret* is so named because the information involved is by its nature harmful if revealed. We are, as we saw in Chapter Three, obliged to avoid harming others unless there is a proportionate reason for risking or permitting the harm. Because the obligation to avoid harm is universal, even a layman is obliged to keep secret the fact that a friend has AIDS lest he be shunned and persecuted unjustly. That obligation exists no matter how the person got the information. Similarly, we are obliged to keep to ourselves information about the private peculiarities of people that might cause them embarrassment if revealed. We might be obliged to keep secret the fact that a person was in the hospital, if revelation of the fact would hurt her business. Even the patient's name can be confidential if revealing it might cause either inconvenience or embarrassment to the patient. The psychiatrist who sold mailing lists of his patients certainly caused them inconvenience and may have exposed them to serious loss of reputation, even though the only thing revealed was the fact of treatment. Unfortunately, that fact has been known to stigmatize an individual in certain groups.

It should be obvious that sometimes the harm that comes from concealing a natural secret outweighs the harm that is being avoided. In these cases proportionality can justify revelation and at times make it a duty. If a friend with AIDS attempts to give blood even after you have argued with him, you have a proportionate reason to tell the Red Cross of his condition in order to prevent harm to recipients of his blood. On the other hand, you would not be justified in telling the Red Cross of an AIDS victim who had no intention of attempting to donate blood. In that case, there is no foreseeable harm. You would have a similar justification for telling classmates that one student insisted on attending class even though he had infectious hepatitis. You would have no justification of generally revealing his infection if he stayed away from class.

The *promised secret* is knowledge we have promised to conceal. Generally, the promise has been exacted because the matter is also a natural secret, in which case the nature of the matter makes the secret stricter. The special evil of revealing promised secrets arises from the harmful effects of breaking promises. Social life depends on people keeping promises, and we depend on social life for nearly all our basic goods. In addition, most of us are wary of the person whom we cannot trust to keep a promise. We leave that sort of person out of many social interchanges.

Here, as in the case of the natural secret, there may be proportionate reasons for revealing the secret. The good to be attained, however, must offset the evil that results from the broken promise as well as from the nature of the information. One will be justified in revealing the intention of someone to kill even though one swore an oath to keep it secret. A layperson might, despite promises, be justified in revealing a friend's diabetes to a health care professional if the friend is not following medical advice and so threatening her health. Once again, it is a question of proportionality, that is, with the need to justify risking or permitting harm by a proportionate good.

The *professional secret* is knowledge which, if revealed, will harm not only the professional's client, but will do serious harm to the profession and to the society which depends on that profession for important services. In many cases, but not all, this secret is recognized by the law so that a professional would not have to reveal "privileged communication" even in court. This means that a physician *cannot disclose* information learned in confidence from his patient unless the patient gives her permission. Clearly, the professional secret is the most serious of all secrets, because its violation can cause the greatest harm.

The importance of the professional secret in health care is best seen by contemplating the consequences if patients lack faith in the confidentiality of their dealings with the health care system. When the law required health care providers to report minors with sexually transmitted diseases to parents (a legal exception to confidentiality), infected teenagers suffered without care and kept on spreading sexually transmitted diseases until the United States had a epidemic. Their distrust of the health care system thus led to a major health problem. A change in the law that restored the principle of confidentiality encouraged young people to go for treatment and cut the incidence of these diseases.

Not only teenagers but all men and women rightfully feel that the condition of their body is private and to be shared with those they choose to help them, but not with anyone else. We do not want to tell our secrets to someone who cannot be trusted to keep a secret. Indeed, with the exceptions noted below, the patient/provider relationship implies a promise of secrecy. For this reason, if for no other, the health care providers must observe secrecy in order to keep their services acceptable to the people who need them.

Society has long recognized the importance of professional secrecy. In order to protect confidentiality, society has even given physicians statutory immunity from testifying about their diagnosis and treatment of patients. The immunity of other health care professionals differs from state to state. In general, society has, for the reasons given below, expected all health care professionals to maintain confidentiality. Unfortunately, the complications introduced by third-party payers, such as Blue Cross, indicate that there is probably a need for rethinking the whole area of professional privilege (Taranto, 1986). We shall say more about this later on.

The professional secret, then, must be kept because of the nature of the knowledge, the implied promise, and the good of the profession and the society.

The Patient's Bill of Rights of the American Hospital Association is quite clear on the obligation of professional secrecy in the hospital setting.

5. The patient has the right to every consideration of his privacy concerning his own medical care program. Case discussion, consultation, examination and treatment are confidential and should be conducted discretely. Those not directly involved in his care must have the permission of the patient to be present.

6. The patient has the right to expect that all communications and records pertaining to his care are confidential.

The application of these statements requires some amplification and explanation.

Confidentiality and Consultation

Unless explicitly forbidden by the patient, a health care professional has a right to consult other health care professionals in an effort to help the patient. In cases of doubt, the permission of the patient or surrogate should be obtained. Among other things, the patient who must pay for the consultation should have a right to decide whether she can afford it. It is understood that the person consulted is bound by the same secrecy. Providers are not ethically free to discuss patients merely to pass the time of day or in a public place where they may be overheard. The hospital cafeteria is not a suitable room for a consultation, let alone a gossip session. Neither are health care professionals free to satisfy their curiosity about patients who are not in their care. A physician not involved professionally has no right to look at the chart of a friend or neighbor who happens to be in the hospital. The principle of confidentiality operates on a need-to-know basis, and that means a *health care need to know.*

Residents, interns, and other students in a teaching hospital are not free to look at charts without the permission of the patient, unless they are directly involved in the care of the particular patient. Some justify a general right to inspect records in terms of a general consent signed by the patient or surrogate on entrance to the hospital. This is a dubious justification since the average patient does not read the form and has no idea of what rights he has signed away. We argue, then, that more explicit permission is required if residents and interns are to ethically examine the records of patients whom they are not directly involved in treating.

Exceptions Required by Statute Law

The exceptions to confidentiality may be grouped under four headings: (1) exceptions commanded by statute law; (2) exceptions arising from legal precedent; (3) exceptions arising from a peculiar patient/provider relationship; and (4) exceptions due to a proportionate reason.

Exceptions are commanded by many statutes for such things as gunshot or knife wounds, child abuse, certain communicable diseases, acute poisoning, or automobile accidents. Some states demand that public authorities also be informed of illegitimate births, birth defects and deformities, cerebral palsy cases, industrial accidents, and chronic drug addiction (Annas, 1975, pp. 115–116). Since each state has its own laws, local statutes must be consulted. In each case, the law presumes that the public good demands an exception and so outweighs the harm of the revelation. It is also assumed that the patient knows that these cases are not covered by the implied promise of the patient/provider relationship.

Health care professionals often find that the assumptions behind these laws are not warrented in a given case. That is, they see more harm than good occurring if they violate confidentiality.

Child abuse laws in many states make mandatory the reporting of suspected abuse whether physical or mental, whether arising from omission or commission. The provider can be torn between conscience and the law, since she may believe that the reporting will only make things worse for the abused child, or that the local child protective services will not handle the situation properly, or both of the above. There is no easy answer to this problem, and in the last analysis the providers must consider both the danger to themselves and to the suspected victim when making a decision.

Exceptions from Court Decisions

Exceptions arising from legal precedent, that is, from court decisions, are harder to pin down since the courts in one state often differ from those in another, and since courts change opinions over time. The famous Tarasoff case[3] held that a psychiatrist should have warned a woman that a patient was threatening to kill her. The court argued that the therapist had to take reasonable steps to protect third parties from the patient.

It is not at all clear that revealing the homicidal tendencies of the patient in the Tarasoff case was necessary or useful. Indeed, two years after the original decision, the same California court that condemned the psychiatrist reworded its ruling so that a professional only had to "exercise reasonable care to protect foreseeable victims." This is more in line with what is the general ethical practice. It rightly assumes that even psychiatrists are not very good at telling who will actually commit murder, let alone whom they will murder. Other courts have relied on this same thinking to say that the psychiatrist need not reveal the ravings of his patients to those who are mentioned as possible victims. Most patients are probably only blowing off steam, and it is estimated that two out of three times predictions of violence are wrong. In other words, flipping a coin might have given better results.

No matter what the merits of the case, many courts have been holding psychiatrists liable if they do not take steps to protect both third parties and the patients themselves. This often leads to the health care workers overprotecting themselves by hospitalizing more people than is necessary and by keeping them hospitalized for longer times. Other mental health workers are playing it safe by not taking any patients who show tendencies to violence. All of these reactions are not in the interests of either patients or the public.

The American Hospital Association's Committee on Biomedical Ethics (1985, p.24) notes:

> Also subject to state law, confidentiality may be overridden when the life or safety of the patient is endangered such as when knowledgeable intervention can prevent threatened suicide or self-injury. In addition, the moral obligation to prevent substantial and foreseeable harm to an innocent third party usually is greater than the moral obligation to protect confidentiality.

While this point should be taken seriously, Chapter Six on death and dying raises serious doubts about the right of the state, let alone medical personnel, to prevent suicide and so to violate confidentiality in the course of the prevention.

Exceptions Arising from Unusual Relationships

The exceptions arising from a peculiar provider/patient relationship occur with family and military personnel who owe a loyalty to their employer as well as to the patient. As long as the patient understands that he is not fully protected by confidentiality, there is no serious ethical problem, unless, of course, the company or military provider in the only one available. The Judicial Council of the American Medical Association (AMA, 1986, pp. 24-25) draws useful distinctions in the industrial context:

> 5.09 CONFIDENTIALITY: PHYSICIANS IN INDUSTRY. Where a physician's services are limited to pre-employment physical examinations or examinations to determine if an employee who has been ill or injured is able to return to work, no physician-patient relationship exists between the physician and those individuals. Nevertheless, the information obtained by the physician as a result of such examinations is confidential and should not be communicated to a third party without the individual's written prior consent, unless required by law. If the individual authorizes the release of medical information to an employer or potential employer, the physician should release only that information which is reasonably relevant to the employer's decisions regarding that individual's ability to perform the work required for the job.
>
> A physician-patient relationship does exist when a physician renders treatment to an employee, even though the physician is paid by the employers. If the employee's illness or injury is work related the release of medical information may be subject to the provisions of workers compensation laws. The physician must comply with the requirements of such laws, if applicable. However, the physician may or may not otherwise discuss the employee's health condition with the employers without the employee's consent or, in the event of the employee's incapacity, the family's consent.

Exceptions Due to Proportionality

The exceptions due to proportionality cannot, of course, be reduced to a few simple rules. Suffice it to say that a great good and generally a public good must be at stake to justify a revelation that will harm the profession and the society as well as the patient. Ordinarily, a professional will not be allowed to reveal information merely for the good of a third party, even if that third party happens to be a patient. In general, the physician may not, without the permission of his patient, tell a wife that her husband has syphilis even though she runs a danger of infection. Nor should the physician inform the husband that the wife is pregnant or intending an abortion. The good of the third parties involved does not, except in rare cases, justify harm to the patient, his trust in the profession, and ultimately the society that depends on that profession. In particular the harm to confidence in the profession and the resulting hesitancy about seeking advice or treatment make it unethical to make such revelations except in rare cases.

The rare exceptions involve more than the good of isolated individuals. It can be argued rather persuasively that there is a proportionate reason for discretely revealing to a wife the fact that her husband *certainly has AIDS*. Here we are dealing with a disease that can harm not only the wife, but children yet to be born and, through dramatically increased health costs, society itself. It becomes hard to justify revealing the suspicion that the husband *might have AIDS*. In the first case we are dealing with the threat of a life–destroying process, in the second with the possibility or some unknown probability of a life-destroying process. As the probability becomes greater, the case for revelation increases in strength. The issue is made more complicated by the fact that warning the wife may be useless and so unjustified since the warning comes too late.

The task of considering all the factors and weighing the relative harms and benefits becomes very complicated in the consideration of exceptions due to proportionality. In practice, the authors believe that the presumption should be in favor of confidentiality unless the case for revelation really shows proportionate goods to outweigh the harm to the profession and the society.

Familial Exceptions?

Medical practice has generally assumed that the provider was free to reveal the condition of hospitalized patients to their families whether or not the family was a surrogate. Indeed, at one time the American Medical Association (Annas, 1975, p.124) stated that "reporting to one spouse information about the medical condition of the other is not a breach of confidentiality." The previous paragraphs have already indicated cases where such revelation would be neither desirable nor ethical. Legally, the position of the AMA is, as Annas says (1975), dubious. Ethically, it is better to insist that spouses of competent patients may not be told without the permission of the patient. The patient who reasonably assumes a promise of confidentiality may have many good reasons for keeping the matter secret from a spouse. The disclosure of the disease may cause anxiety in the spouse, promote smothering behavior, or in some cases arouse suspicion of infidelity. Annas (1975) remarks that permitting the physician to tell the spouse often results in the patient not being told, especially when the news is very bad. Such behavior should not be encouraged. Certainly, the disclosure does not promote trust in the profession.

On the other side are those who argue that compassion for the spouse and family justifies revelation. Except when dealing with surrogates, the permission of the patient should be asked since the relationship is with the patient and the first loyalty is owed to the patient. To the extent that the spouse and family are patients because of their suffering, they should be treated with compassion and concern, but that compassion does not warrant breaking confidentiality.

Most of the previous paragraph would have to be rewritten if the professional relationship is with the family and not the individual patient. In England, for example, the reporting of child abuse is not mandatory, and visiting nurses see their relationship as one with the family and not the individual patient. The English visiting nurses often refuse to testify in cases involving child abuse, lest they damage the relationship with the family. We cannot condemn that stand as long as the terms of the relationship are clear from the beginning.

Exceptions in the Case of Children and Adolescents

Traditionally, it was assumed that health care providers had not only a right but an obligation to report to parents on the health of their children. Increasingly, however, the law has provided for an increasing number of areas where the health care provider either need not or must not reveal the health problems of the child or adolescent to the parents. We have already noted the case of sexually transmitted diseases. Similar reaffirmations of the right to confidentiality exist in the areas of abortion, substance abuse, and contraception but not in the area of sterilization. The law varies from place to place in the United States, but the underlying idea is clear. When confidentiality is necessary for the health of the patient, to protect the patient's rights or for the public health, traditional exceptions that permitted or required that parents be informed become questionable. For a full treatment of the law and the provisions in each state, the reader should consult Morrissey et al. (1986).

Media Publicity and Confidentiality

In recent years the medical problems of prominent people and the drama of new medical technology have often been media events complete with press conferences by physicians, briefings by medical spokespersons, and TV reporters giving their spiels against the backdrop of a hospital. Quite aside from the drama of these media events, some hospitals will give you brief summaries ("she is critical" or "he is in stable condition") of a patient's condition if a person asks. Unless the patient or a surrogate has given informed consent to such revelations, the supplying of information and the publicity may easily violate the principle of confidentiality in health care. In some cases, as noted earlier, even the revelation of the fact that a person is a patient may have harmful effects. Here again, there needs to be a careful balancing of the need of family members to know and the privacy of the patient. Once again, the authors hold that in case of doubt, the presumption should be in favor of confidentiality.

Some will argue that the public has a right to know about public figures, especially political figures whose health is of true public concern. Even if we grant that claim for the sake of argument, it does not follow that health care providers have as a general rule either an obligation or right to supply the information without the permission of the patient or the surrogate. If the public have a right to the information, the sick person and not the health care provider has the obligation to provide it.

Hospital Records, Research, and Confidentiality

A stay in the hospital is or should be meticulously documented in both the financial and medical records of the institutions. Diagnosis, treatment, nurses' observations, progress, and discharge are all reported and stored for future use. Implicitly the patient has given permission for those involved in his direct care to see those records. The permission is on a need-to-know basis. Nurses' aides do not need to see the record and so do not have implied permission to read them.

It may also be argued that the patient has given permission to a peer review board or other quality assurance board since they provide the patient with additional protection. In practice, of course, the billing office has such information that the curious could make rather accurate deductions about the patient's illness. Aside from these individuals and the third-party payers treated below, no one else has a right to see the record without the permission of the patient.

Although the records are made primarily for the good of the patient, they also provide a valuable source of information for health care research. The patient, even if her care is provided at public expense, retains the right to privacy. The records should not be used without the informed consent of the patient. That is, the patient should know that a bit more of her privacy is being surrendered if consent is given. Merely having the patient sign a form on admission is not sufficiently respectful of the patient's right to privacy.

When proper consent has been obtained and research is done on the records, two things should be kept in mind. First, only summary data with no identification should be used in publishing the research. Second, the number of people who see the record itself should be kept to a minimum. Both of these provisions help to protect confidentiality and to remind people of its importance.

Confidentiality and Third-Party Payers

The introduction of third-party payers, whether governmental or private, into the health care system has weakened confidentiality. When we sign into a hospital or have our physician apply for reimbursement through our insurance policy, we give permission for nonprofessional employees to supply the insurance company with information about our diagnosis and treatment. At the insurance company the information is handled by clerks and fed into a computer. While in theory the information is still confidential, a large number of people have seen it in transit, and in practice clever people can get at it with considerable ease.

If that health information came into the hands of life insurers or employers, it could have harmful consequences. For example, some companies refuse to hire people who have had a history of cancer on the grounds that they represent a risk of higher health insurance rates for the company. While this appears to be illegal as discrimination on the basis of alleged handicap, former patients have been injured in this way. In addition, if the revelation involved treatment for a mental condition, chances for promotion or election to public office might be affected. In short, the computerization of health care information represents a potential for harm to patients.

The dangers to confidentiality impose special obligations not only on health care providers but on health care administrators as well. In the first place, all personnel, clerical and nonprofessional as well as professional staff, should be thoroughly oriented with regard to confidentiality. The penalties for the violation of the rule should be both clear and severe enough to demonstrate the seriousness of the matter. In the second place, there should be systems in place to control access to records and to make sure that the need-to-know principle limits even professionals to the necessary minimum.

Confidentiality and the Public Good

When there is not a specific piece of legislation commanding revelation for the public good, physicians can often find themselves in a dilemma. The patient expects confidentiality, and a violation of confidentiality will certainly hurt society. Yet, keeping the matter secret may also harm society. Nowhere is this clearer than in the case of AIDS. Some health care professionals have called for the right to report the AIDS carrier as well as the AIDS victim to those who might be infected. They want the right to inform other doctors about the condition of the patient on a nonconsultative basis. Some even demand that the AIDS patient be quarantined if there is no other way to prevent him from spreading the disease.

The issue is too grave to be left to individual judgment. Furthermore, as we pointed out in Chapter One, the roles of health care providers are determined by society and clients as well as by members of the profession. This society needs to speak through specific legislation which will spell out the exceptions so that both health care providers and patients will know where they stand in the relationship. The legislator must keep in mind that if the exception to confidentiality and the imposition of quarantine lead to fewer people getting treated, we may only have succeeded in hiding the problem rather than in solving it. The experience with reporting venereal diseases of minors should be kept in mind in any legislation on AIDS.

Summary

Professional secrecy is the most obligatory of all secrets, since the violation of confidentiality damages not only the patient but also the sacredness of promises and the good of society and the profession. Professional secrets can be shared in legitimate medical consultations and revealed for proportionate reasons or when there are proper statutory or court–imposed exceptions. There is also an exception to confidentiality in special relationships, which are not true provider/patient relationships.

CASES FOR ANALYSIS

1. Mary is in need of a kidney transplant, and her parents and siblings have been tested for compatibility. Her father is afraid of operations and knows that kidney trouble runs in the family. Before the test, Mary's father tells the doctor that he does not want anyone, especially his wife, to know that he is compatible. He explains that if the family knows, they will pressure him into being a donor. The father turns out to be the only one compatible. Mary asks the doctor, "Are you sure no one in my family is compatible?"

2.   The Smith family was in a car accident, and all five of them were hospitalized as a result. The father was critically injured and in two days it became clear that he was going to die. The wife, who though making good progress was still confined to her room, was told of her husband's deteriorating condition. She insisted that the physician tell her husband, since he was the sort of man who would want to know. The children still in the hospital had not seen their father and kept asking about him. The physician refused to tell the husband of his condition. He died a few days later.

3.   Dr. Xavier has been the family doctor for the Loyolas for over 20 years. He was shocked when Mary, the 16-year-old Loyola, came to tell him that she was pregnant and wanted his help in getting an abortion. Since abortions were against his conscience, he refused. He also informed the parents of Mary's condition and her intentions.

4.   Huntington's disease is a genetically transmitted disease that affects both males and females. Only one gene from either parent is required to transmit the disease to offspring. If a person knows that the disease runs in his family, there is a 50/50 chance that he will have it. Though some tests have been developed to detect the disease, generally people will not know if they have it until the symptoms appear. The symptoms do not appear till midlife. In the United States one person out of 10,000 has it. Thus there are over 20,000 active cases in the United States, and probably 100,000 people who are uncertain whether they have it or not.
       With Huntington's disease there is a continuous and irreversible deterioration of the mental, physical, and motor functions. Clumsiness and forgetfulness are followed by angry outbursts, disorientation, incontinence, loss of speech control, and writhing and twisting of the whole body. Ten or twenty years of suffering leads to death. Victims often commit suicide.
       Dr. Calvin discovers that Mary X., age 40, has Huntington's disease when she comes to ask for help with her loss of memory and outbursts of anger. He does not tell her the truth since there are no medical decisions to be made, but most of all because of the horror of the living death she faces. A few weeks later when Mary's son, age 20, comes in for a premarital blood test, Dr. Calvin wonders if he should tell the son that he has a 50 percent chance of having the disease and so should hesitate about having children.

5.   Doctor Curiosus has a habit of wandering around the hospital and looking at the records of friends who are in the hospital. The nurses have tried to stop him, but he has retaliated by making their lives miserable and belittling them in public at every opportunity. Nursing administration has been notified but has done nothing since it tries to avoid rocking the boat.

6.   At the Oxcrossing Mental Health Center, the administrators have decided to cooperate with a project which will centralize all public mental health records for four adjoining states in a central computer for research purpose. The professional staff objects and refuses to go along unless all identifying information is removed. The administration agrees but is later caught restoring Social Security numbers. The staff

retaliates by listing only vague harmless diagnoses so that the record now reveals little or nothing.

7.   Professor Garrett is in the hospital and explicitly forbids social workers or dietitians to see his medical record. "I do not want them involved in my care," he says. The nurses humor him but allow the social worker and the dietitian to see the records since that is normal hospital policy.

8.   Mary Margaret, R.N., is caring for Mrs. Jones, her neighbor of many years, who has been admitted to the hospital suffering from what appears to be dehydration. In the course of caring for her, Mary discovers that her neighbor is an alcoholic. Intending to help the neighbor, Mary tells her husband and all the neighbors about the problem and warns them not to offer the patient a drink when she comes home from the hospital.

9.   John O., R.N., is a school nurse. In the course of talking to a student in his office, he discovers that the youngster is on drugs and even suspects that the student may be peddling drugs. He reports all of this to the principal.

10.   George has gonorrhea. He does not want to tell his wife but does want to protect her. While undergoing treatment, he asks the family physician to test his wife without her knowing it. When the wife comes in with a bad case of bronchitis, the physician tests her, saying, "I just want to run another test on you to rule out a possibility, a mere possibility, you understand." He finds she has been infected and treats her without her knowing the diagnosis. He merely tells her, "I want you to take these antibiotics as a precaution." In this way he protects the husband.

11.   Dr. Timorous has been requested to examine Mary and Stan Koska to see if there is a danger of them having children with Tay-Sachs, a genetic disease leading to a progressive mental and physical deterioration. Over a period of months, a baby with this disease will go blind, suffer motor paralysis, spasticity, and, finally, rigidity of the muscles. Death occurs in the third year of life.

   The test indicates that Stan has a recessive Tay-Sachs gene. Dr. Timorous tells him this and suggests that he tell his brothers and urge them to have the test, since they too are thinking of having children. Stan feels contaminated and ashamed and refuses to say anything to his brothers.

   Dr. Timorous knows the brothers socially. Though they are not his patients, he has seen one of them professionally in the past. He debates with himself. Shall he send carefully worded letters to the brothers urging the screening? Shall he just keep it all to himself? What is the ethical thing to do?

12.   Dr. Maternus has been the family doctor for the Garrett family for 15 years. He has delivered all six of their children and belongs to the same church as the couple. Recently, during a routine checkup on Tom Garrett, age 3, he noticed suspicious bruises in places that did not fit in with the father's story of the child falling out of bed. Ordinarily, he would report this as suspected child abuse. In this case he keeps it to himself. It is unthinkable that the Garretts would abuse a child. Why start an investigation that will only cause ill feelings?

NOTES

[1]In the appendix to her book *Lying,* Sissela Bok (1979) gives long citations from Augustine, Aquinas, Francis Bacon, Sidgwick, Harrod, Grotius, Kant, Bonhoeffer, and Warnock on the morality of lying. These writers present a huge array of opinions and theoretical approaches.

[2]This definition differs from that given by Bok (1978, p.14) in that it attempts to include wording that takes care of the cases in which a falsehood is justified.

[3]*Tarasoff* v. *Regents of the University of California,* California Supreme Court (17 California Reports, 3rd Series, 425). The case was decided on July 1, 1976.

Chapter Six
ETHICAL PROBLEMS
OF DEATH AND DYING

INTRODUCTION

Few areas in medical ethics are as difficult as death and dying. The topic raises questions not only about when a person is dead, but about the meaning of life and about a person's right to determine when his life shall end. These questions are all basic questions in ethics. They become urgent questions in health care ethics when providers are faced with the necessity of deciding if they will cooperate with those who want to end their lives and whether providers have the right to keep individuals alive against their will or the will of their surrogate. There is even debate about whether it is ethical to prevent a person from committing suicide (Szasz, 1977). The problems are all the more emotionally acute since in life and death situations we are on our guard against camel's noses, wedges, and slippery slopes that may open the door to killing people who want to live. These issues are the concern of Part I. Part II considers more particular problems such as the no-code order and the living will, special problems with feeding and hydration, as well as brain death and the place of ethics committees in the ethics of death and dying.

THE BASIC ISSUES

At the root of nearly all problems about death and dying is not only a fear of murder, but a position about the ethical correctness of suicide and cooperation with suicide.

Since the ethics of suicide is central in both the ethics of the patient and the provider, we shall start with the ethics of suicide. We shall attempt to answer two basic questions: First, is suicide always unethical? Second, is it unethical for health care providers to cooperate with suicide? Once these two basic questions have been answered, we shall then proceed to the large number of questions connected with them: living wills, no-code orders, letting patients die without consent, brain death, ethics committees, and the place of the family in decisions about the termination of treatment.

Suicide

In *The Myth of Sisyphus* (1955, p. 3), Albert Camus wrote:

> There is but one truly serious philosophic question and that is suicide. Judging whether life is or is not worth living amounts to answering the fundamental question of philosophy.

We are profoundly aware that this is true and that our brief treatment of the question is insufficient to answer it. We do agree, however, about two points that are central to this chapter. First, from a purely philosophical point of view, it is impossible to condemn every act of suicide. It follows then that in some cases, patients can be ethical in committing suicide. Second, the health care provider is in no position to judge the ethical correctness of the patient's decision to commit suicide.

Let us start with a common-sense, man-in-the-street definition of suicide as *the intentional termination of one's own life*. This definition will include all those cases where a person wants to kill herself whether she does this by omitting something (passive suicide) or by doing something (active suicide).[1] It does not include cases where the person does not intend to terminate her life, but omits an action or performs an action which she foresees may lead to her death. A person who gives up her food so that others may live is often not considered to be committing suicide, even though she may starve to death. Even if one calls this altruistic act suicide, it would still be ethical in a consequentialist view, since there is a proportionate reason for risking or permitting death. Similarly, in line with what was said in Chapter Three, the person who dies because he has refused treatment in order to avoid a degrading and painful existence may be said to commit suicide but is still ethical. We may say that not all suicide defined as the intentional killing of one's self is unethical by consequentialist or common sense standards. It is necessary, then, to look a little more closely at the reasons given for condemning suicide. These arguments make a *prima facie*, or presumptive, case against suicide but do not in our opinion prove philosophically that suicide is always and in all circumstances an ethical evil.

The notion that suicide is wrong has been supported by a number of arguments. The first argument is religious and theological. It holds that our lives belong to God and are merely loaned to us, so that we have no rights to dispose of our own lives even though we have the right to use them within limits. In this view, we have no more right to kill ourselves that we would have to wreck a rented car. This is a strong argument for those who believe in the basic premises. Even the proponents of this argument, however, must admit that God might, at least by way of exception, grant a person permission to commit active suicide. While they are very hesitant to admit exceptions in cases of active suicide, they do permit some passive suicide. They admit, for example, that a patient is not required to use extraordinary means to continue in existence. As we have noted in Chapter Three, this amounts to saying that in certain circumstances passive suicide can be justified by a proportionate reason. Indeed, these religious writers praise the person who lays down a life for a friend or suffers martyrdom for the sake of religious faith, though they are quite clear that a person ought not to go about looking for martyrdom.

The second argument holds that human life is so precious that to act against it is to act against the greatest of all human goods, or at least against the good on which all other human goods depend. These assertions might appear true in the abstract, as long as one does not specify the specific condition of that life. The abstract consideration overlooks several important truths. In the concrete, life may be experienced as an overwhelming burden and the word "life" may be designating no more than a vegetable existence in a specific case. Further, life can be so painful and so crushing that it renders all other goods impossible. Finally, life can be barely recognizable as human, as in the cases of those who are in a permanent vegetative state. Those who have been in real pain know how pain eats up all other consciousness and abolishes control of much activity even as it makes us insensitive to the feelings of those who love us. When that pain becomes a permanent state uncontrollable by drugs, "life" is no longer the substratum for all other good things. In the concrete, then, life may not be the greatest of all goods. Life may not even be the good on which all other goods depend. In short, life is not an unambiguous reality such that life is always a good. We shall return to this issue in the second part of this chapter.

Those who hold that life is precious and the basis for all other goods recognize the fact of the vegetative state and of pain. Often, then, they will permit as ethical passive suicide for a proportionate reason, even though they reject active suicide, that is, the direct killing of oneself.

The matter cannot be settled merely by permitting passive suicide for a proportionate reason. There is need for a longer look at the value of life and the relative importance of the quality of life. We shall return to this question after we outline the remaining arguments against suicide.

A third argument, this one consequentialist, condemns suicide because it harms the community. This, too, is a bit oversimplified. As a matter of fact not all suicides harm the community. Some suicides may be a positive benefit to the community. We would, indeed, probably be better off if all the criminals did commit suicide. But that is not the real issue.

As we noted in Chapter One, the individual person and not the community is the intrinsic good, and the individual should not be automatically or unnecessarily subordinated to the community. Certainly, the individual must consider the impact of his actions on the society, but the effects on society are not the decisive factor. In short, the harm to the community must be considered in judging proportionality, but the good of the community is on the level of means and is not the intrinsic good. We shall return to this shortly. Thus the mere fact that a suicide might hurt the community does not settle the issue.

A fourth argument proposes that suicide is wrong because it has substantially harmful consequences for other individuals. Once again, we agree that these consequences must be considered, but insist that they are not the only factors to be considered in judging the proportionality of the goods and evils involved. The value of the human person is not solely, or even primarily, dependent on her utility for others either singly or in a group. Thus, the actual and potential harm to the patient can at times be the decisive factor in deciding the balance of good or evil in the suicide situation.

While some writers might theoretically accept the exceptions we have just pointed out, they will argue that in practice suicide should be forbidden because of the wedge principle in either its logical or empirical form. That is, they argue from the long-term consequences of allowing exceptions. Their arguments, based on each of the principles, deserve study.

The empirical form of the wedge principle, which argues that exceptions will lead to the dramatic spread of suicide, seems to have little foundation. Suicide will never become popular for the simple reason that most people are attached to their lives even when they are very difficult. Admitting reasonable exceptions to the general condemnation of suicide hardly seems likely to change this. The 1978 death of 913 people at Jonestown, Guyana, has been used to challenge this assertion, but two facts should be noted. First, Jonestown was a case of mass murder-suicide, since many of the victims were forced to take poison at gunpoint. Second, the entire community seems to have been characterized by a religious frenzy and often blind obedience to the suicidal leader. Under such conditions anything can happen.

The logical form of the wedge principle, which argues that you should be consistent, hardly seems applicable for a consequentialist who consistently insists on the need for considering all the consequences and refuses to rely on oversimplified analysis. We suspect that an emotional need for clear and certain moral rules rather than consistency motivates most objections to exceptions.

This much seems clear: Suicide, though generally an evil, is not universally evil. All major theories appear to allow room for exceptions. Certainly, the consequentialist must admit exceptions because there are cases where the person can quite reasonably decide that, all things considered, continued existence is more evil than the termination of existence. It is for this reason that we contend that the health care provider is in no position to judge the ethical correctness of a patient's decision to commit either active or passive suicide.

Summary: Suicide and the Ethics of the Patient

Both the arguments above and the treatment of beneficence from the patient's point of view (Chapter Three) make it clear that passive suicide is ethical given a proportionate reason, all things considered. The present chapter also argues that even active suicide can be ethical for the patient, granted proportionality of all things considered. To say that it is ethical for a patient to commit active suicide in certain circumstances is not, however, to say that the patient has a right to do so. To put it another way, the ethical correctness of active suicide does not necessarily imply a right not to be interfered with (a liberty right), let alone a right to have others help them (substantive right). It is necessary then to consider first the health care providers' ethics of suicide prevention and then the ethics of cooperating with a suicide.

The Health Care Provider and the Ethics of Suicide Prevention

In Chapter One and Chapter Two we stressed the fact that private individuals, including health care providers, do not have a right to interfere with the activities of others unless authorized to do so by society. In addition, we stressed the fact that, in general, society is justified in interfering and authorizing others to interfere only for overriding social interests.

In the present context of suicide prevention, several points seem clear. First, though the value of the individual is not purely and simply his value to society, most individuals are valuable to society, and society has a legitimate interest in preserving most of its citizens. At times, there may even be a very strong overriding social interest since the individual in question may be particularly valuable to society. Society could, then, legitimately forbid suicide or cooperation with suicide on the grounds that the suicide robbed society of someone valuable. In addition, societies recognize that suicides do affect the rights of others. Spouses and children in particular have important legal claims on a would-be suicide. If the claims to such things as food and shelter are not met, society will be burdened with the support of those left behind by the suicide. For these reasons, many societies have made suicide a crime, that is, an offense against the society.

Sometimes, as in the United States, the society makes cooperating with suicide a crime, although suicide itself is not. This acknowledges that even though a person may be free to commit suicide, the society does not want to encourage it and definitely does not want others helping, since that help can easily turn into homicide, which is definitely to be discouraged. As we shall see, there are cases where society might well authorize controlled cooperation with suicide.

Even though American society does not make suicide a crime, it authorizes medical and police personnel to frustrate and restrain attempted suicides and to initiate a due process which can lead to involuntarily commitment to a mental institution for those who are judged to be a danger to themselves or others. It should be noted, however, that in some states such as New York suicide refers only to self-inflicted harm *and not to a decision to refuse life-sustaining treatment* (New York State Task Force, 1986).

When only danger to the patient is involved, that is, there is no damage to society or spouses and children, this practice of society raises serious questions. Thomas Szasz and the libertarians (those who believe in the maximum freedom compatible with the rights of others) object strenuously. Szasz writes (1977, p. 76),

> The individualistic position on suicide might be put thus: A person's life belongs to himself. Hence, he has a right to take his own life, that is, to commit suicide. To be sure this view recognizes that a person may also have a moral responsibility to his family and others and that, by killing himself, he reneges on those responsibilities. But those are moral wrongs that society, in its corporate capacity as the state, cannot properly punish. Hence the state must eschew attempts to regulate such behavior by means of formal sanctions, such as criminal or mental hygiene laws.

The Szasz position ignores the fact that society might still have a legitimate interest in coercing a person into fulfilling her responsibility to family and others as well as in preventing harm to others. Laws authorizing the prevention of suicide can have legitimate social purposes. There may also be room for a legitimate form of that weak paternalism, discussed in Chapter Two.

This weak paternalism is found in the position of Greenberg (1974), who insists that many who attempt suicide do not really want to die and that efforts to save them are justified. Greenberg, however, notes that a suicide prevention policy should interfere as little as possible with those who after due consideration still want to commit suicide. Thus, the prevention would be temporary, with the purpose of ensuring the patient's autonomy. The position, however, recognizes that in general the state should not interfere unless for an overriding state interest or the protection of the rights of others.

In this context, it needs to be stressed that the prevention of suicide by involuntary commitment requires legal procedures and is not simply a medical question. These legal procedures have been made increasingly strict in recent times since in the past the power of commitment was often abused. This was particularly true when a simple physician with no psychiatric training had sufficient authority in court to assure the commitment.

We shall also see that, despite the laws authorizing suicide prevention, it is not at all clear that even health care personnel can ethically interfere with the so-called passive suicide who is intent on letting himself die. The patient who refuses treatment or refuses to eat or drink may be seen as attempting suicide. Health care personnel, however, do not have a right to force treatment on such a person without a court order. Such orders are not automatically granted. Indeed, the right to refuse treatment and to refuse nutrition and hydration has been recognized not only in the case of terminal patients, but in the case of competent nonterminal cases, as well as being recognized in surrogates for such patients.[2]

The laws on suicide and involuntary commitment of those who are suicidal are not without their problems. Sometimes the law and its application seems more paternalistic than guided by an interest in protecting society. In some cases, the law can be questioned with regard to the lack of full due process or clear norms for commitment. Whether we approve of these laws or not, they are there and must enter into the decisions of health care providers.

COOPERATION IN SUICIDE

It is now time to return to the second of our basic questions: Is it ethical for the health care provider to cooperate in a competent and consenting patient's suicide whether passive or active? In using the word cooperation, we mean to stress that the competent patient has asked for or consented to the cooperation. Where there is an incompetent or doubtfully competent patient or only surrogate consent, we are dealing with an even more delicate problem and we will discuss this separately.

This cooperation may involve either withdrawing treatments that are supporting life or supplying the means of killing. First, the patient may refuse treatment or ask for the termination of treatment in order speed up the coming of death. This occurs dramatically when the patient requests that the "plug be pulled on the respirator" or that blood transfusions be discontinued. It also occurs, though with less fanfare, when certain medicines are discontinued or chemotherapy for cancer is never started. Second, the patient may ask for cooperation in actively terminating their life. For example, "Please, doctor, give me a large enough dose of sleeping pills to kill me" or "Give me an overdose at the next round of medications."

The patient in both sorts of cases may be terminal or nonterminal, with death imminent or not imminent. The patient may be suffering great physical pain or suffering psychic pain from the perceived meaninglessness of life. We shall return to some of these distinctions later in the chapter.

Cooperation in Passive Suicide

The case of passive suicide, where the death results from omitting or terminating treatment, is not condemned in our society even though a consequentialist might see no need for a distinction between passive and active suicide. This is probably because the law recognizes the right to refuse treatment but not the right to be free of interference in committing suicide.

In these cases of so-called passive suicide, the patient or surrogate exercises the right to refuse treatment or demand the discontinuance of treatment in order to speed up dying. As we saw in Chapter Three, the competent patient has a right to refuse or discontinue treatment. Yet a variety of court cases on the subject indicate that there are more complicated emotional and ethical problems for health care providers, depending on whether the patient is terminal with death imminent, merely terminal, terminal and in a permanent vegetable state, nonterminal and in a permanent vegetable state, nonterminal noncomatose and incompetent, nonterminal noncomatose and competent but with difficult life prospects, or even nonterminal noncomatose competent and without difficult life prospects.

When the patient is terminal and death is imminent, no treatment is medically indicated (see Chapter Three), and the competent patient's rightful refusal of treatment does not conflict with the health provider's form of beneficence. There may be an emotional problem in admitting defeat, but there should be no ethical problem. We note that though the patient may not be competent at the end, refusal of treatment may be in the form of a living will or exercised through a surrogate, especially through a surrogate who has a permanent power of attorney for health matters. We shall return to the objections against the living will below.

When the patient is terminal but death is not imminent since the disease or injury is slow-acting, and granted the consent of the patient or surrogate, it appears ethical to omit treatment on the ground that nothing can be accomplished, but not to omit care since human dignity is to be respected even when medicine can do nothing.

The AMA Council on Ethical and Judicial Affairs (1986) takes a clear stand on the issue:

> Even if death is not imminent, but the patient's coma is beyond doubt irreversible and there are adequate safeguards to confirm the accuracy of the diagnosis and with the concurrence of those who have responsibility for the care of the patient, it is not unethical to discontinue all means of life-prolonging treatment.

The treatments include artificially supplied respiration, nutrition, or hydration. We shall return to the special problems of nutrition and hydration later in this chapter.

As we shall see a little later on, this position of the AMA and many ethicians is reinforced by the law in those states which recognize living wills and durable powers of attorney. These legal instruments will be discussed later in this chapter.

Let us look at the reasoning behind the ethical correctness of not beginning or stopping treatment in the case of the consenting patient who is terminally ill. First, the health care provider has no obligation to prolong dying merely for the sake of prolonging it. Indeed, in the vast majority of cases, it makes no sense to prolong life when in point of fact the prolongation of the dying process is the true result. Indeed, when the care is only prolonging the agony of the patient, the continuation of treatment becomes unethical as an insult to human dignity. In such cases, the health care provider would be ethically justified in discontinuing treatment *except when the patient insisted on treatment*. Even here, however, there can be exceptions. When there is a severe shortage of medical resources, the physician might be justified in stopping nonindicated treatment even over the protests of the patient. We say "might be justified," since justification would depend among other things on a new social consensus about the duties of health care professionals. There are still problems in discontinuing treatment when the patient's surrogate(s) objects. We shall return to these questions below.

It should be noted that cessation of life–sustaining treatment does not always bring about a swift and painless death, even though it may speed up the process of dying. For example, if kidney dialysis is discontinued, the person remains conscious and suffers vomiting, internal hemorrhage, and convulsions. The removal of a respirator does not lead to death immediately, and the patient suffers the pain and panic of suffocation. These points will enter in when we return to the question of active cooperation in suicide as a way of relieving pain in the terminally ill.

Cooperation with the Suicide of the Nonterminal Patient

The most emotionally difficult cases arise when the patient refusing treatment is not terminal but will become so when the respirator is unplugged or the treatment is not started or stopped. This can occur when the patient judges that it is not worthwhile living on a respirator forever, or being fed artificially for years. It occurs when the patient does choose not to live at a level below his ideal. In all these cases the treatment is medically indicated from the health care provider's point of view but does not produce a proportionate good from the patient's point of view. No matter what the emotional turmoil suffered by the provider, here (as in Chapter Three) the patient retains the right to refuse treatment. Only a court order or a court-appointed guardian *ad litem* has the right to overrule the patient in these cases. The justice of even such court rulings is not beyond question if the death will not injure society or third parties.

What, however, is to be said of the case where the nonterminal patient not only refuses medically indicated treatment, but asks the health care provider to keep him comfortable while he dies. This was one of the issues in the Bouvia case (see page 136). In that case the patient refused food and drink but asked to be made comfortable in the hospital while she starved to death.

The health care provider can ethically refuse to cooperate in such situations not only on the grounds of individual conscience, if that is the case, but also because the health care professions should not be involved in helping nonterminal patients to shorten their lives significantly. Granted that the provider has no right to force treatment on the patient, the provider has a right to bow out of a suicide attempt, even a passive suicide attempt, when treatment is still medically indicated.

Actively Assisted Suicide

It is now time to return to the problem of active intervention of the health care provider, that is, the case of actively assisted suicide. In the case where the patient asks the health care provider for the means to kill himself or even for the administration of the means, the prevailing health care ethics is clear, even if we admit the patient's competence and right to commit suicide. Traditionally the health care provider has had a *prima facie,* that is, a presumptive, duty not to cooperate, and this for two reasons. First, despite doubts about the complete justice of the law forbidding help to suicides, it is a crime to help a suicide by supplying the means. Second, the health care provider should be devoted to healing. *Active* cooperation in suicide appears incompatible with healing, even if it does promote comfort when nothing else can be done.

Although there is ethically a presumptive obligation against cooperating by supplying the means of death, we recognize the fact that there are cases where neither healing nor comforting are possible. Indeed, in these cases the refusal to actively participate may be equivalent to dooming the patient to useless agony.

Imagine the case where there is no hope of healing and it is no longer possible to control the pain by drugs. The patient's life is a long hell, and we all recognize the reasonableness of the desire to die. Discontinuing treatment may shorten the agony but often at the risk of increasing the agony temporarily. Increased doses of analgesics may lessen the pain, but the pain and the hopelessness remain. The analgesics are often increased to the point where the person is insensible and no more than a vegetable. Finally, even the analgesics do not give relief and only the pain remains.

We would suggest that since the health care professions should comfort when no healing is possible, consideration should be given to professional lobbying for exceptions to the law so that in extreme cases there may be active intervention and cooperation in the suicide of at least competent terminal patients who are in great agony. Physician-assisted suicide, when it aims to protect human dignity and is done with informed consent, may not be traditional, but does appear to further the highest ethical goals.

These exceptions to the law, which recognize that human dignity and autonomy include more than mere life, will have to be hedged with protections against abuse and provide a conscience clause protecting the health care professional. Thus, if the health care provider's conscience prohibits suicide unconditionally, that conscience must be followed and should have legal protection. The safeguards will be similar to those we will discuss in conjunction with the living will.

Thus far only Holland appears to have changed its law, at least in court decisions (Kuhse, 1986). Even in the United States there is increasing agitation for legal authorization of medical assistance in a voluntary, humane, and dignified death by lethal injection. The lobbies include the Hemlock Society in California, and Americans Against Human Suffering to Legalize Physician Aid-In-Dying in New York.

The Dutch case mentioned above involved a competent 94–year–old woman who, in the face of steadily deteriorating physical condition, continuously urged the physician to help her in committing suicide. The reasoning of the court may be summarized as follows. Physicians have a conflict of obligations. On the one hand, they have a duty to obey the law, and on the other, a duty to look out for the best interests of the patient. They cannot be held criminally responsible for following their duty as doctors, that is, to act in the patient's best interests.

The key question is: If it is permissible to *let* some patients die, why is it not permissible to *help* the patient die? The authors believe serious study should be given to this matter even while holding that at present it is illegal if not always unethical to actively help a patient in killing herself.

Letting the Patient Die with Surrogate Consent

Up to this point we have limited ourselves to the case of competent patients who refuse treatment or ask to have treatment discontinued. As a matter of fact, the patient is often incompetent. In these cases, the health care team needs to consult the surrogates about discontinuing treatment for the terminal patient. By "terminal patient" we mean one whose condition will lead to death within a year, or who is irreversibly comatose, or where there is a medical judgment that efforts, including resuscitation, would only prolong the dying process. In all of these cases nothing appears to be medically indicated, that is, intervention will not produce more medical benefits than burdens. Ethically, as we noted in Chapter Three, the health care professional general-ly has no obligation to do what is not medically indicated. The exceptions arise when the patient or the surrogate has nonmedical reasons for continuing treatment. Ethical-ly, however, there is always the obligation not to inflict unnecessary pain on the patient.

The most difficult cases occur when the wishes of the now incompetent patient are unknown and the surrogates insist on aggressive treatment to assuage their own guilt and the physician sees the treatment as prolonging the agony of a dying patient (Brennan, 1986). The law is not clear, and the physician who discontinues treatment in these cases fears suit for negligence. Ethically, however, the obligation is to the patient and not to the family. The answer would seem clear, but the anguish will remain. Certain legal clarifications are needed to protect the patient from unneces-sary pain and the health care team from lawsuits.

The health care team may sometimes ethically continue treatment if the patient or the surrogate insists that there is some legitimate nonmedical good that they seek for the patient, but the health care team may also refuse to treat if it then hands the case over to someone else.

Letting the Patient Die Without Consent

There are cases when the health care provider might let the terminal patient die even without consent from the patient or a surrogate. With the terminal patient there is nothing medically indicated except such activities as will preserve dignity and keep the patient comfortable. The physician is not obliged to do what will produce more harm than good from a medical point of view. Indeed, if treatment, especially aggres-sive treatment, is producing more harm than good, we may even argue that he has an obligation to cease treatment. In practice, however, the health care team needs a con-sent except in rare cases, which will be discussed below.

The New York State Task Force (1986), in speaking of orders not to resuscitate, says that such orders should be issued without consent only if (a) two physicians judge that resuscitation would be futile or (b) there is a judicial finding that a do-not-resus-citate order (DNR) would be consistent with the patient's known wishes or, in the ab-sence of information about those wishes, that the order would be in the patient's best interests. This is a strict standard and makes good sense where there is no consent.

The authors are tempted to propose an argument that holds that, where treating a terminal patient deprives other patients of treatments which will produce more good than harm, a weighing of the consequences seems to create a clear obligation to stop treating the terminal patient and devote the resources where medically indicated. This, however, would be abandonment in the present system of roles that makes the patient/physician relationship personal and independent of outside factors such as the needs of others or of society. In time, society may change the definition of roles and grant health care professionals a carefully controlled right to terminate treatment of the terminal patient when other and viable patients are being deprived of resources. We must stress, however, that the termination of treatment is not the same as the termination of care. More will be said about this under the heading of care for the dying.

The Good of the Patient versus the Good of Third Parties

The previous paragraph presents the case of a terminally ill patient where the interests of a third party seem, at first glance, to be ethically decisive, but on reflection these interests are of ambiguous value. The case raises worrisome questions about the danger of making these decisions not for the good of the patient but for the good of society, the good of the family, or even the good of the hospital or the health care provider.

While both the courts and writers in ethics have rather consistently ruled that a patient is not to be allowed to die because they are or will be a burden to the society or the hospital, the economics of health care are creating pressures to deny treatment in such cases, or at least to deny payment for treatment. In short, the ethics of distribution rears its head. The following facts need to be considered carefully.

A quarter of the $75 billion spent on Medicare is used to maintain the elderly in the last year of life, and most of that is spent during the last month of their lives (Kleiman, 1985). In the case of William Bartling (Gallagher, 1985), the Glendale Adventist Hospital spent more than half a million dollars on seven months of care for one patient. Under the diagnostic-related-group (DRG) system, Medicare paid less than $50,000 of that total. With the threat of this type of circumstance, even the richest hospital in the richest country will have to give more attention to the right of providers to terminate the treatment of the terminally ill.

While we may not wish to terminate treatment for the good of society, our principles in Chapter Four indicate that society may reasonably decide not to pay for treatments which do no more than prolong biological life. We expect that insurance companies and business firms that pay for health insurance will move in the same direction. Though the authors are aware of the alleged danger of "homicide," sound public policy and legal safeguards should be able to deal with the wasteful prolongation of biological life and the danger of homicide.

Cost and the ability to pay would not be ethically relevant in an ideal world, but in the world of scarce resources the economic side becomes relevant even if it should still not be the decisive factor.

When Is it Homicide?

A health care provider might be accused of homicide in the following three situations: First, when the provider deliberately and actively caused the death of the patient.

This would occur when a drug overdose or a poison was administered with the intention of killing the patient. Second, when the provider omitted a medically indicated treatment (one that would cause more good than harm) that the patient or surrogate had consented to. Third, when the provider, knowing that the patient would die without the treatment, did not even present the medically indicated treatment to the patient or the lawful surrogate.

While the deliberate active killing of the patient is homicide, there are questions as to whether it is always unethical when a competent patient, especially a terminal patient, requests it. Neither society nor most individuals appear ready to face this question, but it is a legitimate one. Portwood (1983) and Humphrey (1984), writing under the auspices of the Hemlock Society, argue that in the case of the consenting terminal patient, the provider's active and deliberate killing should not be considered homicide.

When a health care provider deliberately omits a medically indicated treatment that has the patient's informed consent, this is a case of homicide. There is a positive obligation to do what is medically indicated when there is an informed consent. Remember that this does not hold in the case where nothing is medically indicated.

The death of the patient resulting from the fact that the provider never proposed the medically indicated treatment for consent is also homicide, because once again there is a positive obligation to present the medically indicated treatment. Here, too, there is no homicide if nothing is medically indicated.

PARTICULAR ISSUES

Introduction

In this part we will consider no-code and slow-code orders, the living will and the durable power of attorney in health matters, the special problem of omitting feeding and hydration in terminal cases, brain death and the persistent vegetative state, the function of ethics committees, and the place of the family in death and dying.

The No-Code Order

While Part I provided the basic ethical approach to the no-code order, some further investigation is useful in understanding the problem. A no-code order is a written order to do nothing if certain situations arise. Most commonly it is a DNR (do-not-resuscitate order), that is, a written order not to attempt resuscitation in cases of cardiac arrest (Standards and Guidelines, 1986). A slow code, also called a "show code" or merely a "walk slowly code," involves a verbal order to the staff to respond slowly when the patient has a cardiac arrest. Winslade and Ross (1986) note that this is often used to give the appearance of resuscitating, especially to the family. There are also "partial codes," which limit the resuscitation efforts. Each of these codes needs separate consideration.

While hospital policies should be consulted, a no-code order may be ethically issued when the treatment in question or resuscitation is not medically indicated. In other words, a no-code is correct when from a medical point of view more harm than good will be done to the patient by treatment or resuscitation. This will usually be the case when there is no further therapy for the underlying disease process for a terminally ill patient. The order is also justified by the patient's express wish that resuscitation not be attempted. It should be noted that this is a written order for which the physician accepts public responsibility and which should be medically justified on the chart. Granted these conditions and consent, except in the limited circumstances indicated previously, the no-code order is ethical.

The slow code is used to give families the impression that everything is being done for the patient in situations where most of the time a no-code order would be medically and ethically justified. The temptation to issue such an order can be great when a family insists against all reason that a patient be kept alive, even in cases where the patient is brain dead. Nevertheless, the deception involved should be condemned as unethical. The fact that there is no written order, and so a refusal to take public responsibility for the decision is also reprehensible.

We note again that the family may have nonmedical reasons for prolonging the life, even the vegetative life, for a while longer. They may want time for one last relative to arrive to enter into the farewells and the grieving process. There may be legal complications involving the moment of death. When respecting such reasons does not cause the patient additional pain and suffering, the reasons should be given some weight. Certainly they should not be ignored and the family deceived as to what is going on.

The partial code is a written order to omit some medical interventions but to employ others. There may be sound medical reasons to attempt chest compression and electrical defibrillation or to omit intubation. The reasons for these specific orders and omissions should be entered on the chart. Indeed, to avoid any ambiguity, all no-code orders should specify what is not to be done with respect to what illness. Such specification will clarify thinking and accountability as well as help reduce the risk of carelessness.

Care for the Dying

The use of such terminology as DNR, no-code, or slow-code, all of which stress omitting a treatment, might lead to the impression that there is no need to care for the dying. On the contrary, as death approaches and the technical devices of medically intensive care become useless, there is need for humanly intensive care. The dying patient needs the support and comfort of staff and family and friends. Limits on visits should be removed. Even children should after proper preparation be allowed to visit (Jordon, 1987). Long-absent relatives should be encouraged to come so that reconciliations may be made or memories shared. All of this should be provided for in a care-for-the-dying policy which recognizes that death is natural and is, indeed, the last great human experience in this world.

Euthanasia

All of this raises the specter of "euthanasia," which literally means no more than a "good death." It can include, then, death resulting from the justified omission of some treatments and death made easy with analgesics. For some people it conjures up visions of family and health care providers killing off the hopelessly ill in the name of compassion. They cite the case of the nurse who put air bubbles in the veins of homeless old men, or the case of the man who shot his brother who was painfully dying of cancer. Invoking the wedge principle, those who fear "euthanasia" argue that even permitting people to die sets a dangerous precedent. In other words, anything that diminishes respect for life is supposed to lead to murder in the name of mercy. In addition, they often insist that any diminution of respect for life can lead to the horrors of Nazi atrocities. They insist that even when the patient has a living will, it should not be honored since it involves risk of mercy killing. Finally, they assume that one should never give up hope and act as if the patient were surely terminal since there might always be a miracle or a sudden advance in medical knowledge.

Though we sympathize with these fearful thinkers, we have seen no proof that the fears are grounded. Medical homicide has occurred and will continue to occur, but there is no proof that it is a result of letting terminal patients die peacefully and painlessly. There is no proof that it results from allowing physician-assisted suicide under controlled conditions.

Indeed, we believe that the entire area of so-called "medical homicide" needs to be reexamined and carefully distinguished from physician-assisted suicide that has been requested orally or in writing by a competent terminal patient. Certainly, using labels such as "medical homicide" or "murder" or "euthanasia" does not help get at the core of the ethical problem.

The Living Will and Permanent Power of Attorney

Those groups that call themselves prolife tend to reject the living will as being another wedge leading to "homicide." We have seen no evidence of this and believe that the living will solves many problems.

Though the living will is not recognized by statute in all states, it is ethically valid and deserves great respect. Indeed, since both the National Conference of Commissioners of Uniform State Laws and the American Bar Association have approved *The Uniform Rights of the Terminally Ill Act*, we can expect the living will to spread.

The living will is a document signed and witnessed at a time when the patient is clearly competent. It is a patient's written directive to withhold treatment and to administer pain-killing drugs if the person has an incurable injury, disease, illness, or condition, and where treatment would only prolong artificially the moment of death. In short it is a written refusal of treatment for certain limited situations.

The laws which add legal approval to the ethical force of such declarations provide for various safeguards against abuse. *The Uniform Rights of the Terminally Ill Act* (Uniform Law, 1985), for example, requires that the physician who has been provided a patient's living will must make it part of the medical record. It also demands that the physician who is unwilling to comply with the wishes of the patient promptly inform the patient and take all reasonable steps to transfer the patient to another physician or health care provider. The act even goes so far as to cover the cases of pregnant women when it states:

> Unless the declaration [living will] provides otherwise, the declaration of a qualified patient known to the attendant physician to be pregnant must not be given effect as long as it is probable that the fetus could develop to the point of a live birth with continued application of life-sustaining treatment.

Thus, though it recognizes the right of the woman to control her own body, it also recognizes the right of the fetus in cases where the dying mother has not made a decision about this particular issue.

The Uniform Rights of the Terminally Ill Act makes a revocation of the will possible at any time and in any manner without regard to the patient's mental or physical condition. This means that there will be no quibbling about whether or not the patient is competent to revoke the living will.

Depending on the law of a particular state, the living will legislation may contain other provisions designed to prevent abuse. Thus, some provide that the patient must have been judged terminal by two physicians and the will witnessed by people who are not health care providers or beneficiaries of the person's last will and testament. In short, the legislation passed in many states seeks to prevent the more obvious conflicts of interests and dangers to the patient. The same may be said of the Permanent Power of Attorney for Health Care.

Some states that do not recognize the living will do give legal force to the Permanent Power of Attorney in Health Matters. This power of attorney appoints a surrogate for health affairs and gives general direction to that surrogate. It is more flexible than the living will in that powers of the surrogate or agent are not limited to desires concerning life-prolonging treatment. It differs from ordinary powers of attorney in that it is durable, that is, continues even when the person who made it becomes incompetent.

Both the living will and the durable power of attorney in health matters are useful because they provide clear indications of the will of a competent person and help to avoid conflicts among surrogates and debates as to which surrogate has the authority to consent or the correct interpretation of the wishes of the patient.[3]

Feeding and Hydration

In our treatment of the health care provider's formulation of the principle of beneficence in Chapter Three we already touched on the problem of feeding and hydration in the context of the final Baby Doe rule. We now return to the question of whether nutrition and hydration are medically indicated for terminal patients.

Before answering that question, it is necessary to show that the nutrition and hydration in question are generally not matters of sipping liquids or spooning in chicken soup, but of often painful medical procedures (Lynn and Childress, 1983; Steinbock, 1983). A brief look at the methods will show their medical nature.

There are two methods of intravenous nutrition and hydration. Nearly everyone is familiar with the IV or intravenous feeding, where a tiny tube is inserted into a vein in the arm or hand. This method is only temporarily useful for improving hydration and electrolyte concentrations. Often the patient has to be restrained from tearing out the tube. Another IV method involves inserting a catheter (small tube) into a major vein in the chest. This is a more costly method that increases the risk of infection and again often leads to restraint of the patient.

There are also two methods of feeding and hydration by inserting tubes into the intestinal tract. The first method involves shoving a tube up the person's nose and down the throat and then into the digestive tract. It is very annoying to both patients and families and, though cheap, often leads to pneumonia. The second method involves cutting an opening in the abdomen and the insertion of a tube directly into the stomach. The hole needs to be closed by surgery.

We are then dealing with medical procedures, not with simple tasks of everyday living. The question, then, goes back to asking, are these procedures medically indicated, that is, do they do more harm that good for the patient in a given case?

The AMA Council on Ethical and Judicial Affairs gave an official opinion on this matter on March 15, 1986.

> Even if death is not imminent but a patient's coma is beyond doubt irreversible and there are adequate safeguards to confirm the accuracy of the diagnosis and with the concurrence of those who have responsibility for the care of the patient, it is not unethical to discontinue all means of life prolonging medical treatment.
>
> Life-prolonging medical treatment includes medication and artificially or technologically supplied respirations, nutrition, or hydration. In treating a terminally ill or irreversibly comatose patient, the physician should determine whether the benefits of treatment outweigh its burdens. At all times, the dignity of the patient should be maintained.

There are some cases where the feeding is indicated on the compassionate ground that death from starvation is sometimes more painful than death from the particular disease. The patient may be faced with the choice between a slow death from cancer with adequate pain control or a slightly more rapid and more painful death from dehydration and starvation. In such a case, the omission of feeding and hydration would be cruel. For all that, the right to choose the way of death belongs to the competent patient.

Feeding and hydration are not medically indicated in the following types of cases: (1) the procedures are futile since the procedures are unlikely to achieve their purpose; (2) the procedures would be no help to the patient even if successful; (3) the burdens outweigh the benefits (Lynn and Childress, 1983).

Lynn and Childress give the following examples of treatments that are *futile*: (1) the patient has a severe clotting deficiency and has a near total body burn; (2) the patient has severe congestive heart failure with cancer of the stomach, which delivers food to the colon without passing through the intestine and being absorbed. In this case the fluids introduced by hydration will kill by acting on the congestive heart failure while not much of the food is absorbed in any event. In a second class of cases there is *no possibility of benefit to the patient* who has permanently lost consciousness, e.g., in cases of anencephaly, persistent vegetative state, and preterminal coma. In these cases feeding is sometimes done for the sake of the family, but it is not medically indicated. Finally, there are cases where feeding and hydration impose a *disproportionate burden*: (1) the patient's need for nutrition arises only near death, a point at which hydration causes terminal pulmonary edema, nausea, and mental confusion; (2) patients who, though they might benefit in one way, have fairly severe dementia, such that restraints are needed with the result that the patient suffers constant fear and discomfort as she struggles to be free. Life is prolonged but in a captive state.

All of this may be summarized by saying that when hydration and nutrition become medical procedures, the ethics of their omission is based on the ethics of medical indications and not on common-sense notions.

BRAIN DEATH AND THE PERSISTENT VEGETATIVE STATE

All of the judgments required above are complicated by the philosophical ambiguity about the nature of death, by the debate about the criteria for death and the nature of the persistent vegetative state (Cranford, 1988).

The philosophical and even theological ambiguity about the nature of death is clearly seen in the disputes as to whether death is the end of all existence, a reentry into another life on earth, or the passage to an eternity of happiness or punishment. Even a generalized definition such as death as a complete change in the status of the living being characterized by the irreversible loss of those functions essentially significant to it, or death as the irreversible loss of capacity for social interaction (Veatch, 1978), does not solve the problem. We still need social agreement as to which characteristics are essentially significant and what level of social interaction is sufficient. For lack of philosophical clarity, we are driven to legal definitions of death.

Though there is no legal definition accepted by all the states, the Uniform Determination of Death Act (UDDA) has been adopted by many and provides:

> An individual who has sustained either (1) irreversible cessation of circulatory and respiratory functions or (2) irreversible cessation of *all functions of the entire brain including the brain stem* is dead. A determination of death must be made in accordance with accepted medical standards. (italics added)[4]

The Harvard criteria of irreversible coma (Beauchamp and Perlin, 1978) are examples of one set of medical standards. These criteria call first for the elimination of the possibility of hypothermia and coma induced by barbituates and then the application of the following four tests: (1) unreceptivity and unresponsivity even to intensely painful stimuli; (2) no movement or breathing during an hour long period of observation; (3) no reflexes; and (4) a flat electroencephalogram. All of these tests are to be repeated 24 hours later. Other tests are suggested by various groups (Beauchamp and Perlin, 1978). The point to be stressed is that the process of deciding that someone is "brain dead" is not a matter of a single simple criterion.

Where this statute on the rights of the terminally ill is in force, society accepts the irreversible cessation of all brain functions according to accepted medical criteria as the death of the person. The person should be pronounced dead, and there is no need for the permission of the surrogates to cease treatment. Cranford (1982) notes that delicacy requires one to discuss the pronouncement with the family so that they will understand. We shall return to the problem of the family below.

In those states where brain death is not as yet a matter of law, the person cannot be legally treated as dead, but if there is brain death, treatment is certainly not medically indicated since it can do the person no good.

Brain death should be distinguished from the persistent vegetative state. The persistent vegetative state (PVS) results from damage to the cerebral or neocortex which controls the cognitive functions. For this reason it might be called cortical or cerebral death. The body, however, is not dead, since the functions of the brain stem continue in whole or in part. In this state there may still be spontaneous breathing and heartbeat. Persons in a persistent vegetative state are often awake, but they are not aware of what is going on. There is no conscious interaction with the environment and no awareness of the self or the environment (Cranford, 1982). The person in this state lacks and will permanently lack even the minimum that makes life human life. They are, in short, not capable of any human interaction.

The diagnosis of the permanent vegetative state may take three to six months. The diagnosis is not always straightforward and results in varying degrees of certitude or probability that the condition is irreversible. In line with the theory presented in Chapter Three, it should be clear that the lack of certitude is offset by the fact that the good to be hoped for is most often very minimal since there is damage to the higher functions.

People in this state should be treated with compassion and respect and kept free of pain and discomfort, but need not receive either technological support or medical treatment that will produce no improvement in their status.

Since people may persist in this state for years, there is going to be a serious problem with the distribution of resources to their care, and this will affect the decisions about how much and what kinds of care, including feeding and hydration, should be given to them.

The Place of Ethics Committees

Many hospitals have formed ethics committees to help with the ethical problems of the termination of treatment and related issues (Gibson and Kushner,1986). These committees have several missions. First, they are supposed to educate the hospital and its employees as well as the other constituencies of the hospitals. Second, they are to develop policies with regard to the problem areas, especially the problems of death and dying. Third, they are to act as advisory consultants to health care providers and possibly families. In this last role, as consultants, some worry that the committee's decisions, rather than advisory, might be taken *de facto* as binding, and so usurp the role and rights of patients and families as well as of health care providers (Levine, 1984). On the other hand, this third function can be looked at as a support mechanism for decision makers, both lay and professional. This too may be problematic if the committee ends up supporting the institution or the dominant figures in the institution rather than looking carefully at the ethics. Finally, no matter what the intention behind the ethics committee, there is no doubt that the courts have and will make them part of the decision-making process in particular cases. This is a good if it gives decisions a broader base, but it is not an unqualified good if it undermines the rights of patients, families, and professionals. Others (McCormick, 1984) raise issues like the following. Committees can end up diffusing responsibility. When committees seek consensus, they can easily end up avoiding the real point at issue and issuing carefully worded opinions that finesse the problem.

There are also questions about how privacy and confidentiality are maintained as well as about the committee's immunity from civil and criminal liability (Gibson and Kushner, 1986). The committee, in so far as it has members who are representatives of the general public and such non-health care personnel as ethicists, are not covered by the normal professional secrecy. In any event, one cannot assume that patients and families consented to having the most intimate details of their lives discussed by a committee.

At the same time, because ethical decisions in health care ethics involve more than health, life, and death, they require more than medical or nursing expertise. The exercise of the practical wisdom which is at the heart of our approach calls for the wisdom of a larger group, which looks at more than medical and nursing indications. As we note in our treatment of the Institutional Review Boards in Chapter Twelve, it is not always easy to get a representative group whose opinions will approach disinterested practical wisdom. At this stage, then, we think it best to consider the ethics committee as a very worthwhile experiment with all the results not in as yet.

The Place of the Family in Death and Dying

While the health care provider is to make decisions not to initiate or to terminate treatment in terms of medical indications, the patient, if competent, and otherwise the surrogates should be consulted since their feelings, rights, and obligations are involved. The surrogates, moreover, may know of factors that would call for the prolongation of even a vegetative life. There are cases where a woman has been kept in a vegetative state so that the child she was carrying might be delivered. In addition, there are questions of inheritance and even the need of absent family members to say farewell that enter in. For these and similar reasons, the family should be involved even when, were the family absent, the provider would be ethically justified in not initiating or terminating treatment as not medically indicated.

At a certain point in the dying process, the family become secondary patients in need of information about the state of affairs and emotional support. Too often the families are neglected and left to fend for themselves. Yet, in so far as the health care professions are dedicated to relieving suffering, the duty of compassion is in the role of all caregivers. The duty to relieve suffering demands concern for the well and the living as well as for the ill and dying. Families as well as those who are patients in a legal sense have needs which should be respected.

The Value and Quality of Life for the Individual Person

In agreeing that the health care provider may ethically withdraw some treatments from the person in the persistent vegetative state, we have at least implicitly agreed that such a state has no value for the patient. We have, moreover, permitted the health care provider to make a quality-of-life decision on a medical indications basis. This forces us to face the question: What are the minimum factors which give life a value to the patient? To put it another way, what is the threshold of meaningfulness of human life to the possessor of human life?

Biological human life has value as a means, a precondition for specifically human activities of a human person. That makes us face the crucial question: What activities are specifically human, such that lacking these or a reasonable hope of getting them back makes "biological human life" cease to have value for anyone?

Most will agree that life in a permanent vegetative state has no value for the person because there are no recognizable human activities and, indeed, there is a lack of even basic animal activities such as sensation. Having said that, we face vast disagreements. Some demand a maximum, some a minimum of human activity in order for life to be valuable to the person.

There are those who demand a maximum. They see the person as having value only when the powers of intellect and creativity and the strength of the body are at their perfection. To be less than perfect is to be valueless for those who want the maximum. From a philosophic point of view, the perfection of human life does demand all these things. Unfortunately, none of us will ever have all these characteristics in their fullness. It seems ridiculous, then, to demand what is impossible.

Some settle for a minimum in the form of the ability to interact with other human beings (McCormick, 1981). That is all that infants can do, and we find them charming and lovable and rejoice in their pleasure. The retarded and the senile can still interact with others, albeit on an unsophisticated level. We may not want to be like them, but their life still has some value to them. The same can be true for the terminally ill who can still interact with their loved ones.

On reflection we may realize that perhaps even our simplest interactions with others are the most important and rewarding part of our lives. Perhaps loving or snuggling with another person is the best thing in life. To put it another way, emotional and loving contact on even a simple level gives life value to its possessor. Certainly, it is not valueless. The authors refuse to downgrade those who will settle for that as giving meaning to life. We are not wise enough to make the judgment that more is required, nor are we sure that more is really better.

Most of us probably fall somewhere in between those two extremes in our judgments. We will settle for less than perfection but want something more of life than the ability to interact with other human persons on the simplest level. Most of us want or even demand some level of comfort or at least freedom from pain. We are the people who sign living wills and request that treatment be discontinued and no resuscitation attempted when we are terminal and in great pain. Yet, we can no more prove this middle ground is correct than we can canonize either the minimalist or maximalist position as universal principles for all humankind. None of us are wise enough to arrive at objective answers to what are in large part subjective questions.

Although the American College of Physicians (1984) believes the physicians must make judgments about the quality of life, their code stresses the subjective nature of the decision. The following statement in the *Ethics Manual* deserves careful consideration.

> Assessment by a physician of a patient's quality of life can feature prominently in making clinical decisions. It is wise for physicians to be aware of the personal and subjective values that may contribute to such evaluations. Thus, the assessment may vary according to a physician's age, present health, history of personal illness, cultural background, and long-standing knowledge of the patient as a person. Clinical decisions that hinge on assessing quality of life should be undertaken with great care and full cognizance of the subjectivity of the assessment, with full patient participation, or, if that is not possible, with participation of knowledgeable and concerned relatives or guardian. Under ordinary circumstances, a physician's judgment about quality of life should not be unilateral.

We would stress that, in practice, when the desires of the patient are not known, the minimalist position of the value of life should prevail in the physician's decisions.

SUMMARY

From a philosophical point of view, even active suicide, though presumptively unethical, can at times be ethical, especially in the cases of terminal patients in great pain. Health care workers should not cooperate with suicides in even terminal cases by providing drugs or tools for the act, but may cooperate in passive suicides by omitting treatments or procedures when requested to do so by the competent patient or surrogate. No code orders can be correct with those in a persistent vegetative state and with terminal patients when nothing is medically indicated, though there can be non-medical reasons for prolonging life for a short time. At the same time, the increasing pressures on the health care system raise questions about the need to change the law so that health care professions can actively assist in the suicide of competent terminal patients who have requested this help.

CASES FOR ANALYSIS

1. Joe came down with bilateral pneumonia. He was treated with antibiotics and put on a mechanical respirator. After a few weeks the pneumonia was improving and the physician started to wean him from the respirator. Even with a gradual approach, the weaning failed and Joe would demand to be put back on the respirator when he became terrified because he was short of breath. The physician felt that the ultimate chances of weaning Joe were now no more than 20 percent.

Joe, 80 years old and used to being in control, became discouraged and increasingly unable to bear the painful medical procedures (constant intravenous feeding, frequent needle punctures for arterial blood gases, suctioning, and so on). After three weeks of unsuccessful attempts, Joe refused to cooperate. He asked that the respirator be disconnected. "I want to die," he stated.

Despite the pain, Joe is alert and aware and is, in the opinion of the staff, fully competent. His wife and one son keep begging the physicians and the nurses to do something to help Joe recover fully.

2. Elizabeth Bouvia had been diagnosed as having cerebral palsy when she was six months old. At age 10 she had been placed in an orthopedic hospital and remained there for seven years.

She earned a B.S. degree in social work, had been married for a year, and had attempted unsuccessfully to have a child. Her husband, whom she had met as a pen pal while he was serving a sentence in jail, had left her. She had dropped out of graduate school because of difficulties in finding a clinical placement required for her program. As a result of this, the state threatened to take away her assistance for transportation.

At the time of the case when Elizabeth Bouvia admitted herself voluntarily to the hospital on the grounds that she was suicidal, she was a quadraplegic victim of cerebral palsy and confined to a wheelchair. She had limited control of her right hand and needed to be fed. She also had severe progressive arthritis that caused constant pain. Her condition was in no way life-threatening and she had a life expectancy of 15 to 20 years.

She seems to have planned to starve herself to death in the hospital away from friends and relatives. She refused to eat solid food. The physician threatened to have her certified as mentally ill so that he could force-feed her. The hospital also threatened to put her out on the sidewalk. The hospital did seek to transfer her to another facility but was unsuccessful. In the meantime the hospital force-fed her. She repeatedly tore the nasogastric tubes from her nose. The tube was forcibly reinserted each time that she removed it.

She sought legal assistance. The American Civil Liberties Union entered the case and applied for a court order restraining the hospital from discharging her or force-feeding her. Bouvia testified that she was no longer willing to live since she found it disgusting and humiliating to live so dependent a life. She wanted to starve to death while nurses gave her painkillers and kept her clean and comfortable. She had a metabolic condition which caused her blood to become excessively acidic without food. One internist treating her estimated that she could be dead within five days because of the condition.

NOTES

[1]There is a dispute as to whether the difference between active and passive killing is of any ethical significance in the context of euthanasia. See Rachels, 1975, p.78, and Sullivan, 1977 pp. 40–46. Both of these are reprinted in Mappes and Zembaty, 1981.

The terms, however, are descriptively useful, and since society still accepts the distinction as having some ethical utility, it is disregarded at one's risk. At least one of the present authors agrees with Rachels that active euthanasia ought, with suitable safeguards, to be made legal.

[2]See *BioLaw: A Legal and Ethical Reporter on Medicine, Health Care and Bioengineering* (University Publications of America, 1986) and supplements for up-to-date analysis of court decisions with regard to the right of nonterminal patients or their surrogates to refuse treatment or demand the withdrawal of treatment, including the withdrawal of nutrition and hydration.

[3]The Hemlock Society, P.O. Box 66218, Los Angeles, CA 90066–0218 will supply sample copies of a living will and a durable power of attorney based on the California Natural Death Act of 1976. These will be supplied free on receipt of a stamped, self-addressed envelope.

[4]We agree with Bernat, Culver, and Gert (1982) that the first half of this definition is defective and would be clearer if worded as follows: "In the absence of artificial means of support, death (the irreversible cessation of all brain functions) may be determined by the prolonged absence of spontaneous circulatory and respiratory functions."

Chapter Seven
ABORTION

INTRODUCTION

There is probably no more disputed and emotional issue in medical ethics than abortion. The question of abortion appears to pit the interests of the fetus against those of the pregnant woman. Some describe this as a conflict between innocent life and selfishness; others as a conflict between a person's right and ability to control her body and the surrender of that control to an alien invader. Is pregnancy an opportunity for life, or an enslavement of life?

As we suggested in Chapter One, in philosophical ethics the either/or approach is futile and obscures both the complexity of the problem and the fact that there are cases in human life where right and wrong are not always clear. Indeed, while the biological basis for tension between the fetus and the pregnant woman is obvious, many aspects of the opposition between the interests of the fetus and those of the woman are social in origin. Finally, in some situations the abortion issue brings us face to face with the tragic in human life.

We shall attempt to lay out the issues and to isolate those cases where there appears to be no answer, or at least no easy answer, in terms of either personal or health care ethics. First, however, it will be useful to present our view of the relationship of the ethical to religious questions involved and of the separation of the ethical from the legal.

Ethics and Religion

The abortion issue has deeply involved religious groups in controversy. The religious groups rest their case both on scripture or some other sources of divine revelation and on philosophical arguments drawn from reason. The present book is a philosophical treatment and cannot come to grips with theologies based on divine revelation. We can and will, however, analyze the arguments based on reason and point out their strengths and weaknesses. Even the Catholics, who are rather firm in their opposition to abortion, have a long history of debate about the philosophical justification of their position (Connery, 1977). Indeed, despite all sorts of proclamations from the Pope, the Catholics still appear to be engaged in debate as to exactly when you are dealing with an abortion or at least when the fetus has rights (McCormick, 1981).

Law and Ethics

Not everything that is unethical is a suitable object of law. In the first place law ought to be concerned primarily and directly with the public good. It should seek to regulate the behavior of people only when that is necessary or highly useful for the public good or when it is necessary to protect the rights of the individual in the society. In the second place, even such a traditional thinker as St. Thomas Aquinas insists that law should not get too far ahead of the public conscience, lest it lead to contempt for the law. For a similar reason he cautions against making laws that cannot be enforced.

Granted these limits, law is extremely useful and even necessary for defining and specifying ambiguous moral and social problems. The specifications, of course, should be congruent with basic ethical principles and the consensus of the society. As we shall see in the abortion controversy, the law may have given too much specification without enough consideration of all the ethical factors involved.

Of necessity, any consideration of abortion in the United States must look at the questions of whether or not the fetus has rights, and whether these rights should be protected by law. Even if the fetus has rights, there still remains doubt regarding the prudence of laws on the subject, considering their difficult enforceability and the unsettled state of the public conscience. In other words, it is possible to conclude that abortion is unethical and immoral and still hold that it may not be prudent to legislate on the matter.

THE SUPREME COURT DECISION

In *Roe* v. *Wade*, the United States Supreme Court answered, at least temporarily, certain constitutional and legal questions about the legality of abortion in the United States. It quite clearly declared itself incapable of deciding the ethical issue.

In the first place, the Supreme Court decided that the fetus does not have rights in the sense of the Fourteenth Amendment, that is, it does not have a right to the protection of due process of law. Moreover, it did not attempt to settle the question of whether or not the fetus has ethical and moral rights. In the second place, the Court acknowledged the relative right of the pregnant woman to privacy, that is, a right not to be interfered with. The right not to be interfered with in these cases is relative and not absolute, because there can be important state interests involving the protection of health and medical standards as well as the issue of the protection of prenatal life in the third trimester. Indeed, the Court said that states may prohibit abortion of viable fetuses except when abortion is necessary for the preservation of the life and health of the mother.

We do not intend to argue the Supreme Court decision and its consequences, but we note that it does raise the crucial issue of the status of the fetus relative to the right of the mother to noninterference. In our treatment of the ethics of abortion and of a health care provider's participation in abortion, we too must ask: (1) What is the ethical status of the fetus? This may be interpreted as asking if the fetus has rights or has such a connection with the dignity of the human person that we ought to attribute rights to it. (2) If the fetus has any rights, on what ethical basis are disputes between the rights of the fetus and the rights of the pregnant woman to be settled?

Although in line with the customary language of the abortion debate, these questions have been framed in terms of rights, and the underlying question is always one of the dignity of the person and the necessity of protecting that dignity. Indeed, the final question may be: Does the dignity of the human person demand that the fetus be respected even if the fetus itself is not a person?

Why Treat Abortion at All?

It may be objected that the Supreme Court has settled the issue and specified the rights of pregnant woman and fetus. The political agitation that continues seems to indicate that society has not said the last word on the subject. Indeed, though general questions on polls indicate that the vast majority of Americans favor the woman's right to privacy in this area, more specific questions bring out the fact that about half of the respondents want to limit abortions to such cases as a serious threat to the mother's health or incest and rape. In short, the social debate continues and the issues need to be faced over and over.

In the second place, no matter what the health care professional's personal stand on abortion may be, there remain questions of health care ethics such as the relation of abortion to health or the possibility of coercion in performing or refusing to perform abortions. These questions will occupy the final section of this chapter.

The Definition and Types of Abortion

In order to understand the ethical problems of abortion it is first necessary to define abortion, classify the various types of abortions, and specify the range of goods (motives) that are alleged as justifying abortions. This will show that the term abortion does not designate a single reality.

Abortion can be defined as the expulsion or removal or killing of a nonviable fetus, that is, of a fetus which cannot live outside the uterus at that time. The definition is relative since the viability of a fetus depends on where and when the expulsion takes place. A fetus delivered in a neonatal intensive care unit is viable far earlier than one that comes into the world in a shack hundreds of miles from any health care professional.

In biology, the term fetus is applied at the beginning of the ninth week of pregnancy, that is, well into the second trimester. This name change, however, is not of moral significance, and even expulsions early in the first trimester are still referred to as abortions. There is, of course, debate as to when the human conceptus is to be considered a fetus in a moral sense and not merely in a biological sense. We shall return momentarily to the moral status of the fetus. Only when we have determined the moral status of the fetus will we be able to say whether or not the expulsion of the conceptus, the embryo, or the biological fetus is ethically significant.

The abortion can be *spontaneous* (a miscarriage) or the *result of human intervention*. In the first trimester of pregnancy there are many spontaneous abortions. Estimates are that from 15 to 50 percent of all conceptions spontaneously abort. There is really no way of telling the exact percentage since they often occur without the pregnant woman being aware of it. In the second trimester, spontaneous abortions are somewhat more common than natural death among viable fetuses. Even if abortion is an evil, spontaneous abortions in general are not considered moral problems. Exceptionally, a spontaneous abortion might be a moral problem if it could have been prevented by reasonable behavior, or by medically indicated treatment in situations where there was no proportionate reason for permitting or risking the spontaneous abortion. This is in line with the principle of proportionality developed in Chapter Three.

Those abortions which occur because of human intervention may be classified as direct or indirect. The indirect abortion is an unintended side effect that is either risked or permitted when certain things are done. An indirect abortion might result from a medicine taken to cure a disease or from anesthesia or from a surgical procedure. Even if abortion is an evil, the morality of the indirect abortion is the morality of proportionality. It is a question of whether the evil of the risked or permitted abortion is offset by the good resulting from taking the medicine or undergoing the surgery.

In direct abortion, the abortion is the intended consequence. The fetus is to be deliberately destroyed. If the fetus has innate or attributed rights, this is an attack on those rights. If the fetus is a person, this is a direct assault on an individual person who is, as we saw in Chapter One, an intrinsic good in terms of which all consequences are to be measured. Thus, the ethical or moral status of the fetus becomes the issue.

THE MORAL STATUS OF THE FETUS

It is not clear that the biological fetus is a person or that it has rights. As we shall see, simple biological existence does not entail moral status. If it did, all living things might be persons. While something like this position has been proposed (Regan,

1984), it has not been generally accepted in the American tradition. The moral status of the fetus is treated in great detail in Bandesor (1983) and in Shaw and Doudera (1983). With English (1975) and Wikler (Shaw and Doudera, 1983), we believe that there is no completely satisfactory *intellectual* solution to the problem of the status of the fetus. In the first place, ethical principles involve emotions as well as intellect, so that purely intellectual solutions are not always ideal. Second, and even more to the point, we are in an area of opacity, that is, an area where it is impossible to answer the question directly (see Chapter One). Yet the question is crucial, since the problem of the moral status of the fetus involves the basic question of the moral status of human beings and persons in general.

There are, of course, endless arguments about what constitutes a person. Some argue that a fetus is a person from the moment of conception on the ground that the fetus is a human being and all human beings are persons (Noonan, 1970). This stipulation begs the question and is not particularly convincing. Others argue that there is no person before the development of a functioning brain (Brody, 1975). Even if one agrees with that, it does not follow that there is a person present after the development of a functioning brain; other considerations ranging from viability to self-awareness might be necessary (Engelhardt, 1973; Warren, 1973). In short, there is no neat biological answer to the moral status of the fetus.

In the end, the moral status of the fetus is an ethical issue which, like all ethical issues, has its roots in the dignity of the human person, and its expression in the social understanding of that dignity. Thus, the moral status of the fetus will reflect not only the moral status we grant to the retarded, the senile, and children, but the degree to which we want to protect persons or humans in general by forbidding exceptions which might threaten them.

To put it another way, the willingness of a society to attribute or grant moral status and rights to the fetus depends first on whom we already acknowledge as having moral status and rights. The moral status granted the fetus depends on where the whole of society wants to place the outer defenses of the rights already assumed as existing.

We will attempt to show this dependence of the moral status of the fetus relative to the general stand on who has rights by considering three principles which Devine (1978) calls The Species Principle, the Potentiality Principle, and the Present Enjoyment Principle. While this consideration will not settle the issue, it will illustrate the centrality of the question of who has a right to life and how it should be protected.

The *Species Principle* asserts that all biological humans (or all members of the species characterized by "T") have a serious right to life. "T," of course, can stand for such characteristics as being conceived of humans or born of humans or being genetically human. This principle assures the protection of the seriously retarded and those in permanent vegetative states, as well as the permanently insane and small children who have not as yet shown signs of personhood. This principle will also offer protection to the fetus if one accepts "T" to mean being conceived of humans or genetically human.

The *Potentiality Principle* states that all creatures which potentially possess or in due course will possess "T" have a serious right to life. Once again, one may disagree about what constitutes "T." If, however, "T" included the possession of distinctively human characteristics, the principle would protect those fetuses which will come to term and grow into distinctively human beings and ultimately human persons. It would not necessarily protect a fetus who is so severely damaged that it will not live to term and will not develop into full human status, nor would it protect the seriously retarded or those in a persistent vegetative state. The problem here is to decide what are the distinctive characteristics of the human or, more basically, what we want to protect.

The *Present Enjoyment Principle* recognizes a serious right to life only in those who currently possess "T." Here again there are disputes as to what those characteristics are and as to their possession by the fetus. Unless "T" is defined in a fairly minimal way, this principle would not necessarily protect the fetus or the severely retarded or senile old people.

As already noted, these principles and disputes about characteristics involve not merely the problem of abortion, but the question of whom you wish to protect. Thus, the dispute involves the rights of small children, the retarded, the senile, the unconscious, and those in a coma. It is about who or what has rights in general.

The Species Principle

The Species Principle asserts that all humans have serious rights to life. Three things indicate that the fetus is human. First, it comes from humans. Second, it will, if it lives, become in the vast majority of cases recognizably human. Indeed, in the later stages of fetal development (by the ninth or tenth week at the latest) the fetus is already recognizably human. Third, one can with a very high degree of probability show that the tissue is human and not something else. We readily use this sort of argument in granting rights to neonates and small children who have not shown signs of being persons. In view of all three indicators, one can argue from the Species Principle that the fetus has a serious right to life. If you demand greater proof of species membership, not only fetuses, but also neonates and small children may be eliminated from the protection of the principle. Since this is counterintuitive for most of us, society might attribute species membership and a serious, but not absolute, right to life to the fetus, if only to protect the dignity and rights of neonates and small children.

This approach would give the fetus a serious right to life from the moment of conception. Yet not all those who are against abortion want to grant the serious right to life from the moment of conception. As a result, some want to introduce additional distinctions to avoid granting a serious right to life at that moment. For example, they admit the existence of an individual human with rights only after the fertilized egg is implanted in the uterus or only after twinning is impossible. In any event, there is still debate among those who accept the Species Principle.

We know of no theoretical way of settling this type of dispute among the defenders of the Species Principle or any of the other principles. While biological facts are appealed to in each position, by themselves biological facts cannot decide the issue of when the fetus becomes a person. We suggest that, in practice, the wedge principle is invoked in order to arrive at a position. In other words, the rights are attributed even to the fetus as a protection of all others to whom we grant rights. This approach protects the dignity of the human being by attributing the rights which flow from that dignity to others who are not clearly and unequivocally persons. Thus, it is argued that if we do not grant a serious right to life to all beings that are biologically human, we logically open ourselves up to permitting the killing of seriously retarded infants, the senile, and the permanently insane. Indeed, it may be argued that if we restrict the serious right to those who are, in some higher sense, clearly persons, it would be right to kill small children who as yet have shown no signs of personhood. It may even be argued that when you weaken respect for human life on this simplest of levels, you have created a situation which might lead to killing the retarded, the senile, and insane. The logic is correct and, we think, dangerous.

For this reason the authors think that the wedge principle is the principle which best protects human dignity. This is to say that the wedge principle gives the largest outer defense to those to whom we currently accord the right to life. While the authors have not seen convincing proof that the empirical form of the wedge principle is verified by cases of historical atrocities, it seems clear that moving away from the biological criteria provide at least a temptation to go all the way and to act as if the retarded, the senile, and the insane have less of a right to life and to health care. In the past those who weakened the defenses of human dignity went on to negate moral status for women, Jews, Gypsies, blacks, and indeed anyone who was not a member of their "in group."

The respect for human life is, however, lowered by many factors other than deliberate choice. Famine, which creates a competition for survival, lowers the respect for the lives of the weak, that is, those who have the least chance for survival. Indeed, it would seem that scarcity, which makes it more difficult to express the respect for life, lowers that respect as it lowers the expression of the respect. In hard times, when basic resources are particularly scarce, there is a tendency to consider certain kinds of people a burden that can be dispensed with. This tendency is particularly strong when we cannot see the face of the other, or see them as different from us and so less than human. This tendency enters not only into the abortion debate but into a person's attitude toward killing the enemy in war. All this is tragic, and we strive to avoid the situation that creates the tragedy, but the fact remains that we scale down our values when our backs are against the wall.

The Potentiality Principle

The Potentiality Principle states that all creatures that potentially possess or will in due course possess characteristics that are designated as distinctively human or constitute human personality have a serious right to life. At first glance, this principle would grant the fetus a serious right to life since the vast majority of fetuses will, if left to develop, turn out to be clearly recognizable human persons. Unfortunately, the arguments about what is distinctively human or what constitutes personality start at once. The problems are similar to those outlined in Chapter Six when we discussed the value and quality of life. Some demand that to qualify as a person there be a maximum potential for a high level of intellectual functioning. Others assume that all human beings must be considered as persons no matter what level of activity they display. Under some interpretations fetuses with undeveloped cerebral cortices would not qualify as potentially persons and so would have no serious right to life.

In the face of such differences, the wedge principle is once again invoked to settle the issue. This is to say that the lines are drawn in accord with what the writer wants to or has decided to protect. This, as we will show below, depends not merely on subjective whim, but on the *Weltanschauung*, or world view, which forms a person's basic moral outlook. We shall return to the concept of world view later in the chapter.

The authors believe that life has value even for those who can only interact humanly on a very basic level (see Chapter Six), and so we would protect them under the Potentiality Principle even if their potential is very small. This belief would appear to be the dominant belief in American society. Although not always successful, our society attempts to take care of the severely retarded as well as those who have serious mental illnesses. Although they contribute nothing to society and can enjoy little of what most of us aspire to, they still have that minimum capacity for simple human interaction. In all honesty, it must be admitted that none of these positions can be proven or has intuitive validity. We would note, however, it is possible to set the criteria of personhood so high that very few could live up to it. In short, if we demand too much, we will deny serious rights to most existing human beings and set the stage for justified slavery if not for genocide. It is possible to go too far and end up reduced to the ridiculous.

The Present Enjoyment Principle

The Present Enjoyment Principle recognizes a serious right to life only in those who presently possess the specifically human characteristics or are clearly human beings. Once again, there is disagreement about what those human characteristics are and what constitutes a human being or a human person. At one extreme this principle might call upon the unreasonable claim that to be a person one must presently enjoy a high level of intellectual functioning. Toward the other extreme, this principle might define as persons human beings enjoying biological separateness, which would include small children and the retarded, but exclude fetuses.

This can be the most restrictive principle of all since even in its minimum form it denies a serious right to life to the potentially human and so excludes fetuses. As with the other principles, it could in some cases also exclude small children, senile people, and the seriously retarded who do not meet the specific standards set by defenders of this principle (Tooley, 1972).

The wedge principle seems particularly destructive of this position since the Present Enjoyment Principle can easily be interpreted so as to lead to horrible conclusions. In the history of the world we have seen too many cases where Jews, Gypsies, blacks, women, crippled infants, the aged and infirm, as well as those who are merely weak, have been exploited and killed because against all reason they were labeled as less than human or at least as lesser humans and so without rights. The fear of that happening again makes the authors reject most interpretations of the Present Enjoyment Principle out of hand and move cautiously with regard to any definition of human or person which tends to eliminate groups of people whom American society has traditionally and reasonably defended as having serious rights to life. Such a tradition should be guarded and modified only after the most penetrating analysis of all the factors involved.

Summary

Every argument presented thus far has ultimately resolved itself into a wedge argument, that is, into a refusal to make exceptions lest the door be opened to abuses. In point of fact this method of argumentation leads to the conclusion that when there is doubt, we should expand the area of rights in order to protect the value of human life and the rights of persons. To put it another way, the constant use of the wedge principle amounts to building a high and strong wall around the acknowledged rights.

The argument does not, however, settle the issue of who has rights by their very nature. We have then a powerful practical argument rather than a carefully established theoretical basis for an absolute opposition to abortion. This is in line with our general approach of practical wisdom which looks at all implications of an activity in the light of human dignity.

The Species Principle and the Potentiality Principle, when developed by the wedge principle, lead the writers to hold that a fetus has a serious, though not absolute,[1] right to life. Logically, these two principles appear to lead us to say that the right exists nearly from the moment of conception. We hedge regarding the moment of conception because it is not clear that the wedge principle needs to be invoked to cover the period between conception and implantation. To put it another way, it may be possible to allow a few days leeway without undermining respect for human persons. As we have discussed, the attempt to fix a precise moment when the fetus has rights or certain types of rights seldom leads to convincing answers (Bayles, 1984). The effort may be admirable, but it seeks a clarity that is not available. There will always be some arbitrariness since we must draw the line not only in terms of (inconclusive) objective criteria, but in terms of our subjective need for certitude and our desire to build a wall around the rights of those we want to protect. On the other hand, in view of our long tradition of respect for the dignity of the severely handicapped and for all groups, the stand is not unreasonable in our society. Tradition itself has an objectivity in the form of the culture and the values of the entire society.

The conclusion that the fetus has a serious, though not absolute, right to life and logically has it from the moment of conception is not to deny that the pregnant woman too has serious though not absolute rights over her body. Indeed, the conflict between the serious rights of the fetus and the serious rights of the pregnant woman is one of the crucial areas in the debate about abortion. A fair discussion must take into account both sides.

THE RIGHTS OF PREGNANT WOMEN

The Supreme Court decision in *Roe* v. *Wade* affirmed the right of privacy, that is, the right not to be interfered with. It also stated that the right was not absolute but could be limited by the interests of the state in the health of the mother, or the interest of the state in the potential life that is present during the third trimester. In addition to this right to privacy, the woman also has a right to life and a right not to have her health destroyed. It is also alleged (most clearly in the Court's dissenting opinion) that the woman has a right to abort in order to facilitate career plans, avoid poverty, as part of selecting the sex of her child, and to avoid the birth of a defective child.

There has been much disagreement over the right to privacy. While the majority opinion in *Roe* v. *Wade* cited precedent, the dissenting opinion claimed that this right was simply fabricated and had no genuine constitutional foundation. Since we cannot resolve this legal debate, the authors wish to draw attention to one of the fundamental moral issues at stake: Unless there are serious overriding social interests, the decision to have or not to have an abortion is to be made by the pregnant woman or, if necessary, a proper surrogate. Like all ethical decisions, it is to be made in the context of the demands of human dignity as understood and supported by the society. The woman decides under the difficult obligation to consider all relevant ethical considerations, but it remains her decision.

In the current understanding of the abortion debate, we are faced with conflict between various types of rights. First there is the conflict between the serious but not absolute right of the fetus to life and the serious but not absolute rights of the woman to life and protection of her health. Second, there are conflicts between the serious but not absolute right of the fetus to life and the often far from serious and not absolute right of a woman to a wide variety of interests, ranging from the good of the woman's family to the goods of a certain career timetable or a child of a certain sex. The conflicts cannot be settled on a simple individual rights basis, and the impact of such decisions on the respect for human dignity in general must be a continuous concern.

In an ethic based on practical wisdom, which makes the individual human person the intrinsic good, the conflicts between these rights must be judged in terms of the following factors. First there is the question of whether abortion goes against the intrinsic good, the dignity of the individual human person, or if it threatens the rights and thus the dignity of all persons. Thus far, we have only established that the fetus has a serious but not absolute right to life, and certainly we have not established that the fetus is an individual person and so an intrinsic good. Indeed, we have argued for the serious right of the fetus in terms of maintaining limits which protect the rights of other persons when there is a conflict of rights involving more or less important means to the intrinsic good. It must be asked if the proposed good consequences for the woman justify the bad consequences for the fetus and for others who have a serious right to life as well as possibly seriously evil and so overriding consequences for society. It is necessary, then, to consider the various goods which are used to justify an abortion. Sometimes this is called looking at the medical and nonmedical indications for an abortion. Within an ethic of practical wisdom, we are looking at the good consequences which are alleged to justify the evil consequences of abortion. To put it another way, the conflict of relative rights of the pregnant woman and of the fetus must be examined in terms of the consequences for all parties in the conflict, including the society and all who have a serious right to life. Once again we stress that it is not purely and simply a conflict between the rights of the fetus and the rights of the pregnant woman.

The Motives for Abortion

The motives for abortion indicate the range of proposed goods which people seek to obtain by abortion. These goods can be classified under six main headings: (1) abortions that are therapeutic from the woman's point of view, whether as necessary (a) to save the mother's life or (b) on the basis of other medical indications; (2) abortions that are eugenic for the fetus, i.e., the view that a particular fetus is better off dead; (3) abortions that are eugenic from the social point of view, which may include socioeconomic as well as sociomedical reasons and indeed, might be part of a population policy. In this point of view society is considered to better off without this particular fetus being born; (4) abortions for juridical reasons such as rape or incest, though obviously other factors such as maternal mental health are involved; (5) abortions centered on family goods, for example, cases where the family would suffer psychologically and/or economically from the birth of another child or a severely ill child; and (6) abortions for the sake of miscellaneous goods from the woman's point of view, which include everything from lifestyle and career patterns to the desired sex of the baby.

Therapeutic Abortion

Only the first category contains therapeutic abortions, that is, abortions connected with curing or saving the life of the pregnant woman. Some cases in the fourth class, abortions for juridical reasons, may be included here if they also involve threats to the mother's physical or psychological health.

Examples of therapeutic abortions include the case of a woman with certain kidney problems, such that pregnancy could lead to death from uremic poisoning. An abortion in her case could be seen as therapeutic with one life pitted against another. In other cases, the pregnancy might not lead to death but could threaten serious and permanent impairment of the woman's health. Thus, a woman with diabetes might lose her sight if the fetus is carried to term. Here we would see the life of the fetus confronting serious health problems for the woman. Finally, there are cases where carrying the fetus to term is considered a danger to the psychological health of the woman. Obviously the psychological harm might range from mild upset to the onset of a psychosis.

Those who do not grant the fetus a serious, though relative, right to life have no interest in the nature of the reasons given for *therapeutic* abortion, since for them, there is no conflict between the right of the mother and the less significant right of the fetus. Those who recognize the fetus as having a serious right to life must face and resolve not only the conflict of rights but the emotional turmoil and anguish of being in what is often a no-win situation. When we face the dilemma of *the relative right to life versus the relative right to life* we are, indeed, involved in a tragedy where our principles do not give us a way out. If one grants a serious right to the fetus, ethical theory does not give us a clear way of resolving either the ethical conflict or the emotional turmoil. No matter what choice is made, great evil follows. In these situations ethics fails us and we are left with the necessity of choosing in sorrow, knowing that either choice is wrong from one point of view and right from another, equally convincing, point of view. This seems to be part and parcel of the human condition. In such cases one must decide and act on the basis of her understanding of human dignity. Regardless of what decision has been made, she ought to act with sorrow, knowing that a real good has been sacrificed.

When something less than the woman's life is at stake, it seems simple to resolve the conflict since a serious right to life ought to take precedence over a right to some lesser good, such as one's eyesight or one's sanity. This may be true in many cases, but in other cases such an analysis is simplistic, in that it excludes the consideration of goods which are not clearly the object of rights. Consistent with the demands of practical wisdom, the woman must consider the good of the family who might have a blind or a psychotic mother if the fetus is carried to term, just as she must consider what it means to her to possibly suffer that fate. There are important moral consequences no matter what the decision, and there is no easy settlement on the basis of theory. Indeed, this broader consideration of the problems involved forces us once again into the tragic dimension, similar to the life versus life dilemma in that no matter what you do, a great evil will result.

Actions suggested by practical wisdom can only reflect the particular conditions of human life. Practical wisdom cannot always give answers that avoid the tragic. Even absolutist theological positions cannot take away the human condition and remove the emotional conflict which should accompany such important decisions.

Nontherapeutic Abortions

The nontherapeutic abortion causes no personal ethical problems for those who do not grant the fetus a serious right to life. It does create problems not only for those who grant the right but, as we shall see a little later, for health care professionals who are dedicated to life and health.

The first of the nontherapeutic abortions, supposed to be eugenic from the point of view of the child, are generally characterized by the feeling that *this fetus would be better off dead.* This is alleged to be the case where the fetus has been diagnosed as having a serious genetic defect or a chance of being born retarded or the like. The abortion is supposed to be for the good of the child.

This class of cases brings us directly back to the problems of the quality of life and of the right of another, even a mother or father, to make those judgments for a person or for a being with a serious right to life (see Chapter Six). Once again it must be stressed that what makes life meaningful to the individual can go from the simple ability to interact with other human beings to the highest development of the loftiest human potentials. None of us seems wise enough to judge the limits of life for another, and the implications of the wedge principle urge us to approach this question with great caution.

Abortions which are supposed to be eugenic from the social point of view are based on the idea that this fetus, if allowed birth, would be a burden on society. In short, *it would be better for society if the fetus was not born.* The reasons given in these cases embrace not only the chance of serious birth defects, as in the cases given above, but the fact that those defects will cost society a great deal of money. Sometimes it is simply alleged that society has too many people and too few resources to support them. Unfortunately, however, social eugenicism often includes racism of the worst sort. In the United States, for example, there have been cases where government employees were illegally forcing abortions on American Indian and black women in the name of welfare reform.

There are several serious arguments which question the social eugenic approach. First, and most basic, is the fact that society exists for the individual and not the other way around. This limits what society can do even to protect itself. Second, even when, as in Chapter Four, we grant society rights in this area, society itself and not individuals ought to make the decision as to when it is necessary even to neglect an individual in the name of the public or common good. Third, the long-term and not merely the short-term effects of such thinking should be carefully weighed.

Pregnancies resulting from rape and incest, our fourth category, are often put forward as prime candidates for abortion. Sympathy for the victims makes the case particularly emotional. We can all understand why a woman would not want to bear a child that resulted not from an act of love or even passion, but from a cruel and deliberate degradation. Certainly, the effects of both the rape and the pregnancy on the mental health of the individual victim need to be given serious consideration. Perhaps they may even create the equivalent of a life versus life situation.

Our abhorrence of incest creates a similar sympathy coupled with concern about the possibly defective genetic endowment of the fetus and the destructive psychological effects on the victim. Once again, the actual consequences need to be considered, and they may or may not create the equivalent of a life versus life situation.

At the same time, abortion will not undo all the effects of rape and incest and may only create new problems. Most important of all is the question whether or not making exceptions for these cases opens up the way for abuses. Once again we are back to the wedge principle. There are dangers in denying the fetus's serious right to life on the grounds that his father was a criminal, or that the child might be less than perfect or might be a burden to the mother or to society. In addition, the extent of the trauma to the woman is very much influenced by the degree of society's intelligent and sympathetic assistance and if the alternatives of adoption, foster care, and institutionalization are viable. In short, there are many factors to consider even when dealing with the result of rape and incest.

Our fifth class of indications comprises the familial consequences—social, psychological, and economic—of the birth and development of a particular fetus. Let us take the mother of five who has just gotten off welfare and discovers that her 14-year-old daughter is pregnant. She sees reentry into the ranks of the poor plus years of raising the child. Adoption may offer an alternative, but adoption is not always possible. The mother feels trapped and faces once again the agony of living on welfare and the difficulties of a 14-year-old too young to mother a child.

Consider also the case of the parents who already have a Down's syndrome child and are told that they are about to have another. Not only financially, but emotionally, their backs are against the wall. They foresee mental collapse for themselves and severe neglect of the handicapped child they already have. Adoption is not generally a feasible alternative when you are dealing with a retarded child, and they shudder at the thought of putting the child into a substandard public facility. People who consider abortion in such situations face choices where they can never win and settle for what they judge to be the lesser evil, if any of these evils can be called lesser.

Ideally, these conflicts could be removed by superior public care and changed attitudes towards the adoption of the handicapped. In practice, the competition of scarce resources often leaves the handicapped neglected and their parents in the dilemmas we have shown. While the authors are inclined to side with the fetus in these cases, they fully sympathize with parents who seek to protect their family and children.

The miscellaneous category includes a wide variety of reasons for an abortion. These include fear of changes in lifestyle that come about with a pregnancy and the entrance of child into the family. Or perhaps the pregnancy will ruin a career or affect material comfort. The authors doubt that the fetus's serious right to life should yield to such minor goods.

Social Support and the Abortion Problem

Many of the cases mentioned in the previous pages indicate that society's willingness or lack of willingness to help with health care or social services enters into the abortion decisions which women and families make. Simpler adoption laws might make a decision for life easier. Better law enforcement might decrease the cases of rape and incest. A willingness to supply better care and auxiliary services for the handicapped might make families less afraid of bringing a child into the world. All of these good things, however, involve the distribution of scarce resources and all the problems we discussed in Chapter Four. Even the richest society in the world cannot escape the human condition.

Ethics and Tragedy

In line with the consequentialist approach taken in this book which demands proportionality between the good effects intended and the bad effects risked or permitted and sometimes even intended, it should be clear that there is no neat set of answers to the question of a woman's substantive right to an abortion. Nor are there neat answers to the exact extent of the fetus's serious right to life. The life versus life case, however, points up the tragedy at the root of so many cases involving debate about the ethics of abortion.

In the life versus life cases, theory does not permit us to give the primacy to the woman or to the fetus. Two equal goods are in conflict. Though some argue that the woman is a person with full rights and the fetus has only diminished rights, they offer a dangerous distinction and the wedge principle as elaborated earlier should make us hesitate about adopting it.

Abortion, Practical Wisdom, and the World View

In the last analysis, the stand one takes on abortion is not simply a matter of the rights of the fetus and of women, but of a multitude of factors which must be weighted and balanced by practical wisdom as discussed in Chapter One. That practical wisdom considers among other things the emotions and experiences of the individuals in a society. It also recognizes that there is implicit knowledge, including theological beliefs, operating in a society. All of these are combined in an often poorly articulated world view, that is, an accepted and functional view of the meaning of life and activity in the society. The world view contains explanations of evil and good in the whole history of the world.

In our pluralistic American society different groups have different world views. If that world view is fatalistic, people will not struggle to avoid all evil and will often accept pain and suffering as part of life. Those who believe in divine providence may see a retarded child as a possible blessing and not merely as a hardship. Others who see people as capable of solving all problems and doing away with all suffering will not accept any suffering or hardship or inconvenience they can avoid. Each of these groups will have very different attitudes towards life and abortion.

Sidney Callahan (Callahan and Callahan, 1984) adds to the list of world view elements which underlie the dispute. We put her points in the form of questions. Is the individual person's intrinsic worth the center of things, or is membership in the species the more important source of moral worth? Is there purpose and meaning, even transcendent meaning, in the world or do we make our own meanings? Should feminism be only in favor of individual women or in favor of the weakest groups including fetuses? Is all suffering to be avoided or does suffering taken on for the sake of others have significance and value? Granted that the emotions are important in the moral life, which ones are most appropriate and which should have dominance in the abortion debate? Are we to praise rationality and coolheaded control or tenderness and concern for the weak?

These questions are so profound and so difficult to answer that the abortion debate will not end soon. Two points, however, should be stressed. The issues are too important to justify name calling and *ad hominem* arguments. Men and women of intelligence and good will line up on both sides of the debate. They are to be respected even if we find their position abhorrent or stupid. If we lose sight of the need to respect others as a condition for continuing the dialogue, no one will ever win the debate since they will have destroyed the dignity of the debaters and refused to search for needed social improvements which might alleviate some of the tragic situations we have considered.

Second, the issue involves practical wisdom and as such can, at best, only be resolved in a partial fashion by a relative consensus in society. The opacity of the moral dilemmas outlined in this chapter make a clear and certain central philosophical principle impossible. Even "practical" solutions emerging from a relative consensus will be temporary. The material conditions within which the relative consensus developed will become obsolete. Society will change its support for pregnant women, new methods of birth control may even rule out the temptation to consider abortion. We can only hope that our ability to assimilate these changes ethically will allow us to keep tragedy and evil to a minimum. The tragic, however, will always remain.

ABORTION AND THE HEALTH CARE PROVIDER

Introduction

The health care provider must face three sets of problems. The first concerns his personal stand on the morality of abortion . The second involves health care institutional policies on personnel. The third set concerns questions of professional ethics, which exist even for those who have no personal ethical problem with abortion. This third set of problems involves such matters as forced abortions and professional involvement in nontherapeutic abortions.

Abortion and Personal Ethics

The health care provider who follows the approach given in this chapter must decide whether or not a particular abortion is ethical and, in the process, decide whether or not she will cooperate with the woman who wants an abortion. When the provider has decided that the particular abortion is unethical, she should ordinarily withdraw from the case. At times, however, the matter of cooperation is not that simple. Must a nurse withdraw who occasionally tends women in the recovery room after an abortion? Can a physician continue to practice in a hospital which performs many abortions which she considers unethical? The classical principles on cooperation can be applied in situations like these.[2] Thus, though a provider should not perform or directly participate in an abortion she considers unethical, there may be proportionate reasons for taking care of patients under treatment as a result of an abortion. The most obvious reason is to prevent further harm to the patient. There are even proportionate reasons for continuing to work in a hospital that performs a large number of abortions that the health care professional judges to be unethical. Thus, granted that continued association with the hospital is not taken as approval of unethical conduct, the needs of the profession and of patients in the area can often supply the justification for continued association with the group.

Those who see no problems with abortion will have no problems of conscience in this area. Those who see all abortions as *murder* will feel compelled to fight against abortion in any circumstances. Holders of both of these positions must, however, face the problem of institutional policy and its relation to the conscience of those who disagree with them.

Abortion and Institutional Policy

The strong feelings associated with the abortion question can push individuals to promote institutional policies which ban those who disagree with them. Catholic hospitals, for example, might be tempted to ban not only physicians who perform abortions, but those who do not publicly condemn abortion. Hospitals boards, which see the provision of abortions as a mandatory service to women who desire them, may be tempted to deny privileges or employment to health care professionals who are either against abortion or who see the need for deciding each case on its own merit. In short, all sorts of providers may be excluded by health care institutions which feel that they have excellent reasons for their policies.

The authors grant that, as individuals, members of institutional boards must follow their consciences. As members of the board, however, they need to consider four points. First, the institution should have a public written policy. In short, there should be no secret blackballing of potential employees and physicians who desire staff privileges. Second, the policy should be rooted in the publicly stated and carefully articulated philosophy of the institution. In other words, the policy should be relevant to the stated purposes of the institution. Third, the policy should, in so far as consistent with the philosophy of the institution, respect the consciences of the health care providers it employs. Fourth, it should also be in accord with state laws which protect the conscience of health care professionals. In a pluralistic society, at least, it requires a strong justification to exclude those who are against abortion if they will never be involved with abortions. An equally strong justification is required to exclude those who are in favor of abortions if they will never be involved in abortions.

The Nontherapeutic Abortion

Even if the health care provider's personal ethics permits abortion, the health care professional and the institution must still ask whether or not the abortion is medically indicated and therefore within the ethics of healing. In short, there is a question as to whether or not a nontherapeutic abortion is a suitable activity for a physician or a nurse or for a hospital or other health care agency.

The therapeutic abortions—those which are concerned with preserving the life and physical health of the woman—are within the purview of health care providers. To put it another way, if an abortion is medically indicated, the physician or nurse whose conscience otherwise permits may participate. When the abortion is not medically indicated, as is the case with abortions done for social reasons, for eugenic reasons, or for the convenience of the woman, the participation of a health care provider is ethically questionable. Health care providers are supposed to be healing, not passing judgment on the quality of life or the good of society, much less facilitating the nonmedical goals of some patients. To put it another way, traditionally and, we believe, correctly, the professional health care provider is committed to health and not to supplying what the customer wants and will pay for no matter what the need may be. Just as physicians have refused to act as executioners in those states that mandate death by lethal injections which only physician may prescribe, so they should refuse to blur their professional role by participating in nontherapeutic abortions. The tradition, however, seems to have weakened and the mores of the contemporary American society appear bent on making the health care professional a huckster who can do nearly anything a patient will pay for. The authors believe that this can only weaken the health care professions and ultimately harm society.

In practice, there is much dispute as to what constitutes a therapeutic abortion. Some physicians argue that the abortion is therapeutic not only if it prevents or alleviates a serious physical or serious mental illness, but even when it alleviates temporary emotional upsets. In short, the health of the pregnant woman is given such a broad definition that a very large number of abortions can be classified as "therapeutic." Even with this broad definition of health and of therapeutic abortion, many abortions are still nontherapeutic. Abortions to preserve lifestyle or career plans are hardly therapeutic or medically indicated. Eugenic abortions of either type are also not therapeutic.

The abortion problem is just one example of an area where there is need for serious consideration of the role of the health care professional in a society which often acts as if it had a right to purchase every convenience. Is it right to do plastic surgery on people who will not benefit from it? Is it right to patch up athletes and send them back into the game at risk to their health and possibly to their life? Is it right for a health care professional to abort a fetus for the convenience of the healthy pregnant woman? In short, is it right to use professional expertise for nonhealing purposes?

The authors believe that the answer to all of these questions is a clear "no." In our opinion, the health care professional loses professional status and turns into a mere tradesman when medical indications are banished and patient convenience or provider profits made dominant criteria of practice. Thus nontherapeutic abortions remain an ethical problem even for health professionals whose purely personal ethics do not condemn such abortions. Perhaps there is need for a separate group who make no pretense at healing, but handle nontherapeutic abortions, executions, and other services for which the public is willing to pay. Such a separation would not solve the abortion problem, but it would make clear that health care professionals are dedicated to healing and not to death or mere money making.

Coercion and Abortion

The principles of informed consent apply in the cases of abortion as in all medical procedures. Indeed, they should probably apply more stringently not only because such high goods are at stake, but because there are so many temptations to abuse the freedom of the pregnant woman. Indeed, the situations are such that both the Pro Choice and the Pro Life groups are concerned about them. The two situations that call for special consideration are (1) cases where parents are pressuring the young woman to have or not have an abortion, and (2) cases where government employees deceive or even blackmail poor women into having abortions.

Parental pressure is understandable in many cases. The family is often in a highly emotional state since it sees disgrace, expense, and the frustration of dreams if their child has a child before she is able to care for it and before she has "grown up." At the same time, the child often realizes the consequences in only a vague way. The family feelings may be similar even when the case involves not a child but a young adult. The family's feelings can lead to intense pressure for an abortion. The young person is threatened with loss of love and banishment from the family if an abortion is refused. The pressures can become so great that we are probably dealing with coercion where the competence of the young woman to choose becomes doubtful. The health care professional should be very careful in making sure that there is a true informed consent.

Those families who oppose abortion absolutely and who see abortion as murder can create equally great pressures against an abortion. When these families threaten banishment and loss of love if there is an abortion, we are once again in the area of coercion where the competence of the young woman to choose becomes doubtful.

We are faced, then, with a class of cases in which all too often neither the client nor the surrogates are particularly competent. The case is even more complicated in that outsiders are often biased in favor of birth or abortion, so there is no easy and satisfactory appeal to counselors or courts.

In this sort of case, the health care provider whose conscience permits abortion in the case at hand should attempt to reduce the pressure and to have the decision made at a time when feelings have settled down. When there is relative calm, the patient should be honestly informed about the procedures, her alternatives, her risks, and the costs. If the provider attempts to do much more than calm and inform the patient, the health care provider may become yet another force that reduces freedom.

Those whose conscience forbids cooperation in the abortion in question must, of course, withdraw from the case if the patient chooses abortion. Before the patient has made a decision, they too should attempt to increase the competence of the patient and to give the proper medical information required for informed consent. So long as they avoid coercive behavior the providers may in accord with their conscience explain their moral position on the procedure. Those who cannot refrain from coercive behavior should not be professionally involved in such cases at all.

The second class of cases which involve fraud and even blackmail on the part of government employees and health care providers demands vigorous action. In the past, welfare workers and workers in the Indian Service have told clients that their government support would be cut off if they did not have an abortion and consent to sterilization. Since the clients were generally Native Americans or blacks, the deception and blackmail looks alarmingly like genocide. No matter what stand one takes on abortion or sterilization, such conduct is a blatant violation of autonomy and deserves outright condemnation, even if some sort of "good intention" were present. Certainly, health care providers should be on their guard and report any such incidents.

SUMMARY

Even if the fetus is not a human being with all the rights of a person, it can be argued that the fetus has a serious right to life. This argument rests ultimately on the use of the wedge principle in protecting the rights of persons and those we already acknowledge as having a serious right to life. Neither the rights of the fetus nor the rights of the pregnant woman are absolute. When the rights of these parties are in conflict, a settlement is to be sought in weighing the goods and evils to discover who has a superior claim. Often no clear decision is possible, and the moral person is faced with tragedy where ordinary moral categories may no longer apply.

Ultimately, the views on the ethics of abortion depend on the world view of the actors in the drama. Unfortunately, our pluralistic society does not have a universally accepted world view, with the result that the conflicts in this area will continue.

Even health care providers whose personal consciences do not condemn abortions or a particular abortion must be aware that professional ethics would seem to forbid participation in nontherapeutic abortions or in the coercion of consents in this area. Professional ethics demands particular care in guarding against that coercion, which amounts to genocide in the case of minority groups.

CASES FOR ANALYSIS

1. Maruska had her first child at age 14. By the time she was 30 she had five children ranging in age from 16 to 5 years old. Married and divorced twice, she had spent 11 years living off aid for dependent children. During the past five years, however, she had been working in a rehabilitation center, taking courses and advancing on the job even though she had no degree. In the process of all this Maruska had discovered that she was intelligent and capable of controlling her own life. She was also aware of her mistakes and determined to prevent her children from making the same mistakes. When she noticed her 16-year-old becoming overly interested in boys she got her into a state-supported boarding school for poor families. Despite this, the daughter got pregnant. Maruska foresees another child at home, the daughter without education and work, and the start of another cycle of aid to dependent children. Moreover, tests reveal that the child will have Down's syndrome and pose additional burdens on the family. Certainly such a child will have no chance of adoption. The dream of self-sufficiency appears doomed. Maruska brings all this up while in the physician's office with a bad case of the flu.

2.   Ivan and Elena have had three children with Down's syndrome. Despite their efforts at birth control, Elena is pregnant again. Tests reveal that the fourth child will also have Down's syndrome. Ivan works on the janitorial staff at the local general hospital and earns just a little over the minimum wage, which is not enough to put the family over the poverty line. His employer provides family health coverage. With food stamps and occasional help from their family, they barely get by. Elena cannot work since the children require constant supervision and care. In any event she is unskilled and could not get a well-paying job.

Ivan and Elena are loving parents and do not want to put their children into an institution. They doubt whether they can handle a fourth handicapped child. It is not merely a question of the money, but of stamina. The previous winter when Elena came down with the flu for a week, the household almost came apart at the seams. Ivan was even tempted to beat the children when they kept whining for attention.

The couple asks one of physicians at the hospital to perform an abortion.

3.   Theodora and Ambrose have been living together for three years. They plan to marry in another six months when Theodora finishes college and is no longer dependent on her parents for tuition. When she tells Ambrose that she is pregnant, he explodes and says, "Well, you may as well know that I have AIDS. I discovered it just last week. Now I suppose the baby will have it too. Let's call everything off. I just can't take any more." He stalks out of the house. She has not heard from him in two weeks. She decides to have an abortion and approaches you for help.

4.   Jerry and Thomasina, married with no children, live the good life. Jerry, an architect, and Thomasina, a senior systems analyst for a major corporation, have combined incomes that put them in the upper 3 percent of all family units in the United States. They have a condominium in New York City, a second home in the Pocono Mountains, and take two weeks in the Caribbean every winter. They are on the upward slope and things can only get better. In three years they plan to have one male child to carry on the family name. If the conceptus is female they intend to abort it. Thomasina gets pregnant three years ahead of schedule. They decide to abort since taking a leave would block her from promotion to a position that will open up in six months. They come to you for help with the abortion.

5.   Laudator and Desiree have been married for five years. Laudator works as a janitor at the local public school and Desiree has a part-time job in a dress factory. They have no family and few friends. Each is the other's whole life. Because Desiree is a juvenile diabetic, they have practiced birth control lest a pregnancy cause serious harm. In addition, since Desiree's life expectancy is short, they did not even want to adopt since the child might soon have no mother. Now they discover that Desiree is pregnant. The physician tells them that Desiree will almost certainly lose her sight permanently in the course of the pregnancy. She may also die if her kidneys, which have already weakened, give out. The nurse midwife advises an abortion. Laudator, faced with loss of Desiree, wants an abortion. Desiree secretly wants the baby so that when she is dead, Laudator will have someone to love. She thinks that the loss of her sight would be a small price to pay for the child.

NOTES

[1] The fetus does not have an absolute right to life since no one has such a right. One being's rights limit those of another being, and we have social arrangements to resolve conflicts between these rights. When the conflicts are irresolvable, we are faced with the tragic in human existence.

[2] The classical principles vary for consequentialists and deontologists. A consequentialist in line with the principle of proportionality given in Chapter Three would permit cooperation in evil in order to prevent a greater evil, provided that one is not acting directly against the intrinsic good, i.e., the individual person. A formulation of the classical principle from a deontological point of view is found in Ashley and O'Rourke, 1978, pp. 197–199.

Chapter Eight
NEW METHODS
OF REPRODUCTION

INTRODUCTION

Starting with the introduction of artificial insemination and currently ending with the use of frozen embryos, the human race has introduced important modifications into the reproductive process. Undoubtedly, additional methods will be implemented in the near future. Although these methods have brought blessings for childless couples and for those who want children without the inconvenience of pregnancy, they have also created ethical problems, or at least questions about the ethics of the procedures. Some people are against all of the new methods on the ground that they are either unnatural or unsuitable for humans. More specific allegations of ethical problems range from the charge that artificial insemination is unethical since the donor masturbates in collecting the sperm, to questions about whether or not a frozen embryo has a right to be born. Nearly all of the new methods of reproduction create problems, since society must be able to identify the parents if it is to ensure both that the offspring are cared for and that they do not end up as public charges. These questions are accompanied by others about the ethics of health care professionals who are not engaged in healing but in facilitating the questionable interests of healthy people who are capable of having children in the traditional way.

In the pages that follow, we will discuss selected methods of reproduction in some detail, indicating when they appear medically indicated, what ethical problems are raised by the methods, and in particular what social dimensions need particular attention. At the end of the chapter we will discuss the broad and somewhat vague charge that these procedures are unnatural and therefore unethical.

METHODS OF ARTIFICIAL INSEMINATION

Artificial Insemination by Donor

The oldest of the new methods of reproduction is artificial insemination by donor (AID). In cases where the husband lacks a sufficient quantity of sperm or sperm of insufficient vigor to effect an conception, sperm is purchased from a donor and inserted into the wife's vagina by means of a syringe.

Two objections are raised against this procedure. First, it involves masturbation on the part of the donor, and second it involves adultery on the part of both the donor and the wife, since they are having intercourse without being married to one another. Such objections are frequently religious or theological in origin. Officials of the Roman Catholic Church have been particularly vehement on these points, which they phrase in terms of the right of the child to be born as the result of copulation in marriage (Congregation, 1987). Indeed, the Catholics object even to artificial insemination by the woman's husband when the semen has been obtained aside from actual intercourse between the spouses.

From a consequentialist's point of view both objections are pointless. In the first place, there is no evidence that masturbation has any harmful consequences. Second, if the husband agrees to the procedure, the harmful effects of adultery will not occur. Adultery from a consequentialist point of view is condemned because it leads to one or all of the following evils: (1) weakening of the marriage, (2) violence by the injured spouse, (3) doubt about parentage of the offspring and so problems about the inheritance of property and the obligation to support the child. In the case of donor insemination with the competent consent of the husband, none of these consequences are likely to occur and so there is, in the opinion of the authors, no ethical problem.

Although masturbation and adultery do not constitute problems for the consequentialist, unwarranted harmful consequences may occur in the following situations: (1) when the woman is not married, (2) when the donors are not screened, (3) when the donor's identity is concealed, (4) when one donor is used frequently in a given area, (5) banks for frozen sperm and ova are used.

Artificial Donor Insemination and the Unmarried Mother

When the mother in question is not married, there can be questions as to whether or not it is good to deliberately bring a child into a one-parent family or into a family where there is a role model for only one gender. While adoptions by single parents have become more common and can be justified by the fact that an orphan is better off with one parent than with none, the significance of the one-parent and one-gender family needs consideration. Quite aside from the general question about deliberate formation of such families, one needs to ask the following questions about each particular case. Is this woman capable of supporting the child without public assistance? Is she mature enough and emotionally stable enough to provide a healthy home environment? In short, one ought to ask all the questions which social workers consider when investigating candidates for adoption. Indeed, these are the questions that everyone ought to ask before they proceed to have children. It appears clear that legal regulation is required if the interests of children are to be protected.

The authors are particularly suspicious of those cases where the woman desires donor insemination to avoid both the physical contact needed to conceive a child and the emotional intimacy needed to raise a child in a two-parent family. Neither attitude appears healthy and a recommendation for parenting.

Health care professionals have additional problems. Since the artificial insemination is not being used to remedy a defect in the husband, it is not medically indicated, and once again one must ask if the health care provider should engage in nonhealing activities for profit.

Artificial Donor Insemination Without Screening

In many cases, physicians appear to have used donor insemination without doing a health history of the donor and screening for genetic defects associated with the donor's background. Unlike marriage, where pride and passion blind the partners to important health considerations, there is no reason why donor insemination should not be done in a way to avoid the production of seriously handicapped offspring. Further, the health history of the donor should be an important part of the health history of the child. The American Medical Association (1984) has taken a very clear stand on this:

> Relying only on donors' verbal representations of their health without any medical screening is precarious. The donor should be screened for genetic defects, inheritable and infectious disease, Rh-factor incompatibility and other disorders that may affect the fetus.

Concealing the Donors

In addition, physicians using donors often mix the sperm of several donors together and keep no records in order to avoid the possibility of the donor being sued for support. While this may be understandable from a legal point of view it creates some health care problems. Without some knowledge of the parentage and genetic heritage of the child, future health care providers will have to operate without important data. For this reason, there should be a single donor and the health history of the donor should be available. The original fears which motivated concealing the donor have been removed in many areas. Some governments have provided that when the husband agrees to the donor insemination, there can be no paternity suit against the donor. In addition, these laws assume that the husband gave consent unless the contrary can be established. The laws on the subject frequently provide that the children of the insemination can be told the identity of the donor when they reach age 18.

Artificial Donor Insemination and the Danger of Incest

When the sperm of a particular donor is used frequently in the same geographic area, particularly a small area, a danger of incest with attendant genetic problems is created. For this reason, the American Medical Association (1984) correctly rules that "Physicians have an ethical obligation to avoid the frequent use of semen from the same sources."

In this context, it should also be noted that the frequent use of medical students as donors can be seen as a sort of genetic imperialism in which physicians seek to reproduce their own kind at the expense of other groups in society. Quite aside from this, medical students may not be of the best genetic stock, no matter how rigid the screening for training as a physician.

In Vitro Fertilization

In vitro fertilization, or so-called test tube fertilization, is used when for one reason or another the ovum of the woman cannot descend through the oviduct in order to be fertilized. It involves treating the woman with hormones to stimulate the production of ova, then taking ova from the woman by a surgical procedure and sperm from the husband or donor and bringing them together in a petri dish. After conception has taken place and cell division has begun, the conceptus is mechanically introduced into the woman's uterus in the hope that it will nest and grow to maturity. The procedures are expensive and not covered by insurance, so that only those with some wealth can attempt this method. In addition, most attempts do not succeed, so they need to be repeated.

Added complications are introduced if the woman is not married, or if the sperm comes from a donor, or if the fertilized egg is not reintroduced into the woman but put into a second woman who will act as a surrogate mother. We will discuss the problems of the surrogate mother below. Here we will consider only the simpler case.

The objections to in vitro fertilization may be grouped under three headings: (1) the discard problem, (2) the risks to the woman and the offspring, and (3) the artificiality of it all.

The *discard problem* arises from the fact that at least in the pioneering days of the procedure, fertilized eggs which were not introduced into the woman were either discarded or used for experimental purposes. If the conceptus has a serious right to life, the discard would involve abortion and the experimentation would be human experimentation on an unwilling subject. We shall return to the ethics of experimentation in Chapter Twelve.

The discard problem has largely disappeared due to the improvement in techniques, which now use fewer eggs and increase the chances of nesting and a baby being born by introducing several fertilized eggs into the woman's vagina. The optimum number appears to be four fertilized eggs. The additional fertilized eggs are then frozen to provide material for additional attempts if the first implantation does not succeed. This has the added advantage of reducing the number of surgical procedures necessary to obtain eggs, but the freezing of eggs creates additional problems (discussed later in this chapter).

Risks to the Mother and Child

The risks to the woman can be calculated, but the risks to the potential offspring are largely unknown. The risks to the woman include the risks of treatment with hormones, the risks of the operation (laparoscopy) and the anesthesia, the risks of damage to the uterus at the time of insertion and the risks of ectopic gestation, i.e., a pregnancy outside the reproductive system, and the risks of amniocentesis (discussed in Chapter Ten on the ethics of testing and screening).

The largely unknown risks to the fetus complicate ethical judgments in this area. The fact that defective fetuses are often detected by amniocentesis and then aborted only further complicates the issues. Indeed, the research which could clarify many issues is itself the subject of debate and regulation (Abromowitz, 1984). Even though we lack the information needed to make definitive judgments in this area, we should not lose sight of the fact that the dangers to the fetus are ethically relevant.

We do know that there are an increasing number of healthy children born as a result of in vitro fertilization and that many childless couples are willing to undergo the risks and the expenses associated with it. It would appear that the risks in general are not as great as some originally feared. The risk in an individual case, however, remains a relevant ethical factor.

Surrogate Mothers

There are cases where a fertile woman cannot bear a child because of some other defect in her reproductive system. In these cases it is possible to do an in vitro fertilization and then implant the fertilized egg in the uterus of another woman, who will delivery the baby and allow the baby to be adopted by the couple who supplied the egg and the sperm. More common are the cases where the woman has no fertile eggs. In these cases, the woman's husband artificially inseminates the surrogate, who agrees to let the initiating couple adopt. These surrogates may be recruited by newspaper, lawyers, or various profit and nonprofit groups interested in promoting surrogate motherhood. In practice, the surrogate mother has her health care expenses covered and is paid a fee. These fees plus the uncertainty of who is responsible for the child and worries about coercion raise serious ethical and legal objections to the use of surrogate mothers. Other objections of less importance are discussed by Robertson (1983) and Krimmel (1983).

In 1983, the American College of Obstetricians and Gynecologists (ACOG) issued a nonbinding set of guidelines entitled "Ethical Issues in Surrogate Motherhood"

(Robertson, 1983). The guidelines note that the surrogate faces all the physical risks of pregnancy and its long-term health effects and even the remote possibility of death. There is also a danger of psychological harm when the surrogate is separated from the child. A consideration of all these risks must be part of the decision to participate. In addition, it is not at all clear whether the surrogate mother alone or the surrogate plus the adoptive parents should make decisions about the fetus. Included are decisions about smoking and using alcohol during pregnancy. There may be particular problems if the surrogate decides to abort the fetus over the objection of the adopting parents. ACOG also raises questions about the dedication of couples to parenthood when they wish surrogate motherhood only as a convenience rather than for medical reasons. The guidelines particularly warn physicians against accepting payment for recruiting or referring potential surrogate mothers.

Though the fee may be viewed as compensating the surrogate for the inconvenience and risk of being pregnant, it is in fact a payment for the purchase of a baby. Robertson (1983) says that it is quibbling to question whether the couple is purchasing a service or buying a baby and holds that they are really buying the right to rear a child. No matter what may be said of that, most states have laws against selling babies and others make adoptions illegal if money is paid for anything other than legitimate expenses. The commercial nature of the transaction appears in typical contracts (Krimmel, 1983), which provide genetic tests of the fetus and state that the surrogate must have an abortion if the child is defective or keep the child herself. In the famous Baby M. case (see pages 174–176), the contract also provided that the surrogate took all risks, including the risk of death, and that she would be paid nothing if she miscarried before the fourth month, and only $1,000 after the fourth month, even if the child was stillborn. If the surrogate handed over a live, healthy baby, she would be paid $10,000. The surrogate abdicated her legal right to abort unless the physician said it was necessary for her health. The surrogate also agreed not to smoke cigarettes, drink alcoholic beverages, or take medications without written consent from her physician.

Such provisions indicate that the fee is a payment for a healthy child and not for the rental of a uterus. In short, payment is rendered only for a satisfactory product. One can easily imagine a contract that had the same provisions about sex and eye color. No matter what one thinks is quibbling, it all looks too much like buying and selling a product and so treating a human being as a commodity, an object in commerce. Although the motive for all this may be a desire to share one's love with a child, the fact remains that the presence of fees—often large fees—makes the transaction very dubious despite some court decisions that have upheld the surrogate contract.

Because this is a grey area and best not left to the courts, legislation permitting and prohibiting or otherwise regulating surrogate motherhood has been introduced in many states. Among other proposed regulations are those that permit the surrogate a cooling-off period during which she can rescind the contract and requirements for counseling before the contract is solved. Between legislative battles and conflicting court decisions, we can expect a decade or more of struggle to resolve the problems posed by surrogate motherhood.

Where the surrogate donates her services, as one sister might do for another, the problem of buying and selling babies is obviously not present, though the far more serious problem of responsibility for the child remains.

Responsibility for the Child

The ethical problem connected with responsibility for raising the child is well illustrated by the following case.

Mr. and Mrs. Xavier contract with Mrs. Loyola to bear a child that will result from artificial insemination with Mr. Xavier's sperm. Mrs. Loyola delivers the baby, who turns out to be seriously retarded. The Xaviers pay Mrs. Loyola's delivery expenses but refuse to adopt the baby. Since the contract between Mrs. Loyola and the Xaviers is not enforceable in the particular state, the Loyolas are left with a defective baby that they do not want. The Loyolas then sue Mr. Xavier for child support on the ground that he is the genetic father. A blood test reveals that Mr. Xavier could not have been the father. Investigation reveals that Mr. Loyola is the father. Loyola had intercourse with his wife at the time of the artificial insemination.

In this case, no one wanted the child and it was not immediately clear who the father was. As a result the responsibility for raising the child was blurred and settled only after medical testing and legal proceedings. It should be noted that another set of complications would have occurred if the Loyolas did not want to give up the child. In this case Mr. Xavier could have sued for custody.

Some people argue in favor of surrogate motherhood on the grounds that it is just another form of adoption. Indeed, since one of the adopting parents is the natural father of the child, it is argued that it is a very suitable form of adoption. This is simply not true in the absence of clear regulation. Davis (1985), writing in a British context, raises important points that are equally applicable in the United States. First, there is no careful screening of the suitability of the commissioning couple who want to adopt the child of the surrogate mother. Not everyone should be allowed to adopt or to use the surrogate mother route. Second, there is no careful screening of the surrogate mother, thus increasing the chances that there may be unnecessary births of defective children. The mere fact that a surrogate is willing to carry the child does not mean that she is a suitable biological and gestational mother. The surrogate may have both genetic problems and habits which threaten the health of the fetus. Until such problems are taken care of by legal measures, the adoption analogy is unjustified.

All of these difficulties could be mitigated if not solved by clarifications of the law (Annas, 1984). Indeed, nearly all the new methods of reproduction require such clarification. Annas correctly notes that the specification of responsibility should not be left simply to contractual agreements since society has an interest in deciding who is responsible for what. The task may not be simple since there are 50 sets of state laws which cover the problems. In 1986, Annas reported on Kentucky court decisions which approved baby sales if the price was agreed on *before conception* and gave the surrogate mother the right to cancel her contract up to the point where she gave up her parental rights. Further complications were introduced when the court decided that the donor of the egg would be the natural and so the legal mother, and the sperm donor the natural father if (1) the surrogate had contracted to have the baby by IVF and (2) tissue typing confirmed the genetic links between the child and the gamete donors. It is not at all clear whether the rights of the child are really protected or even considered.

Rights of the Surrogate

Though the good of the child and in particular the protection of the child's future is the main concern, consideration must be given to the surrogate or gestational mother. While the surrogate may agree to give the child up for adoption, she may form such an attachment to the child that she decides to keep it. At this point, she may be coerced into giving up the child by threat of an expensive lawsuit or other harassment. While the law favors the gestational mother (Cohen, 1984), the surrogate may not be able to afford a lawyer and so the surrogate may be effectively blackmailed. Ethics obviously forbids this, but we need law to protect the surrogate.

Taub (1985) believes that the surrogate is most likely to suffer psychologically when the child is given up. Indeed, the psychological dangers are such (Parker, 1983) that Taub believes an Institutional Review Board (see Chapter Twelve on research ethics) would not permit surrogate motherhood if it was being carried out as a research project. This aspect of the problem certainly requires more careful study.

We must also face the fact that the presence of payment may tempt financially distressed women to agree to surrogate contracts against their best interests. Winslade (1981) discovered that 40 percent of the volunteer surrogate mothers were unemployed or on welfare. This is an additional reason why ethics would seem to forbid the payment of money other than for reasonable expenses.

Cohen (1984) suggests that the surrogate mother could be better protected if the states passed laws permitting revocable birth agreements just as they now permit revocable adoption agreements. Such a law would forbid payment for anything but expenses and would leave the child with the gestational mother pending the settlements of any disputes.

Embryo Transfer

In embryo transfers the process starts with in vitro fertilization with the conceptus being implanted in the surrogate to be flushed out later and implanted in the would-be mother. As early as 1984 there was a firm offering embryo transfers for profit. Though the success rate had been very low, the company anticipated a market of about 50,000 cases a year in the United States alone. The cost was estimated to be $4,000 to $7,000 per attempt.

Even when embryo transfer is not a blatantly commercial venture, several points need to be considered. The risks to the conceptus are greater than in ordinary in vitro fertilization since there are two transfers of the conceptus. In addition, the medical necessity or advantages of such a procedure are not at all evident. In any event the technique is still experimental in the human and the success rate very low. Quite aside from the crass monetary and highly experimental aspects, the procedure appears unethical, unless when the experimental stage is completed, the additional risks are offset by newly discovered medical or health benefits.

Frozen Embryos and Sperm Banks

Embryos are sometimes frozen at the time of in vitro fertilization in case the first implanted embryos in the woman do not nest and reach birth. The frozen embryos are a reserve which can be used rather than subjecting a woman to another operation to obtain ova. This technique could, of course, be used by people who wish to postpone reproduction for some time but worry that their semen or ova may not be suitable at a later date. In these cases the stored frozen embryo is introduced into the vagina of the biological mother or a surrogate at a future date when a child is desired.

The techniques are still experimental and the embryo is at risk of being destroyed during either the freezing or the thawing process. Only about 60 percent of the embryos are recovered, and one experimenter reported that he had achieved success, that is, helped the couple achieve a live birth, only twice in 30 tries.

The Rios case has shown that serious problems can result when there are no legal provisions to cover such problems as the right of the frozen embryo to be born and, in case the parents die, the rights of other than the parents to adopt the embryo and inherit from its estate (Ozar, 1985). In 1981, the Rioses, a very wealthy couple, had one fertilized egg implanted in the wife while two were frozen. The implanted embryo spontaneously aborted, but Mrs. Rios was not ready for another implantation. Some time later the Rioses adopted a child. The husband, wife, and adopted child were all killed in an airplane crash in 1983.

According to the law of both Australia, where the conception took place, and the United States, where the Rioses were citizens, if the conceptus were born alive it could inherit the parents' wealth. It is not clear, however, whether, in the absence of a will, the child would be the child of the woman who bears it or the woman who supplied the egg. Similarly, is the child the child of the sperm donor or of some other father? If the donors, in the Rios case the married couple, are dead, who makes the decision as to whether the child will be born and as to who will have custody when born?

Laws on in vitro fertilization and related matters such as frozen embryos enacted by the Province of Victoria in Australia, the site of much research in this area, are informative (Singer, 1985). The law provides that only parents who are married may be treated and then only as a last resort and after at least a year of other treatments. The use of donated sperm, eggs, or embryos is also to be a last resort either when there is no reasonable hope of a pregnancy or when without the donation the woman would risk a child with a hereditary disorder. No payment may be made for sperm, eggs, or embryos, though related expenses can be covered.

In the case of frozen embryos the law provides that if the woman who donates the egg is incapable of receiving the embryo, *she and the sperm donor* may consent to the embryo being given to another woman. If that consent cannot be given because the donors are dead or untraceable, the Minister of Health may order the hospital to make the embryo available as a gift.

While these legal provisions specify certain things, they bypass serious philosophical and ethical issues. Does the frozen embryo have a serious right to life? If it does, who has the obligation of fulfilling that right, especially when the "parents" are dead? On the other hand, do even married couples have a right to have children by any means? These are questions that should be answered before more comprehensive laws on the subject are passed. In the meantime, it seems best to delay further implementation of the techniques that cause more problems for society than they solve.

The Charge of Artificiality

It is not clear if those who condemn the new reproduction as artificial do so because the artificial is inherently evil, because it risks harmful consequences, or because it involves venturing into the unknown.

The approach of practical wisdom used in this book emphasizes the consideration of all consequences and balancing the burdens and benefits in the light of human dignity. In the context of the new modes of reproduction, we can anticipate some problems because we know something about the problems involved in adoptions. Similarly, because people do not want just a child but a certain type of child, we can anticipate trouble with surrogate mothering when the "right" type of child is not produced (Krimmel, 1983). Unfortunately, more often than not we lack even analogical evidence about both the presence and the absence of risk. In these cases we are not dealing with the probability of an evil, but with fear of the unknown and *all the evils that could be there.*

The fear of the unknown is widespread, but it is not a justification for doing nothing. If humankind had refused to venture into the unknown because of what could happen, we would have made no progress and would still be living a very primitive existence. We are ethically justified in venturing into the unknown in order to obtain real goods. Indeed, granted the nature of human curiosity, we are probably justified in venturing into the unknown just because it is unknown.

If we take the artificiality objection to be a deontologically based argument, we are then faced with the need to distinguish between what is ethically and what is unethically artificial. Nearly all of modern medicine with its elaborate testing, complicated transplant surgery, and man-made medications is certainly artificial. Nature did not provide these directly to us. Yet, few would argue that the testing, surgery, and medications are unethical. Humans have merely used their natural talents to produce things that, while not found in nature, do come from our nature as thinking, problem-solving beings. Unethical artificiality must be something more than merely the man-made.

Ethics and the Unity of Procreation and Love

Some of the thinkers who object to nearly all the new forms of reproduction do so on the basis of a required unity between love and procreation, that is, between the unitive and procreative function of sexual intercourse.

While the union of love and procreation is undoubtedly a nice romantic ideal, we must face the fact that the ideal is not always possible in the case of infertile couples. We will shift our attention, then, from the nonobligatory ethics of the ideal to the more basic ethics of what is permitted in view of the consequences. It should be noted that many of us who currently walk the earth may have been the result of less than the ideal intercourse. Despite that, our existences are not necessarily blighted, nor has society been severely injured.

The Roman Catholic Church does not see the union of love and procreation as an ideal, but as mandatory, and indeed as something that the offspring have a right to. While we do not wish to venture into the realm of theology, several philosophical points appear relevant to the present discussion. The 1987 Roman Catholic position paper on the new modes of reproduction holds that a child has a right to be born of loving intercourse between a man and a woman who are married. When the reproduction takes place without that intercourse (penetration by the male organ), or without the marriage, it is to be condemned. This is true even when the husband's sperm is artificially introduced into the wife.[1]

The insistence on ordinary copulation seems to sacramentalize the mere physical act of penetration rather than treating it as a means to reproduction. In addition, by saying that the child has a right to be born of such intercourse, the position paper leaves us wondering how a child has a right before he is even conceived and on what basis one would establish a right to be born of loving intercourse. It might even be difficult to establish that the child has a right to love, let alone to a beginning in loving intercourse.

While there are undoubtedly strong theological arguments behind the Roman Catholic position paper, the philosophical arguments are not overwhelming or universally accepted by even Catholic theologians.

THE ETHICS OF THE HEALTH CARE PROVIDER

The health care provider is supposed to do what is medically indicated, granted the informed consent of the patient. The first question, then, is whether the new reproductive modes are medically indicated. This involves asking whether or not it is aimed at making up for a defect in the reproductive organs of the people involved or is merely a way for healthy people to avoid some of the inconveniences of reproduction. When the new reproductive mode makes up for a defect in the human reproductive system, we are dealing with a medical problem and the question becomes one of proportionality, that is, whether or not more good than harm will be done from a medical point of view.

There will be particular doubts about medical indications if the treatment includes provision for the abortion of fetuses which are found to be defective or probably or possibly defective in the course of the pregnancy. Indeed, if abortion is unethical except where some serious right of the mother is threatened, such eugenic abortion and its inclusion in the surrogate mother or in vitro fertilization agreements should be condemned.

If the new reproductive mode is merely a way for healthy people to avoid the inconveniences of reproduction, we are not dealing with a medical problem at all, but with the sale of a service to whomever is willing to pay for it. This would occur in the case of the single man or woman who wants a baby without having what they consider the mess and emotional involvement of intercourse. The woman will want donor insemination and the man will want to hire a surrogate mother. There would also be a desire for a surrogate mother when the woman wants a child but sees a pregnancy as interfering with her career. The case is similar with the parents who want to store a frozen embryo as a safeguard against a future loss of fertility. In all these cases, it is convenience rather than medical indication which is at the root of the request. For this reason, the involvement of health care professionals is at least inappropriate. It can easily be unethical since some of the procedures involve risks that are unnecessary in the case of healthy people. Performing an operation to procure eggs for in vitro fertilization when there is no health problem does not meet the requirements of proportionality for a health care provider.

The problem is more serious than merely a question of medical indication versus convenience. There is also a question of whether a health care provider should cooperate in activities which, if not illegal, are problematic and possibly unethical. As noted earlier, single-parent families are less than ideal. It is questionable if health care providers should help in creating more single parent families.

There are serious problems when the husband has not consented to donor insemination, since here the evils of adultery reappear. It is not ethical for health care providers to facilitate adultery. Further, when the husband has not consented, there are legal problems about who is responsible for the child, since in this case it is easy for the husband to disavow the child and to prove that he is not the father (Annas, 1984). To create such a situation hardly accords with the most basic of obligations to do good and avoid evil.

Since the use of surrogate mothers generally involves payments that might violate the slavery laws or others laws involving adoption, the health care professional should be particularly careful. That care would appear to call for health care professionals having their own legal counsel in these matters. More importantly, the provider should beware of involvement in situations where the offspring may be the victim since the assignment of legal responsibility is not always clear. In short, there are such risks involved that it would take a very serious reason to justify cooperation even when the reproductive procedure might seem medically indicated. In other words, the presence of medical indications in the adult patients does not mean that the provider can disregard the good of the offspring and of society.

Although medicine and the health care professions have generally and correctly concentrated on the good of the patient, the good of society needs particular consideration in the case of the new modes of reproduction. A defective child is generally a burden on society as well as on the parents. The health care providers should certainly do all they ethically can to avoid the conception of such children. As noted above, the physician has an obligation to screen donors of semen for genetic defects and other disorders that affect the fetus. The other disorders might include drug addiction, alcoholism, AIDS, and herpes. It seems clear that surrogate mothers and host mothers who hold embryo transfers in the intermediate stage should also be screened, on the grounds that there is no justification for exposing the offspring and society to unnecessary problems. Once again, legal provisions for screening would seem to be in order.

We will go a step farther and say that the health care provider would be unethical if he aided the reproductive activities of people who are obviously unfit to be parents or where there might be special problems for the children. For example, drug addicts, alcoholics, child abusers, and a whole army of emotionally unstable individuals are obviously unfit to be parents. In cases of doubtful competence in parenting, we need more information about consequences before we can give either definitive approval or definitive condemnation of either a class or individual case of a new mode of reproduction.

A Question of Distributive Justice

The new modes of reproduction involve more than risks to children and society. They cost money and they use scarce health care resources. Those that involve in vitro fertilization and surrogate mothers generally involve a great deal of money and large amounts of medical resources. Since these are not covered by health insurance, let alone Medicaid, the new modes of reproduction will be the privilege of those who are comfortably off. This raises the question of social or distributive justice. The conclusions of Chapter Four are applicable here. First, the central task of health care is to meet the needs of human dignity such as maintaining and restoring health as well as alleviating pain. Second, society has a duty to provide its members with access to an adequate level of health care that fulfills basic needs. Third, society must in the interests of social contributions permit individuals to purchase more than the care adequate for basic needs. Ideally, the additional care should be purchased only when the basic needs of all have been met.

In view of these conclusions, the authors argue that *ideally* no resources should be diverted to the new modes of reproduction until the basic health care needs of all have been satisfied. In practice, this is not possible granted the rights of individuals to dispose of their own resources.

In any event, we argue that the new modes of reproduction cannot be considered necessary for basic health care needs. For this reason there should be no direct government support or insurance coverage for the new modes of reproduction, particularly in those cases where the new mode is used only for the convenience of the patient and not to remedy or bypass a physical defect. In these cases the services do not constitute health care or any essential good. It would be foolish to spend public monies to gratify an individual's or couple's desire for convenience.

The use of public monies or insurance to pay for even "medically indicated" services does not appear to be part of what constitutes adequate health care. In the first place, the services do not remedy the defect in the person, but merely bypass it. The defect, moreover, is a problem only when the persons want children. The defect does not lead to sickness or death or serious impairment of day-to-day functioning. It does not seem right to devote public funds or insurance funds to the treatment of such a defect while there are far more serious problems which call for resources.

We do not think that there is any injustice in society deciding that people do not have a right to these particular services. Indeed, the case of the new modes of reproduction raises the question of the justification of all sorts of health provider activities, which may be profitable but do not make good sense either in terms of the healing function of the professions or the shortage of resources.

CASES FOR ANALYSIS

1. Mr. and Mrs. Baldinucci, citizens of the United States, were in their thirties and had been married for 10 years. Mrs. Baldinucci had a congenital defect which prevented her from having children. The Baldinuccis were well-educated professionals, easy in their relationship and respected in their community. They had grown impatient with the groups attempting to find them a child for adoption. At this point, they approached a agency, which offered to find an English surrogate mother for a fee of $9,000.

Mr. Baldinucci went to England to give sperm. The surrogate mother was inseminated by a nurse. In a television interview the surrogate claimed that she conceived with the second insemination attempt. She voluntarily gave up her parental rights for a fee and left the hospital some hours after the birth of the child and had not seen the child since. Since the child had been abandoned, they applied for a custody order to protect the child. The Baldinuccis then applied for guardianship of the child. The court, considering only the interests of the child, granted them custody on condition that they return to Britain if the court should so order. There was, of course, no way to enforce this condition since the couple had no property in England. The couple then returned to the United States with the child in their custody but not legally adopted.

There are doubts as to the citizenship of the child and her rights to inherit. She is at best the illegitimate daughter of Mr. Baldinucci, the natural father, and has no legal claims on Mrs. Baldinucci.

The gestational mother received the sum of $30,000 for her story, which appeared without her name but with a picture. The agency which had arranged the agreement refused to pay the surrogate her fee since she had made so much off the story.

2. Mr. and Mrs. Kinderless, married 10 years, have discovered that Mrs. Kinderless can never have children. They go to Lawyer Baby in order to procure a surrogate mother. Lawyer Baby charges them $25,000, of which $10,000 will go to the sur-

rogate mother upon the birth of a healthy child, while the remainder will cover the expenses of the birth and legal fees. The lawyer sets things up with Mrs. Theresa Avila, whose husband agrees, although he was at first unwilling. The Avila family is a happy one, though of modest means. The $10,000 will certainly come in very handy.

Mrs. Avila has an uneventful pregnancy. She is in excellent spirits and goes around talking to the baby within her. She delivers a healthy baby but refuses to give it up for adoption since it looks so like her first child that she grew immediately and deeply attached. Her husband, while admitting that the sperm came from Mr. Kinderless, also feels the child is his since he has lived through the pregnancy. Mr. Kinderless sues for custody of the child on the grounds that he is the natural father and that the Avilas do not have the finances to give his child a good home. He also sues for damages for breach of contract.

3.   Ms. Rapacious, a single woman, has already been a surrogate mother on two previous occasions. Indeed, for the last two years, the major part of her income has come from this activity. This is her third transaction in the business and she is nearing the time of delivery. She has met the would be parents and senses their anticipation and anxiety. She believes that she can get an extra $5,000 out of them. When the couple's lawyer balks, she threatens to hold on to the baby. The couple comes up with an additional $5,000.

4.   John and Mary, a childless couple, feel that only a child can save their marriage. They do not, however, want to interrupt their careers with a pregnancy. They start thinking of a surrogate mother as a solution to their problem. The marriage counselor tries to convince them that their marriage has basic problems and a child will only make the marriage more difficult. Indeed, the counselor argues that it would be very unfair to bring a child into a family that is bordering on the edge of a breakdown. Despite this advice, John and Mary go to a lawyer and pay for a surrogate mother, whom they have not met.

Rosha, the surrogate mother, age 34, had recently been discharged from a state mental hospital and had a long history of alcoholism and drug addiction which compounded her problems. Both of Rosha's parents were diabetics and one of her brothers has mild Down's syndrome. The surrogate contract calls for her to refrain from smoking and drinking and taking drugs during the pregnancy, but her previous history gives little assurance that she will abide by these provisions. Her husband had reluctantly agreed to the surrogate contract.

5.   In what came to be known as the Baby M. case, Mary Beth Whitehead, married to Richard at age 16, agreed to be a surrogate mother. The contract specified that the wife of the adopting couple was infertile and provided for the payment of $10,000 for a healthy child. Mary Beth already had two children of her own, but was inspired by the infertility of her sister, who she hoped would conceive if she herself became pregnant.

In accord with the agreement she was artificially inseminated with the sperm of William Stern, married to Elizabeth Stern. When the child was born Mrs. Whitehead did not want to give up the child; she refused to sign the adoption papers and fled to her parents' home in Holiday, Florida. She had the child there for four months until the court gave temporary custody to the Sterns. Mrs. Whitehead said that at the end something took over and overpowered her so that she could not give up the child. Her obstetrician says that during her three days in the hospital she was distraught and constantly crying.

The Sterns sued in New Jersey to enforce the agreement, to strip Mary Beth of all parental rights, to win custody, and to prevent Mary Beth from having any visitation rights.

Mr. Whitehead had served 13 months of active duty in Vietnam. On discharge he became a truck driver for construction and sanitation companies. He was injured in an accident and blinded in the left eye. In December 1973 he married Mary Beth, who was eight years younger than he. The following year they had their first child, Ryan, a boy. In January 1976, they had a daughter. In 1978, Richard fell asleep at the wheel after drinking and hit three poles. He lost his driver's license and truck driver's job. He entered Alcoholics Anonymous. At this time Mary Beth took a job as a dancer and bartender in her sister Beverly's bar for a few months. Over the course of their marriage she had also earned money cleaning houses, running coatcheck counters, and selling ski equipment in department stores at Christmas. The couple had separated for six months at one time. During at least part of this period Mrs. Whitehead was on welfare. In 1983 they declared bankruptcy. At the time of the trial Mr. Whitehead was working for the sanitation department at an annual salary of $28,500. They were still in financial trouble and failed to make a lump sum payment on a house they had bought in 1985 from the sister, who then sued to foreclose.

Witnesses testify that Mrs. Whitehead is an excellent mother and no one even remotely suggests that she neglects or abuses her children. Proof of such would be necessary to declare her an unfit mother.

One mental health expert testifying on behalf of the Sterns diagnosed Mrs. Whitehead as having "mixed personality disorder." Another did not confirm that but described her as impulsive, overly dramatic, self-centered, and in need of psychotherapy.

The Sterns put education and careers ahead of marriage and children. They had dated for five years before marrying in July 1974. They were in their late twenties at the time of marriage. He had a doctorate in chemistry and she in human genetics. Right after the marriage Mrs. Stern began medical studies and decided to put off pregnancy till she finished her residency, at which time she would be 36. By the time she had finished her residency, the couple had rejected the idea of having their own children. During the previous years Mrs. Stern had suffered several symptoms of multiple sclerosis, such as brief numbness in her toes and legs and blurred vision. She diagnosed herself as having multiple sclerosis. The Sterns saw pregnancy as a risk of aggravating the symptoms. The condition was not independently diagnosed until they were in the middle of the custody battle and the doctors considered the symptoms mild. Some neurologists would urge a woman with her symptoms to have a child if she so desired.

Mr. Stern felt a great need for a child and said he loved this child more than he loved his wife. The depth of the need seems to spring from the fact that he lost all his relatives except his parents in the Nazi camps in World War II. There was a need, according to one doctor, to show love to someone to whom he was biologically related.

NOTES

[1]Probably the most sweeping condemnation is to be found in a Roman Catholic document issued by the Congregation for the Doctrine of the Faith, *Instruction on Respect for Human Life in its Origins and on the Dignity of Procreation. Replies to Certain Questions of the Day,* Vatican City, 1987.

This document is not consistent throughout and is, in the opinion of the authors, purely theological rather than a theology backed up with philosophical reasoning. Indeed, it suffers from a sort of theological positivism, since its footnotes refer not to scripture and tradition, but to other papal documents.

The document rests on respect for the human embryo as a person from the first moment of conception, even though it admits that the Church has never taken a metaphysical stand on the personhood of the fetus. A secondary principle asserts the right of the child to be conceived through the marital act (copulation inside marriage) and the unique right of the parents to conceive the child through, and only through, the marital act.

While the document speaks of the spiritual nature of the marital union, it appears to fall into a sort of "physicalism" when it insists on the copulative aspect of procreation. In the last analysis, it appears to put the biological over the personal.

Chapter Nine
THE ETHICS
OF TRANSPLANTS

INTRODUCTION

The problems connected with organ transplants are material for the drama of life and death and the romance of new technology. The problems also involve ethical decisions for donors and recipients, as well as for members of the health care team and ultimately for society as a whole. The answers to some of the ethical questions shift with changes in the state of the art and the changing level of risk involved. The answers may also change as the availability of organs increases or decreases, or as society is more or less able or willing to pay for transplants. The underlying problems remain the same. When is it ethical to donate an organ? When is it obligatory to donate an organ? Is it always ethical for the patient to accept an organ? What are the medical criteria for the allocation of organs? What should society pay for in the area of transplants? These are the principal concerns of the present chapter.

Many transplant procedures also pose questions about the ethics of experimentation. Finally, there are questions of informed consent involving patients and donors, or the surrogates of the deceased in the case of cadaver transplants. The questions of informed consent in experimental procedures will be treated in Chapter Twelve.

In the pages that follow we will first consider the ethical problems of the donor and the recipient and then move on to the more complicated problems of the health care team and of the entire health care system.

THE ETHICS OF ORGAN DONATION

The Ethics of the Living Donor

The ethics of the living human donor are strongly influenced by the question of whether the donation involves a renewable resource such as blood or bone marrow, or paired nonrenewable organs such as the corneas or the kidneys, or nonpaired non-renewable organs such as the heart or the liver.

Today there are few ethical problems with the donation of such a renewable resource such as blood, since there are no real dangers to the donor and few to the recipient if the blood has been properly screened for such things as AIDs. On the other hand, bone marrow transplants involve risk to the donor and involve some pain. These facts, plus the varying rate of success, make the calculation of proportionality a little more complex than in the case of blood donation.

The donation of a nonpaired, nonrenewable organ such as the heart or the liver from a living donor spells death for the donor. The donation of such an organ inter vivos (between living persons) would be unethical except in rare cases, unless one approves of altruistic suicide. The rare exception arises when a living donor gives his heart as he is simultaneously about to receive a heart and lungs from a third party. The exception arises because in this case the donation of the heart does not entail death.

The Living Donor of Nonrenewable Paired Organs

The only nonrenewable organs that we have in pairs are our corneas and kidneys. The donation of these are not per se unethical, though attended by risks which need to be justified by proportionality. As we saw in Chapter Three, there can be no proportional reason for risking harm if there is a harm free or less risky alternative available. In the case of transplants, the less risky alternative of cadaver donations can raise ethical questions about donations inter vivos. This is to say that the alternatives remain a part of the consideration of the proportionality needed to justify taking risks. Whether or not the cadaver donation is a true alternative depends on such factors as availability and the success rate of cadaver transplants in a given institution.

The exact nature of the alternative changes with the state of the art and is sometimes debated hotly among experts. Today the alternatives are such that there would seem to be few if any cases where it would make sense for a living person to donate a cornea. The supply of cadaver cornea has increased to a point where the need for a living donor is rare.

The case of kidney donation is more complicated since cadaver kidney's are in short supply and the success rate with cadaver donations is not at this writing equal to the success rate of inter vivos donations between matched relatives. That advantage, however, may be lost as immunosuppresant drugs and better matching take away the advantage of having a donation from a living relative.

Proportionality in Transplants

For the sake of exploring the ethics of the living donor of a matched nonrenewable organ, let us assume that a kidney donation inter vivos offers the best hope in a given case. What are the factors that must enter into the ethical calculation of proportionality? Since the transplantation of the kidney involves an operation with general anesthesia, there is risk of death and of blood clots that can do serious damage (Starzl, 1985). The donor, having given his back-up kidney, has increased the risks to himself if anything should happen to the remaining kidney. These risks might be significant if the donor is a relative. In those cases the family history often indicates that the donor too is at risk. Other abilities or disabilities of the particular donor will also enter into the calculation. For example, a hemophiliac (a bleeder) risks more than a healthy person when there is question of a major operation. A single person has less at stake than a married man with 10 children. A donor who can afford excellent medical care if anything goes wrong is in a different position from the person who has no way of getting adequate care. All of this becomes part of the equation.

The size and nature of that risk versus the possible good to the recipient are crucial factors. If the potential donor comes from a family with a history of kidney problems and the transplant has a low chance of success, the ethical balance changes. The living donor must consider these medical burdens and benefits. In addition to the medical factors, the donor must also consider all her obligations to family, friends, society, and self in deciding if potential goods to the recipient outweigh the potential harms to all the other people who will be affected. The donor, like patients in general, must consider the proportionality of the consequences, *all things considered.*

Both the donor and the health care professional have their decisions further complicated by medical controversy about the use of the immunosuppressant cyclosporine versus careful matching with traditional immunosuppressants (Department of Health and Human Services, 1986). There are also problems with patients who have had or rejected a previous transplant or who have been exposed to foreign HLA antigens through blood transfusions. Patients who have been sensitized are difficult and at times impossible to match. The National Task Force (Department of Health and Human Services, 1986) noted that half of all those awaiting cadaveric kidney transplants in the United States were already sensitized. Only greater organ sharing with groups that have participated in serum-sharing programs can hope to meet the needs of many of these sensitized patients. This is not the place to discuss such technical matters in detail, since research may alter the debate from day to day. It should be clear that the state of the art in such areas dictates the medical feasibility and so the ethics of many transplantations.

The Living but Terminal Donor

The possibility of transplanting from terminal patients and, in particular, from anencephalic infants raises a host of questions (Capron, 1987). The basic question, however, is simply whether or not it is ethical to terminate the life of the donor in order to supply an organ or tissue to a patient. The answer would appear to be a clear "no." The fact that the anencephalic infant[1] is going to die in a short time does not mean that it is dead or without dignity and rights. Treatment may be ethically terminated and the dying process shortened for the sake of the infant, but the actually killing of the child in order to get its tissues is impossible to distinguish from murder no matter how noble the intent. Thus, neither the patient nor the surrogate has a right to consent to such a transplant.

Transplanting Fetal Tissue

Animal experimentation with the transplantation of fetal tissue has created the possibility of new treatments for diseases due to brain deterioration. While we will return to the issue of fetal experimentation in the chapter on the ethics of research, a few remarks are in order with regard to the use of tissue from live fetuses (Mahowald et al., 1987).

This is a complex issue and would require a chapter of its own for adequate treatment. We confine ourselves to two remarks. First, in line with what has been said in the chapters on abortion and new modes of reproduction, great care is necessary in any area where widespread adoption of a practice can lead to disrespect for human dignity and human life. Second, in the present case, even if the tissue is from a dead fetus, the informed consent of parents should be required, lest fetal tissue be treated as so much throwaway material that has no dignity. This is no more than an extension of our culture's centuries long insistence upon decent burial and other signs of respect for the dead. In the authors' opinion even such small protections of human dignity should not be disregarded.

Selling Organs

Some people are morally repelled by the idea of selling blood or organs. They see it as degrading to make even a part of a person an object of commerce. The National Organ Transplant Act of 1984 (Public Law 98–507) goes so far as to forbid the sale of organs in interstate commerce, and some states ban payment for specific organs. The usual arguments in favor of the law may be summarized as follows. First, selling organs will make it harder for the poor to get expensive organs and so make equality of access to treatment more difficult. Second, the poor will be tempted to sell their organs in time of great need and will be exploited. Third, organs should be looked on as a national resource. Another argument (Murray, 1987), while not condemning sale outright, sees donation of organs as such a strong bonding agent in society that the sale of organs should be strongly discouraged. These arguments demand some comment.

Viewing organs as a national resource is dangerous if it implies that the organs belong to the society rather than the individual. Since it seems clear that the organ belongs to the individual, it would follow that *prima facie,* that is, presumptively, *it is ethical to sell the organ whenever it is ethical to donate the organ.* At the same time, the social bonding function of donation points up goods such as dignity and self-respect that are obtained by donation and not by sale. Since the social bonding, that is, the increase in felt community union is particularly beneficial, the balance of good would generally favor donation over sale. A consideration of additional problems with sale reinforces this general conclusion.

The first problem that might result from widespread sale of organs involves the exploitation of the poor. The second involves a distribution of organs in accord with the ability to pay rather than on the basis of need.

The problem of exploitation of the poor arises from the fact that those in need may be tempted to sell organs without consideration of the alternatives and without concern for the long-range health consequences. The problem exists even in the sale of blood, but is not as serious since blood is a renewable resource. Organs, however, do not renew themselves with the result that a donation is a serious matter. The temptation can be very great when an advertisement in the newspaper offers huge sums for a kidney. This is particularly true when the organs are to be imported from poor nations in which even modest sums by American standards may seem enormous to the donor. At the same time paternalistic "protection" of those who are allegedly exploited poses its own ethical problems. From the poor seller's point of view, being "exploited" may be a lesser evil than seeing his children suffer from malnutrition or go without proper shelter.

Granted that, all things considered, selling the organ might be the greater good for the impoverished organ seller, it is still based on an exploitation of the seller's extreme need and so should not be encouraged. It is not, however, the selling itself that is wrong but the exploitation. In so far as this exploitation results from conditions supported by society, society should change the conditions or at least regulate the sale of organs to prevent exploitation through coercion or price gouging. The right of the seller, however, should not be completely denied when lesser measures will provide protection.

If the selling of organs spreads, a strong market for organs may develop, the price may soar, and the distribution of organs would be based on the ability of the few to pay the high prices rather than on medical need. Assuming that organ transplants are socially defined as part of adequate care, this adds to the complications of the humane distribution of organs, which will be discussed below. It is obvious that the health care system already works to favor those with more resources. This is true even in England and other countries which have systems of socialized medicine. As noted in Chapter Four this is not necessarily unethical if the system provides adequate but not necessarily maximum care for all.

With Andrews (1986), we note that the dangers that might occur from selling organs can be controlled by laws that prohibit brokering organs and make sure that the sale was truly voluntary.

The social bonding argument, which stresses important human and community benefits that arise from the donation of blood and organs, rests on and seeks to promote a series of important values. First, it sees the body as belonging to that class of things that are sacred and so not really suitable for trade or ordinary barter. Second, it stresses the noncontractual bonds which arise from gift giving and serve to create healthy noncontractual obligations between families and whole societies. Third, both these values are valuable counterbalances to commercialized and bureaucratic life which can break down the sense of both individual worth and communal solidarity.

We believe that all of these points argue against the sale of organs, but not to the extent that make sales per se unethical. The social bonding arguments do, however, give us an ideal to strive for. We conclude that though the sale of organs cannot be considered necessarily unethical, caution is in order.

The Ethics of Cadaver Organ Donation

The ethics of organ donation after the donor is dead is obviously much simpler than the ethics of donation inter vivos. There are, however, legal and ethical problems. The Uniform Anatomical Gift Act makes it legal for a person to will his body or body parts for medical research or for transplants. Legally, the valid consent of the donor gives the person authorized to receive the gift the right to possess the organ for the uses specified by the donor. Peters (1986, p.248) holds that this right of the person authorized to receive the gift is "paramount to the rights of others and is preempted only by the rights of coroners, medical examiners, and physicians to conduct autopsies under conditions described in the state's death laws...."

Cadaver donations include not only kidneys, but such single organs as heart, liver, lung, pancreas, and spleen. The list will undoubtedly grow as the sciences and medical techniques advance.

In general, there is no dispute about the ethical correctness of a person donating organs for use after death. Indeed, such a donation is not ethically neutral but praiseworthy as a service to one's fellow humans with no risk of danger to one's self. None of the major religious groups forbid cadaver organ transplants as long as due respect is shown the body of the deceased. There are, however, problems if a person's religious or philosophical position considers such donation as involving a unwarranted mutilation of the body and so disrespect for the dignity of the human body. Such beliefs bind the donor and, as we shall see later, question laws that provide for automatic harvesting of organs without the permission of the dead person or the surrogates.

Is There an Obligation to Donate?

Here as elsewhere in this chapter a distinction must be made between an obligation to make a donation between two living persons (inter vivos) and an obligation to will all or part of one's body for the help of others, whether that be by way of transplant, blood transfusion, or a harvesting of chemicals in the body.

While risking one's life, even laying it down for another, may be an altruistic ideal, it is not an obligation. There is no natural or legal obligation, contractual or otherwise, to sacrifice an organ for the good of another person even when the principle of proportionality is satisfied. One individual is not subordinated to another individual even in the areas of life and death. Yet, when the risk to the donor is minimal and the potential benefit to the recipient is great, the person who refuses to help when asked is hardly worthy of praise. This minimal risk is the case with regard to blood transfusions, but certainly not the case with respect to kidney donations.

Granted that a donation inter vivos is not obligatory, we may ask if a person is obliged to donate a cadaver or parts of it. At first glance there would appear to be an obligation to donate the cadaver or cadaver part since the donation can do a great deal of good with no possible harm to the donor. Not to donate would appear to be a form of indifference to the welfare of other human beings. It might even be taken as denying the dignity of the other.

In practice, the complexities of human feeling make this *prima facie,* or presumptive, obligation problematic. Supported by some religions, individuals can have strong feelings about mutilation and so would oppose donation. In particular the sensibilities of the survivors may make the would-be donor hesitant to sign over his body. Others may feel that the whole process of transplantation is unnatural and to be discouraged. In short, the symbolic meanings of the body and of organ transplantation are factors which prevent us from arguing conclusively to an obligation to donate. These same factors must be considered when we return to the question of whether or not society ought to abolish the requirement that informed consent be obtained for even cadaver organ donations.

THE ETHICS OF THE RECIPIENT

The would-be recipient of an organ transplant is most often in a desperate condition. No matter how serious the condition, there are still ethical demands on the recipient. Obviously, the recipient must consider whether the transplant will produce more harm than good, all things considered. Granted that the recipient has been properly informed by the health care team, the effects of the transplant on the quality of life and on family and society must be taken into consideration. The expense of the transplant and the equally expensive aftercare, often not covered by insurance, are very relevant factors. Unfortunately, the financial effects on others are also ethically relevant. This would be particularly true if the transplant promises no more than a few months of tortured life but guarantees agony and poverty for the survivors. At the same time, it could make good ethical sense if the transplant is funded and will produce useful knowledge for other victims of the disease. That is to say that the patient can ethically volunteer to be a subject in an experiment as long as undue burdens are not placed on survivors. Indeed, without such unselfish volunteers, medical science could not advance.

Granted that the recipient has a proportionate good to gain, she and her family and physicians must respect the autonomy of the potential donors. Families in particular can bring such pressure to bear that donors can be blackmailed into the procedure against their wills. This might well be the case of a sibling or parent who does not want to donate for fear of the damage to their own health, but is given no peace until there is a consent. While such pressure is humanly understandable, it is unethical and the health care providers should guard against it. Indeed, the danger is so great that to ensure freedom from all duress, the Australian Law Commission recommended that the consent be given in the absence of family and friends and with the help of an independent medical advisor (Steinbrook, 1980).

Even in life or death situations, it will still be unethical for would-be recipients to bribe physicians or hospitals to give them a privileged position on the waiting list. There have been rumors of rich families buying their way to the top of the list with enormous donations to hospitals licensed to do transplants. While money may talk loudly in such situations, it also eats away at the integrity of the health care profession and destroys any reasonable ethical basis for the allocation of very scarce resources.

THE ETHICS OF THE HEALTH CARE TEAM

The following statements of the AMA Council on Ethical and Judicial Affairs (1984) present the principal ethical concerns of the physician and the health care team.

(4) Full discussion of the proposed procedure with the donor and the recipient or their responsible relatives or representatives is mandatory. The physician should be objective in discussing the procedure, in disclosing known risks and possible hazards, and in advising of the alternative procedures available. *The physician should not encourage expectations beyond those which the circumstances justify.* The physician's interest in advancing scientific knowledge must always be secondary to his primary concern for his patient. (italics added)

(5) The transplant procedures of body organs should be undertaken (a) only by physicians who possess special medical knowledge and technical competence developed through special training, study and laboratory experience and practice, and (b) in medical institutions with facilities adequate to protect the health and well-being of the parties to the procedure.

(6) Transplantation of body organs should be undertaken only after careful evaluation of the availability and effectiveness of other possible therapy.

A few comments on each of these provisions will help to clarify the issues involved.

The first concern involves informed consent in an emotional situation where the wishful thinking of both patient and family, as well as enthusiasm of health care professionals, could easily lead to misunderstanding. The Guidelines insist that the patient comes first, even in research situations, and that informed consent be respected. This is not always as simple as it seems. In the Baby Fae case, where a baboon's heart was transplanted into a child, it appears that the parents were not told of the source of the organ. This was a relevant, if emotion-laden, fact and could have affected the parents' decision. It was also a relevant fact from a medical point of view, since the fact that the organ came from another species increased the chances of rejection.

The necessity of proposing alternatives and their chances of success is particularly important in transplant cases, since they generally involve serious decisions in areas where there is little scientifically established certitude. It is not always clear that a kidney transplant will be more helpful than the continuance of dialysis, or that a heart transplant will increase the quality of life for all recipients even though it may increase life expectancy. Christopherson (1982) and Caplan (1985) note that the scientific basis for transplanting a baboon heart into a child was suspect since peers were not given a chance to evaluate all the factors. In any event, the AMA Guidelines see a transplant as the last option. The patient needs to know the facts even if they are grim. The physician needs to face the facts even if they run counter to the interests of her research.

When a cadaver transplant from a presently living patient is anticipated, the physician shall continue to give the donor the same care as usual. This warning is issued lest the health care team be tempted to speed the death in order to get the organs as early as possible or in time for a particular transplant. In addition, the donor shall be declared dead by at least one physician other than the physician of the recipient. This is in order to avoid both the reality and the appearance of a conflict of loyalties.

The stress on competence, training, and adequate facilities might seem obvious. It is there since there are ambitious men and women who, in their eagerness to make medical history, might overlook these basic protections for the donor and the patient.

All of this says nothing of the crucial ethics of the proper distribution of health care in this area. We shall return to the ethical obligations with regard to the allocation of organs and transplant operations a little later in this chapter.

Relationships with Surrogates and Families

There are additional problems when the would-be donor is brain dead and is kept breathing so that the organs can be harvested while fresh. It is the opinion of the authors that this sort of cadaver maintenance can be ethical if done for only a short period of time and if families of the dead person and the third-party payers are not billed for the extra time in the hospital. If the breathing is to be prolonged for a longer time, thus increasing the bill and prolonging the agony of survivors, we believe that explicit permission of the survivors is required as well as explicit and legal arrangements obligating the researchers or recipients to pay for the continued care of the cadaver until the transplant is performed. Without such agreements, the transplant team might end up stealing money from the family and the insurance company, neither of which should be unknowingly forced to pay for keeping a cadaver in good shape for a transplant.

The health care team also has ethical and legal obligations with regard to the way in which they approach, or do not approach, the family for permission to take the cadaver organs for transplant. On the one hand, the health care professional, aware of the good that may be accomplished with a transplant, may disregard the feelings and needs of the anguished and grieving family. On the other hand, ignorance of the law and oversensitivity to the feelings of families may cause the health care professional to violate the will of the donor and the requirements of the law . We will examine first the problem of required requests for organs and, second, the case where the donor card is disregarded.

Some states have laws which require that the family be asked for a donation. These laws put the health care provider in a position in which it is impossible to utilize real judgment as to what should be done in a given case. While the laws are well intentioned in trying to increase the supply of organs, they may not promote professional sensitivity and ethical conduct. The feelings of the family may be morally decisive only if the deceased has not made her will clear. When the patient has made her desires clear, they must be respected. More will be said of this when we treat other efforts to increase the supply of organs.

In this context, it should be noted that when there is a valid donor card, there is legally no obligation to ask the permission of the family. If there is a card forbidding donation, an attempt to get the family to overrule the negative decision of the deceased is reprehensible. The will of the patient should rule. Many hospitals, unfortunately, have a policy requiring the permission of the family, even when there is a valid donor card. This practice gives the family the false impression that they have a right to overrule the deceased's organ donation or refusal of a donation (Peters, 1986). In practice, it may lead to the actual voiding of the donation and a decrease in the number of organs available.

At the same time, there is still the need to be sensitive to the feelings of the family. Peters suggests the following political compromise (p. 260).

> The family of the medically acceptable declared donor should be informed that the hospital is about to take the necessary steps to give effect to the decedent-authorized donation. The family is not asked to consent to this activity since such a request is both unnecessary and inappropriate. The family is simply informed, as a matter of courtesy, about standard hospital procedure.

Questions of the family should be answered. If the family still objects to the donation, Peters suggests that it should be asked to sign a written declaration of dissent, which will request the recipient to decline the gift. The declaration should give the reasons for the family's objection. In these circumstances, Peters feels the waiver of the recipient should be automatic.

The authors believe that Peters' attempt at a political middle ground may unduly complicate the whole process. Indeed, it appears to put the family through even more agony. Granted that the family should always be told, we do not see why the intended recipient should be informed of the family's wishes and respect the wishes of the family rather than those of the deceased donor. The body belonged to the donor, not to the family.

When the organs, fluids, or body parts are taken for experimentation or for research, there are additional problems both with regard to consent and to payment for the commercially valuable results of the research (Andrews, 1986). In this context, we merely note that researchers cannot presume to use even cells or fluids let alone whole organs merely because that patient has signed a general consent for treatment on admission to a hospital. As with all truly ethical consent procedures, specific information is required. In the present case that would include a separate form giving specific information about the experiment or research and the ownership of valuable results.

Increasing the Supply of Organs: Ethical Problems

In the face of the shortage of organs and the urgency of many situations, there are proposals to increase the supply of organs by improving the recruitment of volunteers and by changing the legal requirements for surrogate consent. The methods proposed pose their own ethical problems.

We have already mentioned the problems caused by laws or hospital policies which require nurses and physicians to seek family permission for the donation of cadaver organs. Others suggest that hospitals should be required to ask about consent to organ donation at the time of admission. Such inquiry would hardly be comforting to the patient, who would rather not think of being a cadaver at that particular moment. Moreover, the patient and his family have enough decisions to make regarding treatment or cessation of treatment without being involved in another emotional situation. Again, delicacy and a respect for the freedom of the patient and family seems to dictate at least a reasonable hesitation about such a request at the time of admission.

The supply could be increased if the hospitals obeyed the law and accepted the donor card provided for in the Uniform Anatomical Gift Act as proof of desire to donate. Unfortunately, as we just mentioned, many facilities will not act on the basis of the donor card but require the consent of the family. Whether this is because of the fear of lawsuits or respect for the feelings of the family, they not only reduce the supply of organs available, but override the will of the patient which is legally entitled to respect.

Since the volunteer method is not sufficiently successful, various laws have been passed to facilitate the harvesting of organs for transplant or other purposes by modifying the need for consent.

A 1968 Virginia law (Lombardo, 1981) provided the medical examiner the right to hand over unclaimed or unidentified bodies to a transplanting physician, who requested them in a case where the patient was in immediate need of an internal organ transplant. Others wish to pass laws permitting health care groups to harvest organs from cadavers as long as neither the person nor the surrogates have rejected such use of the body. Some would add that the consent should not be presumed when the patient belongs to a religious group known to object to mutilation of the corpse. This proposal is based on a notion of presumed consent, since studies show that the vast majority of people are in favor of organ transplants, even though very few sign up for them.

Such proposals are a strong departure from the American tradition and need to be examined for their long-range consequences as well as their nature. First of all the assent is not truly presumed. The presumed consent is too much like the negative option used by book and record clubs. If you don't reject the selection of the club you get the book or record and the bill. The system depends on the fact that people in general are too lazy or lackadaisical to reject the offer. This is not a true presumption of consent but an exploitation of human weakness. The same is true of the negative option contained in the presumed consent theory as applied to cadaver organ donations. Once again, human weakness is exploited. In addition, the so-called presumption in organ donations may also exploit human ignorance. If people are not clear that they can say "no," they will not say "no." Indeed, rather than providing for an informed consent, the "presumed consent" to organ donation is an uninformed and exploitative nonconsent.

More serious yet is the implication in the law of presumed consent that society has the right to control the disposal of bodies not only for the public health, that is, for sanitary reasons, but for therapeutic reasons, that is, for curing particular individuals. The present writers are wary of such an extension of political power, especially when it is being handed over to individuals and institutions in the private sector. Our experience with the donation of whole blood indicates that over time education and social bonding will increase the supply of organs. Where at one time much of the blood used in the United States was purchased, by 1982 only 3 to 4 percent came from paid donors. Indeed, 70 percent was provided on a purely voluntary basis with no strings attached. Perhaps 25 percent was given through "blood credit" programs, where it was donated for special uses or specific people . Education, good organization, and widespread altruism explain the dramatic change.

THE HEALTH CARE PROVIDER'S ETHICS OF DISTRIBUTION

In the present section we will first study and comment on the ethics of the actual means of distributing organs in the United States and then proceed to a discussion of the public policy and the obligations of society. Health care professionals, because of their expertise, are involved in distribution and should be involved in the formulation of public policy.

The pages that follow will illustrate the technical complexity which dictates certain aspects of distribution, as well as the conflicting social values which must be reconciled or at least prioritized in developing an ethic and a public policy on the distribution of organs. In particular we will see the strains between equity, need, efficiency, and the limits of resources.

The Actual Distribution of Organs

In practice, the actual distribution of organs both from cadavers and living donors has often been governed by publicity, that is, by the ability of patients or surrogates to recruit donors or, as one might suspect in a market economy, by the ability to pay.

Distribution by media occurs when some person, generally a child, manages to get such publicity that they obtain an organ without going through channels. Media people are aware that in choosing to publicize the need of one child rather than another, they often "decide" who will live and who will die. That "decision" is made without any knowledge of who has the greatest need or the greatest chance of profiting from the transplant.

In time, as the organization of organ donation and transplants increases, distribution by publicity should, as a general rule, be eliminated as much as possible in a free society. Yet, though distribution by publicity is not desirable, it may be tolerated at this stage of medical history. First, the publicity raises the public's awareness of the need for transplants and so in the long run should increase the supply of donated organs. Second, frequently the media plea brings in more volunteers than those required for the case being publicized.

Like it or not, the ability to pay for at least the cost of the transplant has been a factor in distribution of transplants. Arthur Caplan (1985) has noted that at one large medical center you could not even get on the waiting list unless you had $100,000 to $150,000 in advance. In such a situation neither need nor equality of opportunity is the primary guide to distribution of donated organs. Such a norm of distribution has nothing to recommend it, though, as we have seen and shall see again, the possibility of reimbursement is still a factor in the allocation of health care.

Location, too, can become a basis for distribution. Because local health care facilities are established to fill local needs, many institutions give priority to those who are part of the area they serve. No one of these methods of allocation is ideal, yet we cannot label as unethical either the recipients or the health care providers who benefit from the existing situation. The patient has a primary obligation to self. Similarly, the health care provider has a primary obligation to the particular patient (American Medical Association, 1984). Even granted these primary obligations, there can be unethical methods of getting organs.

There are times when physicians in their zeal for their patients have surreptitiously conducted unethical searches of existing data banks whose contents were supposed to be confidential (Caplan, 1983). This violation of confidentiality gave the physician's patient a clearly unfair advantage over others who needed a transplant.

From the point of view of the health care system and of society, distribution by publicity and personal privilege does not maximize the good. Those who are in charge of tissue banks in particular have had to think through the question of priorities. As we saw in Chapter Four, the problem is not simple.

Medical Criteria for Microallocation

Some would argue that organs should be distributed on the following basis. The first priority might be given to those who are hospitalized and critically ill, with a lower priority given to those who are stable and at home. The hospitalized and critically ill, however, are not necessarily those who will received the greatest long-term benefit from a transplant. If the transplant grants only a few years of very reduced quality of life accompanied by great depression, it may be a very inefficient use of resources. Indeed, one may ask if it is even medically indicated.

The American Medical Association (1986), speaking of the allocation of health resources in general, states: "Priority should be given to persons who are most likely to be treated successfully or derive long term benefit." The Massachusetts Task Force on Organ Transplantation takes a similar position when it proposes that the first screening of candidates be on the basis of *clinical suitability with reference to the benefits to the patient in terms of lifestyle and rehabilitation rather than simple survival.* Clinical suitability or the medical indications in terms of these benefits then becomes a crucial element in the distribution of organs.

Criteria of medical or clinical suitability have looked to such items as the absence of other life-threatening diseases, age, and the absence of severe emotional and psychological difficulties. Before discussing these and other proposed criteria or clinical suitability, it will be useful to note technical factors which influence both clinical judgments and priorities.

Technical Factors

Priority according to need plus hope of rehabilitation often has to yield to the limits imposed by time, compatibility of tissue, and the availability of the right personnel and facilities.

In the first place, tissue compatibility is important for the success of the transplant. For this reason, many centers make the issue of compatibility primary. In the second place, while kidneys can be stored for several days, hearts and livers must often be used within hours. In the case of hearts and livers, then, the ability to harvest and implant the organs rapidly becomes an important factor in distributing the organs. Because the liver and heart must be used so rapidly, there is no time for tissue typing and matching. In practice, it is necessary to know the recipient before these organs are removed. Finally, not all hospitals have the same record of success in using organs, with the result that the skills of the transplant team becomes a relevant factor in setting priorities for allocation. It does not make much sense to allocate a kidney to a very sick person if the surgeon available has a poor track record.

A little reflection on the facts given in the last paragraph indicates that even rational allocation must deal with random factors such as the time and place of death and the place of the person needing the transplant. These random factors are in large part not under the control of any human agents with the result that the ethics often involves simply doing the best you can, all things considered. Allocation also has to deal with both objective and subjective judgments about the relative skills of surgeons and hospitals as well as the needs of patients. Such judgments, because they cannot be neatly justified, further complicate the already complicated ethics of distribution.

Criteria of Clinical Suitability

While a transplant procedure is in the experimental stage, additional criteria may be necessary in order to control the experiment and to maximize the chance of success. Originally, to be considered for a heart transplant at many centers, the patient had to meet the following criteria (Christopherson, 1982): (1) the patient had to be in a physical state where he led "a bed to chair existence" and had an estimated life expectancy of less than six months, (2) other major organ systems had to be free of disease, (3) there had to be strong family support, (4) the patient had to have a history of following medical orders, (5) there had to be no history of psychiatric illness or substance abuse, (6) the patient had to be under 50, (7) the patient had to be capable of real informed consent, (8) the patient, his family, or community had to be capable of paying for such expenses as travel, living away from home, and the like. This last criteria points up the fact that geography and the ability to overcome its limits is another one of those random factors that affects the distribution of health care. Several of these criteria need comment, since there have been ethical disputes about them.

The Criterion of Family Support

If ultimate rehabilitation is a key part of the screening process, the appropriateness of strong family support as a subcriterion for selection is well illustrated by the Baby Fae case (Caplan, 1986). Baby Fae was at first denied a transplant since the parents did not appear capable of caring for her during the long recuperation period that would follow the operation. Since good care during that period is essential if the procedure is to be worthwhile, the surgeons correctly did not wish to add to the risk factors and turned down the application for a transplant. After much public outcry, alternate and more capable guardians were found and the transplant operation performed. The principle behind all of this is clear. Physicians should not allocate scarce resources to those who seem unlikely to benefit from them when they have other patients who have a chance or a better chance to benefit.

When we are dealing with scarce resources, and granting the attainment of the basic health care demanded by human dignity, the outcomes should be maximized as much as possible. Though the principle is reasonable, there was and can be debate as to whether the support of parents is the crucial element in maximizing the results. Parents, after all, are part of the natural lottery. Yet the support of the family is often crucial to the recovery of the patient and so becomes part of the medical decision-making process even though it grants an advantage to those with supportive families. Such inequalities are like those introduced by the presence of genetic inequality. They are facts that cannot be done away with and *when relevant to outcomes in the use of scarce resources* they should be given weight.

There remains a question, however, as to whether a physician has to give priority to a person who is not her patient. After all, the physician is responsible to her patient, not to the other. Once again the ethics based on loyalty to the patient comes into conflict with maximizing the results of procedures using scarce resources. The American Medical Association (1986) holds clearly for the physician's patient.

2.03 ALLOCATION OF RESOURCES. A physician has a duty to do all that he can for the benefit of his individual patient. To expect a physician when treating a patient to make rationing decisions based on governmental or other external priorities in the allocation of scarce health resources creates an undesirable conflict of interest with the primary responsibility of the physician to his patient.

While we cannot disagree with the AMA, we find the statement lacking since it does not recognize the fact that there is a team involved in transplants, and various agents in the process are not directly responsible for the physician's patient. For this reason and in view of scarcity, social policy or hospital policy or organ center policy may make the maximization an obligation, even though the ethics of the health care provider in the one-on-one relationship does not, with rare exceptions, look to anything but the maximization of the good of the patient under the physician's care. To the extent that the treatment is paid for by the society, the society may impose reasonable conditions on the distribution of resources in this area as in so many others. Unfortunately, at this stage in history, there is as yet no satisfactory balancing of the obligations to the individual patient with the obligation to distribute the scarce resources in a reasonable manner.

Ageism

As the procedure becomes less and less experimental, questions are being raised about the use of age 50 as a cut-off age for suitability. Dr. Thomas Starzl of the Presbyterian-University Hospital in Pittsburg has been fighting this limit for liver transplant patients and by the mid-1980s had already accepted 20 candidates for the operation who were over 60. He and the ethics advisory committee at Presbyterian Hospital distinguish between age and general health on the ground that age does not stand for specific medical criteria. Some people are poor candidates at 30; others are good candidates at 70 or older. The point is well taken. The consideration of medical criteria is relevant, the consideration of age alone may be no more than ageism.

Ability to Pay

The ability and willingness of the patient, family, or community to pay is hardly a part of a medical indications policy. It is, however, a reasonable criterion for the health care institution and the health care providers. These institutions and individuals cannot exist without income. If the individual or his family cannot pay, it becomes a question of whether or not society will pay. This in turn is a question of the way in which a society prioritizes certain values in formulating public policy.

Whether the community is both able and willing to pay is, as pointed out in Chapter Four, a function of all the needs of society and individuals, and not merely a question of the need for health care, let alone the need of this particular individual for transplant. A transplant may or may not be considered part of adequate and humane treatment to which everyone has a right and which society must fulfill.

While questions can be raised about the appropriateness of some of the criteria, they illustrate the complexity of the problems which must be examined in allocating experimental transplant procedures. At this stage in both medicine and medical ethics, we are far from having definitive answers. As we have said, considering the nature of the problem, it is not likely that there are definitive answers.

Economic Costs and the Distribution of Transplants

Various task forces have attempted to formulate foundations for public policy for the distribution of organs and transplants. The difference between the National Task Force on Organ Transplantation and the Massachusets Task Force on Transplantation are illustrative of the issues that have not as yet been resolved.

The National Task Force on Organ Transplantation (Department of Health and Human Services, 1986, p. 11) writes:

> In order to insure that patients in need of an extrarenal organ transplant can obtain procedures regardless of ability to pay, the Task Force recommends that private and public health benefit programs, including Medicare and Medicaid should cover heart and liver transplants, including outpatient immunosuppresive therapy that is an essential part of post-transplant care.
>
> A public program should be set up to cover the costs of people who are medically eligible for organ transplants but who are not covered by private insurance, Medicare or Medicaid and who are unable to obtain an organ transplant due to lack of funds.

These recommendations involve mandating private health insurers to include more in their policies as well as extending financial aid to everyone who is not covered by some program. The report unfortunately does not provide careful study of the costs of such recommendations.

Transplants are so expensive that few individuals can pay for them. A single liver transplant might cost as much as $250,000. The follow-up costs of counseling and other psychiatric care plus the continued use of immunosuppressant drugs are often not estimable. Both the high costs of transplants and the unknown follow-up costs have rightfully made insurance companies and the government reluctant to pay, lest the cost of health care increase even more (Caplan, 1983). The experience with the enormous costs of government-funded dialysis is used to back up this hesitation. The dialysis program, which was originally to cost only $400,000 a year, ended up costing $2,000,000,000 a year as early as 1982. In subsequent years the costs continued to skyrocket.

As long as resources are limited, not everything can be authorized. This is particularly true where it is not clear that the transplant produces medically justifiable results. The mere fact that a transplant extends life does not justify it. As we saw in Chapter Six, mere vegetable existence is hardly desirable. When we are not dealing with basic health care, the costs too are factors which must be considered by society in deciding who shall get and who shall do without. As long as resources are scarce, society must, in accord with the system of priorities mentioned in Chapter Four, ration its direct support of health care services which are not at that stage part of basic health care.

In view of facts such as those given above, the Massachusetts Task Force (1984) adopts a less idealistic and more realistic approach. A few of the key recommendations from the Massachusetts report illustrate the differences (pp. 10–11).

2. The decision of when extreme and expensive medical technologies, like heart and liver transplants, should be generally available should be made only after the clinical, social and economic consequences of introducing the procedure, including cost effectiveness, ethical implications and long term effects on society, are studied and reviewed by a publicly accountable body. . . .

5. Patient selection criteria should be public, fair and equitable. Primary screening should be based on medical suitability criteria made available to the public which are designed to offer transplantation to those who can benefit the most from it in terms of the probability of living for a significant period of time with a reasonable prospect for rehabilitation. If there are insufficient resources to transplant all who can so benefit, selection made from the medically suitable group should be based primarily on a first-come, first-served basis.

This approach stresses efficiency and a balancing of costs against social and economic consequences as well as against clinical benefits. It does not leap to the conclusion that because transplants can do a great deal of good that everyone has a claim to one no matter what the level of benefits to be obtained or costs to be incurred. The authors favor this approach because it is both realistic and recognizes that more is involved than mere medical indications.

Transplants and Nonimmigrant Aliens

The status of nonimmigrant aliens further complicates the problems. What priority should be given to citizens of another nation who come to the United States for a transplant? The question is particularly poignant since there are thousands of Americans awaiting transplants, some of whom will die before an organ becomes available. Some professional groups want to provide a quota for such nonimmigrant aliens, others do not.

The Task Force on Organ Transplant (Department of Health and Human Services, 1986, p.95) recommends that:

non-immigrant aliens not compromise more than 10 percent of the total number of kidney transplant recipients at each transplant center, until the Organ Procurement and Transplantation Network has had an opportunity to review the issue. In addition, extrarenal organs should not be offered for transplantation to a nonimmigrant alien unless it has been determined that no other suitable recipient can be found.

Eight members of the Task Force objected to allowing even the 10 percent quota for nonimmigrant aliens in the case of kidney transplants. They argued that the organs come from United States residents and that kidney transplants are paid for by the taxpayers so that Americans can reasonably expect to be given priority.

This argument is not unreasonable, and American society may decide that it will not pay even indirectly for noncitizens or nonresidents. This decision would be all the more justified if the society also decided that such transplants are not even part of basic health care. At the same time, such social decisions would leave many of us morally uneasy, since their basis is nationalistic rather than humane or even utilitarian. The recommendation which allows for the 10 percent quota at least admits that nationality or resident status is not the dominant moral consideration.

Medically one's exact legal status is not a relevant factor, but membership may be a relevant factor in the social distribution of goods. At present there seems to be no easy answer to the ethical importance of legal status.

Summary

Careful distinctions must be made between the donation of renewable and non-renewable parts as well as between those that come in pairs and those that do not. The living donor may not donate a nonrenewable, nonpaired part since, except in rare cases, this is equivalent to a unjustified suicide. Other donations may be made for a proportionate reason. There is no obligation to donate organs inter vivos, but cadaver donation should be seen as an ideal to be encouraged. It is desirable that organs be donated rather than sold, but selling cannot be condemned out of hand.

Would-be recipients of organs should be on their guard against blackmailing or coercing donors. The recipient should look at all the factors when deciding whether to ask for or consent to a transplant.

Proper consent which respects the will of the donor and the feelings of families is essential even in cadaver organ donations. Legal schemes for increasing the supply of organs which disregard the feelings of families or are disguised forms of manipulation should be avoided.

Distribution by publicity may be tolerated because it provides some overall educational benefits for society as well as individuals. In the long run, a medical indications policy needs to be developed and enforced within the limits of the rights of citizens. Until society specifies that transplants are part of the minimum human and adequate medical treatment to which all have a right, economic factors must still be considered. Membership factors may also be valid factors in distribution.

CASES FOR ANALYSIS

1.   Peter Canisius, a widowed and childless college professor, age 40, had coronary bypass surgery 10 years ago. He made a fine recovery and returned to work with a very high level of involvement in both college and community affairs. In the last year his health has deteriorated badly. He has developed congestive heart failure, which does not respond well to medication. His physician and consulting cardiologist feel that another bypass operation will not restore him to the level of functioning he desires. The physicians recommend a heart transplant and have Canisius placed on a waiting list at a medical center. Canisius has a family history of clogged arteries and veins so that the transplant, even if successful, does not guarantee more than a few years of life. If he has to wait a long time for a transplant, it may be necessary to put him on

an artificial heart to keep him alive. This artificial heart causes additional psychological and physical problems.

With the artificial heart in question, the patient is equivalently chained to a large piece of machinery, which sometimes causes damage to the blood with subsequent damage to other parts of the body. For an active person like the professor, a long confinement while waiting for a transplant will almost certainly involve depression. There is, of course, no guarantee that a transplant will become available for him. Though of modest means, the professor's insurance will cover the operation and 120 days in the hospital. He can get 80 percent of the other expenses from his $250,000 major medical policy.

2. Robert di Nobili, age 25, has lost 50 percent of his kidney function due to diabetes, which has also left him blind and with severe neuropathy in his legs and feet. His general condition is deteriorating so rapidly that he probably has no more than a year to live. Robert's father wants to donate his kidney, if he is compatible. Dialysis is no option in the mind of the father since he feels that Robert could not take it psychologically. The family has a history of both diabetes and liver problems. The transplant will help with the kidney problem but will not reverse or stop the progression of the other effects of the diabetes.

3. Entrepreneurial Hospital Inc., located in a medium-sized city, has been preparing for its first heart transplants. The team is not fully trained as yet, but the chief surgeon, Dr. Corazon y Hartz, has had a great deal of experience at a major medical center before coming to Entrepreneurial. St. Isadore's Hospital, some 30 miles away in a large metropolitan area, has had two years' experience with heart transplants and a fully trained team.

John Locumtenens, a local patient, has been awaiting a transplant at St. Isadore's for over three months when a heart becomes available locally. His physician with the informed consent of John asks Dr. Hartz to do a transplantation.

4. Mrs. Simpatico, a registered nurse, had cared for Joseph Foi for three weeks and had become attached to him and his devoted family. Joseph, who was only 30, died. The hospital has a policy which requires nurses to ask the families of all dead patients for organ donations. Both she and the family are very upset about the death. Joseph's young wife and three children need comfort and not decisions at this moment. Mrs. Simpatico does not ask for the organ donation, even though the hospital has a long waiting list. When the nursing supervisor discovers this omission, she reprimands Mrs. Simpatico and puts a warning in her personnel file. "One more incident like that," says the supervisor, "and you will be fired. A policy is a policy and it is not up to you to make exceptions."

5. Two men on the same service are awaiting a keratoplasty (cornea transplant) because of chemical burns on their eyes. One is an alcoholic street person with other serious health problems. The other is a prominent lawyer with a wife and three children. A donor's eye becomes available and by coincidence both men's circular segment of the cornea match the donor's. The physician makes his decision on the basis of "first come, first served" and transplants the cornea to the alcoholic.

6. Mary, age 4 months, has been diagnosed as having liver pathology and other congenital defects. The liver pathology will threaten her life within a very short time unless she receives a liver transplant. Her father, owner of the local TV station, is able to get national media attention and a donor is discovered within two weeks. John, also age 4 months, has the same liver condition, but is otherwise in good health. Friends rally around the family and raise the funds for a transplant, but no donor is found. John dies in six months.

NOTES

[1]The anencephalic infant is born without all or most of the cerebral hemispheres. It is a fatal neurological defect, and most afflicted infants will not survive more than a week. The condition is sometimes misdiagnosed because it sometimes overlaps with other conditions such as the affliction of hydranencephalics, who survive somewhat longer because their skulls are intact.

Chapter Ten
THE ETHICS OF TESTING AND SCREENING

INTRODUCTION

The present chapter is concerned with the often overlooked ethical problems of tests used in diagnosing the complaints of patients and in screening symptomless populations for the presence of a defect or illness. Though the same techniques may be used in both testing and screening, we distinguish the two by saying that testing is for the diagnosis of an individual with symptoms, while screening is for case-finding in a population without symptoms.

The ethical problems of testing involve not only charges of overtesting, but problems of accuracy. These problems are in turn connected with the problem of informed consent in testing and in particular with the question of whether or not there is an obligation to tell the patient of the limits of the test and its utility as well as about its risks, if any.

While the problems of testing carry over into the area of screening, that is, case-finding, there are additional ethical problems when the screening is for the purpose of public health or employability rather than for the good of the individual. These additional problems involve the confidentiality of test results, the risk of the loss of a job, the denial of insurance, or even prosecution for a crime. Second, mass screening may stigmatize an entire population, as was allegedly the case with the testing of blacks for sickle cell anemia. Finally, from the society's point of view, there are questions

THE ETHICS OF TESTING AND SCREENING

of the cost/benefit ratio of case-finding by screening. In short, are the benefits of screening sufficiently great to justify the cost of finding a case? This problem is especially acute when health care resources are scarce.

TESTING

The Central Question

While problems with cost/benefit ratios and stigmatization of groups are extremely important, the central question from the patient's point of view is: *Will this test and the subsequent treatment lead to more good than harm, all things considered?* From the view of the health care professional, the central question is similar, but not identical. *Will this test lead to treatment which, from a medical point of view, will benefit the patient enough to justify the costs and risks of both the tests and the treatment?* This is, of course, the medical indications principle developed in Chapter Three.

To answer the central question given above, both the patient and the health care professional must first ask the following questions: First, how accurate is this test? Second, what are the risks of this test relative to the severity of the illness? Third, is there a treatment for the disease so that it is possible to improve life?

The third question is particularly important. If there is no possible treatment and no possible improvement of life, there is no justification for the cost and risks of the test. The mere desire to confirm the diagnosis is not a justification for the tests. In other words, even an accurate test is not automatically justified by the fact that it improves diagnosis. *In health care practice, as opposed to research, the question must always be whether or not the test can lead to benefiting the patient.*

The Accuracy of Tests

In view of all of the above, the first thing to be determined is whether or not we are dealing with an accurate test. Since it is impossible to discuss all tests and since new tests are constantly coming into existence, we shall confine ourselves to the general nature of the problems and illustrate these with historical examples.

The widely used tests for serum cholesterol provide a clear example of the problem of accuracy (*Medical Letter*, 1987). Different laboratories testing the same sample often come up with quite different test results. This is due in part to different laboratories using different methods. Even when the same method is used, however, the results can vary significantly. One survey, for example, indicated that for all laboratories and all instruments using enzymatic methods, the results for a single sample varied from 197 to 397 mg/dl. The correct result was supposed to be 262.6 mg/dl.

These differences have consequences. According to the National Institutes of Health Consensus Conference Guidelines for the interpretation of the results, one of the lower readings given above would call for no treatment, a higher reading would call for treatment with diet alone, and a yet higher reading for treatment with both diet and drugs. Some of the treatments with drugs have unfortunate side effects. Unfortunately, the health care professional does not know what the readings mean unless they can be related to the method on which the Consensus Guidelines were based. As a result of inaccurate testing, treatment may be omitted where required, or the wrong treatment given.

Studies of medical and even university laboratories indicate that such problems may be widespread. Mendelsohn (1981) noted that Centers for Disease Control studies of even the better laboratories are not encouraging. Between 10 and 40 percent of the laboratory bacteriological testing was unsatisfactory; 12–18 percent made mistakes in blood grouping and typing. Hansen et al. (1985) found that less than 10 percent of the laboratories had acceptable performance for testing barbituates, amphetamines, cocaine, or morphine. They found error rates as high as 100 percent for other drugs analyzed. The results are all the more surprising in that many of the samples were mailed from drug treatment centers, so that the labs should have been alerted to the nature of the samples. The failures may be due to various causes such as laboratory perceptions of what results are expected, costs, carelessness, personnel problems, methodological design, poor specimens, and even reimbursement patterns (Ingelfinder et al., 1981). The point to be made is clear—errors in testing are frequent and many of the errors are due to negligence or even culpable ignorance. The situation is serious since such errors can lead to unnecessary and even dangerous treatment or to the omission of necessary treatment. Not only those who perform the tests, but those who use the results have a serious ethical obligation to make sure that they are dealing with accurate results.

False Positives and False Negatives

Many tests, like those for serum cholesterol, look for the relative amount of a substance in the blood. Other tests, like those mentioned in the previous paragraph, look for the presence or absence of a chemical or an antibody. Tests of this second type should be both sensitive and specific. A test is sensitive if it yields few or no false positives. It is specific if it yields few or no false negatives.

A false positive is a result that says the condition is present when it is actually absent. For example, the test might indicate that the patient has AIDS when as a matter of fact he does not. On the other hand, a false negative says the patient is free of the condition, when in point of fact the condition is present.

The consequences of either false positives or false negatives can be extremely serious. The false negative gives false security and leaves the illness untreated. The false positive can torture patients and expose them to unnecessary and even dangerous treatments. Sometimes, as in the case of AIDS, the false positive is an apparent death sentence that can lead to both despair and suicide. If the test results are not kept confidential, they could also lead to isolation and loss of employment.

Both types of error can also expose the health care professional to malpractice suits.

The issue of false positives is particular acute in testing for HIV (AIDS) infections (Mayer and Pauker, 1987). In the mid-1980s, testing started with an enzyme immunoassay. Since this test had a relatively high rate of false positives, good procedure called for it to be done several times. If there were repeated positive results on the enzyme immunoassay, more complicated and expensive tests were needed to confirm the diagnosis.

The Western blot test was one of the more common confirmatory tests and was, indeed, the standard against which new techniques were evaluated. Unfortunately, the testing methods had not been standardized, interlaboratory variations had not been carefully studied, and the criteria for interpretation varied from laboratory to laboratory and even from month to month (Mayer and Pauker, 1987). In some studies of healthy adults, these factors led to a high rate of false positives at several large commercial testing firms. The confirmatory test is, then, not perfectly sensitive when used with low risk populations. This will have important consequences for the ethics of screening.

The problem of false negatives is illustrated by a test which accurately indicates presence of a disease but not the absence of the same disease. Thus a brain biopsy for herpes simplex encephalitis (see Chapter Twelve) is valid when positive, but tells us nothing when negative, since it may have missed the focal point of the infection and so detected nothing.

Problems with both false positives and false negatives arise from such usual procedures as tonometry to test for glaucoma (Fortress and Kapp, 1985). Writers like Robin (1984) question the value of the test, since he claims early treatment has not been proven to stop the advance of the disease and alleges that treatment with conventional drugs produces no clear-cut improvement. In the case of such a test with a high percentage of false positives and no clear cut treatment, the authors consider the test unethical, quite aside from the unnecessary anguish it causes.

The Interpretation of Tests

Test results generally require interpretation in terms of the health care professional's experience and the history and symptoms of the patient. These interpretations are not a question of scientific fact, but the results of more or less probable deductions and of the interpreter's "feel" for the tests. There is room, then, for error.

Even as common a procedure as an X-ray requires interpretation, and experts can and do disagree about the meaning of the same X-ray plate. In one case the internist saw a broken femur in the X-ray, while the orthopedic surgeon saw no fracture when the plate was placed properly on the screen. Such fallibility of interpretation is a major reason for second opinions in serious cases.

The cervical Pap smear, a commonly used method of detecting the earliest possible stage of cancer of the uterus, requires interpretation, and various doctors examining the same specimen can disagree. One study showed disagreement in as many as 40 percent of the cases (Robin, 1984, p.180). This obviously leads to a large number of false positives and false negatives. The false positives have often been confirmed by examination of the uterus after it has been surgically removed, at which point the truth is of little help to the patient. While the Pap smear is credited with saving the lives of countless women, it is not an infallible test.

Surprisingly enough, the interpretation of a test also involves disputes about the assumptions behind testing and about the way their results can be summarized (Hlatky, 1986). The clinical presentation of the test, the age and sex of the patient, the presence of more than one disease, and the interaction of the disease with the test all cause complications in interpretation.

The variation in interpretation points up the fact that medicine is an "art" as well as a "science." The "art" side, of course, can be highly subjective and loaded with the values of the interpreter. Thus, the interpreter may be disposed to accept any "positive" test results as a mandate for treatment, no matter what the rate of false positives or the risk of misinterpretation.

The Risks of Testing

The risks associated with a given test must enter into both the patient's and the health care professional's judgment of proportionality. This judgment of proportionality includes, of course, a consideration of the alternatives available.

The issues are well illustrated by the methods of prenatal testing. Although these tests have been discussed frequently and heatedly because of their connection with abortion, they can pose ethical problems in and of themselves. There are three principal techniques: ultrasound, amniocentesis, and chorionic vili biopsy.

Ultrasound is a noninvasive technique in which sound waves are bounced off the uterus and, with the aid of a computer, produce a picture of the woman's uterus and its contents. This appears to be the safest technique, and up to now there is no evidence that it is dangerous to the fetus. Until research shows the nature of any possible effects, the test needs more justification than mere curiosity. In time, it may prove so safe that it can be done routinely.

Amniocentesis is a surgical technique which involves penetrating the abdomen and uterus of the pregnant woman with a hollow needle in order to take a sample of amniotic fluid from the amniotic sac. Ultrasound is generally used to guide the needle. The fluid obtained is cultured and then examined. It should be noted that in 10 percent of the cases no fluid is obtained and that 10 percent of the fluid does not yield a culture.

This test has risks for the woman. There are cases of death and complications such as vaginal bleeding or puncture of the bladder. The rate of complications varies greatly from hospital to hospital and physician to physician. Indeed, there are extreme variations in all effects depending on the way in which the ultra sound is used to guide the needle (Katayama and Roesler, 1986). The same is true of risk to the fetus. A spontaneous abortion may result from the procedure. If part of the fetus is touched by the needle, it necroses (dies). Rh-immunization may also occur if the mother is Rh-negative and the fetus Rh-positive. Once again, the test needs to be justified by a proportionate reason and should not be performed routinely. Certainly, it is not justified to satisfy parental curiosity about the sex of the fetus.

The age of the pregnant woman is often taken as a sufficient medical indication for this test. Age, however, needs to be combined with other factors that would indicate high risk, since it can be argued that age alone is too crude an indicator of the risk for a particular woman or fetus. Let us illustrate. Studies indicate that the risk of a Down's syndrome baby increases with age. The statistics in that study included healthy women and women in poor health, as well as women with a history of such births or with relatives who have the disease. The risk for a particular woman to be tested depends on all of these factors and not on age alone. Age alone, then, may not be a sufficient indicator of a need for the test. What indicators should be used is debated in medical circles. A series of letters to *The Lancet* (July 26, 1986), for example, illustrates a considerable range of opinions among British physicians. In any event, both the medical and ethical evaluation of the test needs continual monitoring. In time, the risks may even be so reduced that routine usage could be justified.

The third technique, chorionic vili biopsy, does not involve surgical penetration of the abdomen and uterus and so is much safer than amniocentesis. In this technique, the entrance is made by way of the vagina and a sample is taken from the chorion, which has the same cellular material as the fetus. At this stage of its development, the test cannot detect everything that is detectable by amniocentesis. On the other hand, it can be done earlier and the results are obtained faster.

As with amniocentesis, it should be noted that samples are not obtained in every case. Even though this test might appear to be safer than amniocentesis, there is a worldwide fetal loss rate of 4 percent even when the procedure is performed by experienced obstetricians (McGovern, 1986; Wass, 1986). Certainly, at this stage it is not for routine use.

It should be noted that in many cases where these three prenatal tests can detect a defect or disease with some accuracy, they cannot detect the severity of the disease. Thus, it is possible to detect neural tube defects including spina bifida, but it is anyone's guess as to how serious the condition is in any particular fetus (Kolata, 1980). Similarly, amniocentesis can detect Down's syndrome, but cannot tell us whether or not the retardation will be mild or severe. This is an important point since in many cases the diagnosis of Down's syndrome leads to the recommendation for an abortion.

The danger of the tests or of the treatments based on tests which have false positives or false negatives means that many of the tests should not be used routinely. When they are used, they need to be justified by a proportionate benefit to the patient. The patient must have the information needed to judge if there is a proportionate benefit, all things considered.

The Cost of Tests

For some time, health insurance and third-party payment has pushed cost into the background, so that the patient does not often ask about cost and the health care provider does not mention it. Lately, the rising costs of health care have made it important to think about the costs of tests. Certainly such measures as Diagnostic Related Groups (DRGs) have made providers and health care administrators much more sensitive to the issue. After all, if you are not going to get paid for every test you make and if you risk losing money if you make too many, caution is in order. Patients will become equally sensitive if higher deductibles have to be paid out of their own pockets. In any event, the era in which cost was no object in health care seems to be drawing to an end.

Here, as earlier in the book, we wish to stress the fact that not merely financial cost, but physical, psychic, and social costs must be justified. The anxiety caused by testing, especially by false positives, must not be overlooked in making the ethical judgment about a particular test. In addition, the fact that some tests carry risks means that these costs, too, need to be justified.

In health as in every other aspect of life, we must husband our economic resources. So we must ask if the money expended on health produces results proportionate to the expenditure. This question of proportionality between cost and benefit becomes particularly acute when we are dealing not with tests done for diagnostic purposes, but with those done *routinely* as part of the examination of a *healthy person*. This would be the case in the annual physical. In 1980 the American Medical Association abandoned its long support of the routine annual physical (Mendelsohn, 1981). Many hospitals have long ceased demanding routine chest X-rays on admission. This tells us that the medical profession has rethought at least some of routine testing in terms of cost/benefit. As we noted in Chapter Four, patients who are forced to pay for larger and larger sums for testing may also begin to reevaluate their willingness to pay and so the value of the tests to them, no matter what their value to the health care provider.

The Charge of Overtesting

Physicians have been charged with overtesting, that is, using more tests than are necessary for the good of the patient. This may be due to a desire to know as much as possible about a given case whether or not the additional data will help the patient. As we have already noted in the consideration of costs, therapeutic rather than merely diagnostic accuracy is needed to justify the tests. Critics in the popular press claim that overtesting is due to the health care providers' efforts to protect themselves against malpractice suits. The professionals are alleged to feel safer if they can prove that they did *everything possible* and not merely everything necessary. Though this fear of malpractice due to a failure to test appears relatively groundless (Fortress and Kapp, 1985), the fear is still operative. Overtesting exists and can become so extreme that either the hospital or the physician's colleagues in a group practice have been known to bring greater pressure to bear on the offender. That is to say that there are cases of collective judgment by qualified peers that a physician is overtesting. Short of such a collective judgment, it can be difficult to decide when a physician is guilty of overtesting.

Robin (1984) asks whether even the collective judgment is valid, since he believes that overuse is not merely a problem of individual abuse, but a built-in fault of the entire health care system. While he makes a very strong case for this, and despite various review procedures mentioned in Chapter Eleven, we are still left with only the collective professional judgment as even a rough norm of overtesting in most cases.

We must consider that there is room for wide variation in the use of tests, both by medical speciality and by individual physicians. Internists by the nature of their work use more tests than surgeons. A consulting specialist who deals with difficult cases may use many more tests than a primary care physician. A naturally timid or cautious physician may also tend to use more tests. Thus, there is no sharp line to mark off overtesting from prudent testing. The collective judgment norm given above is broad, possibly biased, and, according to Robin, not easy to apply, but it is the best we have.

Testing and Informed Consent

Tests can sometimes involve more than minimal risks, and even routine tests cost money and require time of the patient. At least some of the elements of informed consent may enter into testing. The patient should be told the purpose of the test and the benefits, if any, to be gained by it, as well as the side effects and the risks, if any, beyond the minimum risks of everyday life. The authors have found that some physicians and nurses are evasive when asked what is to be gained by the test. Indeed, sometimes explanations of even a rudimentary sort are forthcoming only when the patient says, "Well, let's skip the test."

The patient should also be told the costs and the amount of time the test may require. One should not assume that every patient is willing to pay any amount or put up with any inconvenience for a marginal increase in the accuracy of diagnosis. In the cases of inefficient laboratories the patient may waste hours waiting and the patient's time is valuable. Indeed, the time may be more valuable to the patient than any benefit the health care provider can bestow.

The fact of costs should not be overlooked just because the patient has insurance that will pay for the test. Indeed, one way to test the necessity of the test may be to ask if it would be done if there were no insurance and the person could not pay for it. This, of course, fits in with our idea in Chapter Four that heightened cost consciousness is necessary if we are to mitigate, if not solve, the problem of health care allocation.

Even when a health care professional sees benefits from a test, the patient may not agree. For example, a patient may refuse a diagnostic procedure such as cardiac catheterization on the grounds not only of cost, pain, and danger, but also because she will not consent to any further treatment no matter what the result of the test. There comes a point where some patients just say "enough is enough" and refuse treatment and tests that might lead to treatment. That may seem puzzling to some health care providers, but there are, as we have pointed out in Chapter Two and Chapter Three, more than medical factors involved in making reasonable patient decisions.

The variability of interpretation and the heavy subjective component in this also raise a question as to whether ethics demands that patients be told the chance of testing errors and not allowed to believe that they are dealing with certitudes. For example, since the presence of exposure to AIDS is not detectable for a number of months after exposure, a negative test result may give an unjustified sense of security.

When it is not merely a question of the limits of a test, but of the fallibility of interpretation, should the patient be told and encouraged to get a second opinion? To put it another way, does respect for the dignity of the patient demand more disclosure than currently demanded by the principle of informed consent?

While revealing such chances of error will undoubtedly make the health care provider's job more difficult, it might also serve to demystify the whole process of health care. Neither of these effects is particularly harmful. Indeed, as we have suggested in Chapter Four, stripping health care of its cloak of scientific omniscience may help in reducing health care costs. In addition, patients who know that they are dealing with less than scientific certitude will be psychologically freer to exercise more autonomy and exact a greater degree of accountability from health care providers.

ETHICAL PROBLEMS OF MASS SCREENING

The previous section concentrated on the problems that arise from the use of tests not only in diagnosis but in routine screening of individuals. In this section, we consider related and additional problems that arise when tests are used for mass screening. In mass screening large numbers of apparently healthy people are tested in order to detect the few people with what is sometimes a relatively rare condition. Everyone has encountered mass screening during so-called Health Fairs conducted at shopping malls or by hospitals. At these, everyone is invited to have their blood pressure taken. Sometimes there are instant detection blood tests for diabetes and in the past there were chest X-rays for TB detection.

There are two sets of problems connected with mass screening. The first set is an extension of the problems of routine testing. The second set concerns stigmatization of certain populations, special problems of confidentiality, and the constantly recurring question of the proper distribution of health care resources.

False Positives in Mass Screening

The first set of problems arises from two facts. First, mass screenings with symptomless populations often produce higher rates of false positives. Second, when there is no truly effective treatment for the condition detected, the tests are medically useless.

The example of AIDS testing illustrates both points. Suppose that both tests mentioned in the first part of this chapter have been used to detect and "confirm" the presence of AIDS. If the joint false positive rate were 0.1 percent when symptomless women were tested, 10 women without the disease would be falsely identified for each one that was correctly identified (Mayer and Pauker, 1987). If there were only a single stage testing program, say, using equipment in a physician's office, the joint positive rate has been known to go as high as 0.5 percent and stigmatize 50 disease-free women for each true case actually detected.

The fact that AIDS is a stigmatizing disease for which there is no cure means that the mass screening cannot be justified on the basis of patient benefit. Indeed, a false positive rate that puts many people in a state of unnecessary agony raises further questions about the legitimacy of the screening. Finally, as we will see below, even screening for the protection of others may not be easy to justify.

Robin (1984) raised the same problem of false positives with regard to testing for pancreatic cancer. Similar questions can be asked about other forms of cancer screening, such as using mammography followed by various forms of chemotherapy and surgery (*Lancet*, 1984). Even the optimistic studies (Rodes et al., 1986) only say that their results *suggest* that improved survival in breast cancer screening programs is in *large measure* due to the ability to detect lesions before they become palpable. This study detected only 167 malignant lesions in the 10,187 asymptomatic patients tested. Again, the success rate of such screening raises disturbing questions about its appropriateness, even before we look at the cost factors.

Cost per Case Detected

In mass screening programs cost can be a particularly relevant factor. In the case of mass screenings there is a question not only of the cost of the individual test, but the cost of each case detected. Thus, though an individual test might cost only $3, it might cost $10,000 for each case detected. At the height of the agitation over drug testing in government and business, the Department of Defense spent $52 million dollars on two sets of tests on 3.6 million employees. Since only about 92,000 users were alleged to have been detected, it cost $500 to detect each alleged user. We stress that these were alleged users since, as noted, the test are not always perfect. There are then cost/benefit problems as well as questions about the distribution of health care resources.

The cost/benefit analysis might favor the drug tests in question if the end result was a proven improvement in health or efficiency or security. If there were no such improvements, the tests would have to be judged unfavorably even aside from the issue of stigmatization and civil rights, which we will discuss shortly.

In one instance, 21,071 people were screened for Tay-Sachs disease and 24 *at risk* couples were discovered; three pregnancies were monitored and one fetus was aborted. "At risk," of course, refers to the possibility of these couples having a child with Tay-Sachs disease and not to the fact that the couples could get the disease.

The program, which used less expensive batch methods of analyzing blood samples, cost $100,000, not counting the time of volunteers (Goodman and Goodman, 1982). If other methods of analysis had been used, the out-of-pocket costs could have run to $250,000, or $10,400 for each at-risk couple discovered.

While Tay-Sachs is a particularly horrible fate for a child and his parents, there is still a question of whether or not, from society's point of view, the money could have been used to better advantage. It could have been used for other ends, for example, providing basic health care to a large number of others, or it could have been used more efficiently, for example, the government-financed screening program could have used the more economical method of limiting testing to high risk pregnant women and then testing the husbands only if the woman were positive.

Something similar can be said of the mass screening involved in premarital blood tests for syphilis (Polonoff and Garland, 1979). Since the laws requiring those tests were passed, the use of antibiotics has radically reduced the rate of syphilis in the population. Less than 1 percent of all cases of syphilis were detected by premarital blood tests. In 1978, when only 123 cases were discovered by this method, it is estimated that $80,000,000 were spent on the tests. This means that each case detected cost $650,000. Once again, we ask if there are not better uses or at least more efficient uses of public funds.

Similar problems of cost per case detected arise with routine mass screening for AIDS, that is, for exposure to the AIDS virus. While there is a wide variation in estimates for the cost of cases detected by tests on a marriage application, they ran from $18,000 to $110,000 per case. The costs of counseling and follow-up are not included in these figures. Yet, there was no cure for AIDS and there was doubt as to whether mass screenings would only drive the high risk groups underground, compounding the problem.

The monetary costs of testing plus the debates about the utility of the testing pose serious questions about the ethics of allocation. We shall return to this later in this chapter.

Stigmatization

The second set of problems connected with mass screenings involves stigmatization. Stigmatization refers to placing a mark of infamy, disgrace, or reproach on a person or a group. Goffman (1963) refers to stigma as the situation of a person who is disqualified from full social acceptance. He also refers to stigma as an attribute or undesired differentness which is deeply discrediting. He also gives three classes of stigma, all of which can enter into health care (p. 4).

> First there are the abominations of the body—the various physical deformities. Next there are blemishes of individual character perceived as weak will, domineering or unnatural passions, treacherous and rigid beliefs, and dishonesty, these being inferred from a known record of, for example, mental disorder, imprisonment, addiction, alcoholism, homosexuality, unemployment, suicidal attempts and radical political behavior. Finally, there are the tribal stigma of race, nation and religion, these being stigma that can be transmitted through lineages and equally contaminate all members of the family.

The process of stigmatizing a person or group often involves emotion, taboos, and social prejudice rather than reason. Thus, it can occur no matter how good the intentions of those doing the screening. So serious are the felt effects of stigmatization that those at risk may prefer ignorance to knowledge when knowledge can lead to them being outcast. Indeed, so serious are the effects of the stigma when known that most make a serious effort to conceal them.

In the health care context, this effort to ignore or conceal can be particularly strong and very reasonable when there is no effective treatment for the condition that is the object of the screening. Confidentiality becomes increasingly important in these cases. We shall return to this problem shortly.

At the start of the AIDS epidemic, the fear of the disease was enormous and in direct proportion to the ignorance about it. Those who had the disease or who had even been exposed to it were often shunned, even by physicians and nurses in the hospital. They had been stigmatized. An attempt at a mass screening for the disease, even in populations at high risk, would have carried the risk of stigmatization and isolation even while there was no hope of a cure. No wonder the gay community, a high risk group, fought mass screening.

When awareness of a condition detected by the mass screening may lead not only to stigmatization, but to the subsequent loss of a job, refusal of health or life insurance, or, in the case of drug screening, trouble with the police, the objections to it become even stronger. Compulsory testing for drug usage certainly falls into this category. Here there is an invasion of the privacy of the body plus stigmatization that requires the gravest justifications. For this reason, health care providers should be wary of involvement in such testing. We shall attempt to draw more careful distinctions below when we discuss confidentiality.

Stigmatization and Genetic Screening

Sometimes, as in the case of Tay-Sachs disease, the screening is not a therapeutic but a preventative health measure designed to obtain information useful in genetic counseling, that is, for advising people about the chance that they will produce defective offspring. Those who object to abortion will, of course, object to screening that leads to abortion as a method of avoiding the defective child. Even when abortion is not anticipated, the health care provider should weigh the stigmatizing effect of an unfavorable test on both individuals and groups. The individual who learns that he has an incurable defect such that reproduction is not advisable may feel degraded. If the defect becomes known, the person with the defect may be left out of the marriage market and become a second class member of his group. Finally, when the screening involves ethnic or racial groups who are at high risk, there is danger of the entire group being stigmatized. This appears to be the case with screening for sickle cell anemia among American blacks and Tay-Sachs disease among Eastern European Jews. The most devastating case of all occurs when there is no cure for the disease, as is the case with Huntington's disease (Rosenfeld, 1984; see the case on this disease in Chapter Five).

In the case of Tay-Sachs disease, the Goodmans (1982) note that there was a special problem with the "apparent scientific confirmation of age-old prejudices about racial debility, clanishness and the like." In addition, the stigma discouraged marriage and reproduction between Eastern European Jews at a time when fertility is below replacement and the outmarriage rate is approaching 40 percent.

The problems of mass screening can only increase in the future as science discovers "markers" for patterns of genes associated with such diseases as heart attacks, emphysema, Altzheimer's disease, diabetes, and certain cancers. If tests for such markers are made standard procedures before life and health insurance can be issued, those stigmatized by the "marker" can find themselves uninsurable, or insurable only at a very high cost. This is particularly serious in the case of health insurance, where a person might end up with no insurance, and possibly no health care, because of a "marker" for a disease that may never appear or appear only 20 or 30 years later.

Confidentiality in Screening

The principles developed in Chapter Five obviously apply here. There are, however, special problems when the screening is not for the benefit of the patient, but for the benefit of the insurance company, or, allegedly, for the public health and safety. We shall return to the public health and safety issue shortly.

Even in these cases, the ethical problems are not major if the patient voluntarily consents to the screening and has been informed of the following: first, the specific persons to whom the results will be revealed; second, the actual risks of false positives; third, the potentially harmful consequences such as loss of a job, denial of entry into the country, or refusal of insurance. Finally, in the event that a test is positive, the person should have the right to be retested by an independent laboratory. This seems particularly important when even top-rated laboratories such as the Civil Aeromedical Laboratory of the Department of Transportation have been known to be sloppy in their procedures and even fraudulent in their results.[1]

While it is difficult to imagine many cases of a truly voluntary consent, when there are such serious harmful consequences, we must allow for the possibility. The health care professional, of course, should be on her guard against involuntary screening disguised as voluntary. The more serious problems arise with involuntary testing and the cooperation of health professionals in such screening.

Health care professionals should not take part in involuntary screening except when it is legally and ethically justified. It takes extremely serious reasons to justify even unwilling cooperation with unjustified involuntary testing.

We must ask, however, when involuntary testing or involuntary testing disguised as routine testing would be ethical and legal? We will divide our discussion into testing that is involuntary because mandated by law and that which is involuntary because some private group such as a corporation has the power to force the test on employees or prospective employees.

Involuntary Testing and the Public Good

Granted the protection of confidentiality, involuntary testing mandated by law would be legal and ethical only when necessary for the public health and legally enacted. Granted enactment of the law, the screening could be necessary for the public good if it could detect a serious threat to public health and *lead to effective preventative measures*. If there is no treatment available for the disease, or if there is no legal way to prevent the spread of the disease, the testing can hardly be called useful, let alone necessary for the public good. As the AIDS problem has demonstrated, it is one thing to detect a carrier of AIDS and another to convince the victim to avoid infecting others. Third, proposals to stop the spread of disease by quarantine need to be scrutinized carefully, since the most serious questions of civil rights are involved. A person cannot be deprived of his privacy, livelihood, and freedom to travel without due process of law, even when the public good is at stake. Indeed, since it is hard to keep the results confidential, useless tests expose people to the danger of stigmatization on the basis of tests that may have false positives. The danger of stigmatization needs to enter into the justification of even necessary tests.

Despite the potentially paternalistic nature of the law, we see no problem with legally mandated testing of newborns for conditions that should be detected and treated early. Such testing and treatment leads not only to the improvement of the quality of life, but to enormous savings to families and to society.

Compulsory Testing for Private Purposes

The ethics of compulsory testing of employees and prospective employees depends in the first place on whether or not the condition being detected is relevant to the business. Thus, drug and alcohol abuse can be relevant not only to safety and efficiency, but to the ability to resist temptation in handling drugs and large sums of money. On the other hand, it is not immediately obvious that AIDS is relevant to the functioning of a business except indirectly through its impact on health insurance premiums. Indeed, a case can be made that testing for AIDS and eliminating those who test positive is discrimination on the basis of handicap rather than on the basis of job-related factors.

The ethical health care professional will carefully study the relevance of testing before deciding to cooperate with a company that requires tests. When the tests are subject to a large number of false positives, which can cause serious impacts on the worker, the health care professional must see to it that the testing program is scientifically sound so that no unnecessary harm is done.

Testing and The Ethics of Allocation

The cost of tests on the basis of cases detected and the relationship of cases detected to cases successfully treated poses the problem of social allocation. When the tests are basically useless since they do not lead to effective treatment or prevention, they are clearly wasteful and should not be paid for out of public funds. Indeed, the government might well spend money educating the public to the sham of such screenings. In other cases, the screening, though expensive on a case-detected basis, can lead to some real good for some few individuals. The question then becomes: Is such screening part of the basic health care to which every individual is entitled? Or to put it another way: Is our human dignity disregarded if we are not screened for potential diseases or for diseases we might transmit to our children? Put this way, the question calls for a negative answer. Our dignity does not demand every possible health service. At the same time, and in line with our principles in Chapter Four, the society may decide that such screening is part of the basic health package to which every person is entitled. At the present time, cost consciousness about health care seems to militate against this, but the possibility remains. Public education as to the dangers and limits of testing and screening should make the society and individual health care consumers less anxious to submit to or pay for tests and screening. In short, the future decisions in this area should be based on increased awareness of what testing and health care can and cannot accomplish.

SUMMARY

In treatment situations, tests are ethically justified only if they can lead to an improvement in the patient's quality of life. The accuracy and interpretation of the tests, their tendency to give false positives and false negatives, and the availability of effective treatments enter into the justification of tests. Some tests are dangerous and need to be justified by proportionate benefits to the patient. The costs of tests must also enter into the decision if health costs are to be constrained. Overtesting by individual health care professionals is difficult to establish, though there is a suspicion that the entire system may lead to wasteful testing. The nature of tests raises questions about the duty to give patients more information about tests, so that they can accept or reject them in terms of the patient's priorities and values.

Voluntary screening may be ethical if the subject is told who will have access to the results and what harmful consequences may result. Involuntary screening by government needs justification in terms of the public good. Involuntary screening by private groups needs justification in terms of relevance to goals of the particular organization. In all screening, the danger of stigmatization, the high cost of cases detected, and the dangers to confidentiality need special consideration. The cost factors of mass screening often pose problems in fair allocation of health resources.

CASES FOR ANALYSIS

1.   Magdelene, a nursing student, is taking part in a health fair at the Uptown Mall. She takes blood pressures with a cuff that has not been calibrated in a long time. Despite this she suggests that those with borderline and high readings visit their personal physicians. She also does simple accuchecks for blood sugar, and makes refer-

rals where indicated. She has no idea if the machine has been calibrated and what the margin of error is. She has no idea if any of people she refers will go for help, if she has needlessly alarmed them, or if she is wasting her Saturday afternoon at the Mall.

2.   Dr. Propaideutic, a country physician, has invested in office blood testing equipment and a stress test machine, which he wants to pay off in a hurry. He uses the equipment routinely since many of his patients have never had a full check-up. He does not worry about the accuracy of the machine, though there have been articles about the need to calibrate them. He does not worry about overuse, since Blue Cross and Blue Shield and Medicare will just refuse to pay him if he overuses the tests.

His early experience has been that the tests generate other income since they unearth problems which require additional treatment. Besides, the patients appreciate the convenience of having the test right there rather than traveling 30 miles to the nearest city with a regular laboratory.

3.   Mary Einfuhling works as a medical technologist in a large commercial laboratory which has just started to do drug testing for the Azziz manufacturing company, the major employer in her small town. She is very aware that some of the tests used to detect drug usage are insensitive, that is, give false positives. Urine tests used to detect marijuana use will give positive results if the person had used ibuprofen, which is found in such over the counter drugs as Advil and Nuprin. Some cold remedies, such as Contac, will also cause the subject of the test to show up as an amphetamine user. Good procedure would call for expensive additional tests to discover what the person had actually taken.

The owners of the laboratory have told Azziz of the limits of the tests, but additional tests are not done. Quite a few people were fired after the first tests were reported to the company. Now Mary comes across a positive test for her boyfriend, who she knows never takes anything stronger than a cold remedy or an antibiotic prescribed by his physician. She falsifies the test result.

4.   A for-profit hospital which has just moved into the area wants to demonstrate community awareness and to attract business. It decides to sponsor colorectal cancer screening or, more accurately, the free use of hematocrit kits. These will detect the presence of bleeding that is not visible to the naked eye and indicate the need for additional examination for possible cancer of the colon.

While the cost of the individual test is small, the cost of mass screening may be high in terms of the number of cases detected and successfully treated. There is then a question of whether or not the screening really makes good sense. In 1978 the Consensus Development Conference on Mass Screening for Colorectal Cancer concluded that there was insufficient data to prove that the test reduced mortality in a screened population. The report also indicated that the benefit/cost risk indexes could not be calculated and recommended that the uncontrolled use of the method outside of special evaluation studies may not be of benefit to patients. Robin (1984) notes that nothing has changed since that time.

Despite this, the marketing department pushes the tests, even though some of the medical staff object that the campaign may deceive the public. Others on the medical staff disagree.

NOTES

[1]The scandal connected with this laboratory is described by Walt Bogdanich, "Testing Debacle: Federal Lab Studying Train, Airline Crashes Fabricated Its Findings," *Wall Street Journal* July 31, 1987, pp. 1 and 16. It would appear that some of the technicians did not even know how to use the sophisticated equipment.

Chapter Eleven
ENFORCING STANDARDS IN THE HEALTH PROFESSIONS

INTRODUCTION

Traditionally, the learned professions, including medicine, were supposed to control entrance into the profession and to police themselves. This obligation is twofold. In the first place, there is the obligation to maintain and improve the quality of health care. In the second place, there is the obligation to police the profession in order to protect the public from dangerous and unqualified practitioners.

The obligation to maintain and improve the quality of health care is acknowledged in ethical code provisions like the following from The American Nurses Association:

> 5. The nurse maintains competence in nursing.
> 7. The nurse participates in activities that contribute to the ongoing development of the profession's body of knowledge.
> 8. The nurse participates in the profession's efforts to implement and improve standards of nursing.
> 11. The nurse collaborates with members of the health professions and other citizens in promoting community and national efforts to meet the health needs of the public.

While not so explicit or broad ranging, at least one principle of the American Medical Association applies here:

> V. The physician shall continue to study, apply and advance scientific knowledge, make relevant information available to patients, colleagues and the public, obtain consultation, and use the talents of other health professionals when indicated.

The obligation to police, which includes the obligation to blow the whistle, is recognized in varying ways by the following excerpts from the codes of health care providers.

The American Nurses Association:

> 3. The nurse acts to safeguard the client and the public when health care and safety are affected by the incompetent, unethical or illegal practice of any person.
> 10. The nurse participates in the profession's effort to protect the public from misinformation and misrepresentation and to maintain the integrity of nursing.

The American Physical Therapy Association (1987):

> 7.1 Physical therapists are to report any conduct which appears to be unethical, incompetent, or illegal.

The American Medical Association (1980 version):

> A physician shall deal honestly with patients and colleagues and shall strive to expose those physicians deficient in character and competence, or who engage in fraud or deceptions.

The American Medical Association (1986) is more explicit in its Current Opinions of the Council on Ethical and Judicial Affairs:

> 9.04 DISCIPLINE AND MEDICINE. A physician should expose, without fear or favor, incompetent or corrupt, dishonest or unethical conduct on the part of members of the profession. Questions of such conduct should be considered, first, before proper medical tribunals in executive sessions or by special or duly appointed committees on ethical relations, provided that such a course is possible and provided, also, that the law is not hampered thereby. If doubt should arise as to the legality of the physician's conduct, the situation under investigation may be placed before officers of the law, and the physician-investigators may take the necessary steps to enlist the interest of the proper authority.

These citations express professional obligations first to maintain and promote standards of care, and second to police the profession and to protect the public from incompetent practitioners.

PROMOTING QUALITY

The maintenance and promotion of standards theoretically falls within the responsibilities not only of individual health professionals but of such professional groups as the hospital's medical staff committees on credentials, on tissues, and on medical records as well as of government mandated Professional Review Organizations, which must oversee Medicare and in some states Medicaid as well. In theory, too, peer review by the board which oversees state licensure might also have some weight here. In practice, things are not quite so simple.

Hospital utilization review procedures are concerned with the allocation of hospital resources in an effort to provide high quality care in a cost-effective manner. Their focus is on cost considerations, such as overutilization, underutilization, and inefficient scheduling of resources, rather than directly on the quality of care.

The credentials committee examines the qualifications of those who apply for staff privileges. The tissue committee examines and evaluates the tissues removed during surgery to see if the surgery was really medically indicated. The medical records committee not only examines records for completeness, but is also to act as a judge of clinical care as this is reflected in the records.

Professional Review Organizations (PROs), which replaced the Professional Standard Review Organization (PSRO), were federally mandated to determine whether the care given to Medicare patients is of sufficient quality and delivered at a reasonable cost. State and Medicaid programs may also use PROs. As with utilization review, the PROs' primary concern with cost and focus on meeting professional standards does not assure that they are truly determiners of quality, let alone sources of improved quality.

In practice, the boards that control state licensure are, at best, involved primarily in setting standards for entrance and occasionally for disciplining those who violate the standards. Some nursing boards require evidence of continuing education, but this is not true of medical licensing boards. The licensing boards are not involved in ongoing study of the quality of the physicians' or nurses' performance and do not require reexamination. It should be noted that even the specialty boards which certify a physician in a specialty do not, with the exception of the Family Practice Board, require reexamination at periodic intervals. In any event, there is a question as to whether all of these committees and groups constitute adequate ways of judging and improving the quality of medical care.

This question grows even larger when we realize that these boards are interested in technical competence rather than total competence, which would include the ability of the professional to relate to people and to treat them with due respect for their dignity as human beings.

Judging Quality

Even if these groups demanded continuing education and had formal reviews of practice, this would not necessarily assure the maintenance or improvement of the quality of health care. There is in the first place no agreement as to what are the criteria of quality health care. In the second place, even if we had agreement about the criteria, there would still be grave doubts about our ability to apply the criteria.

Three broad criteria could be used to measure the quality of health care: (1) inputs, (2) process, and (3) outcomes. The input analysis would look at the preparation of the health care professionals and their credentials as well as the availability of state of the art equipment and facilities. Process analysis of quality would consider what the health care professionals did or did not do. They would be judged in terms of procedures and protocols that are approved by the appropriate bodies or at least by an informal consensus of professionals. The third method, outcomes analysis, would look at the results of the health care. It would ask if patients got better and how soon, as well as whether the health care system as a whole lowered mortality rates or the rate of infection. As part of the evaluation of the quality of health care, the rates in one country or part of a country might be compared with the rates somewhere else.

Each of these methods rests on assumptions that are debatable (Jonas, 1981). The input method assumes that the right credentials and right equipment equal quality care. The credentials, however, do not tell us if the practitioner graduated at the top or the bottom of the class or are well trained in the use of the latest equipment. The process method may unearth mistakes, but it does not ask if the approved and accepted methods are themselves sound. In short, it assumes that the accepted methods are normative. The outcome method assumes that there is some common method of comparison of results. Unfortunately, one hospital may have a higher death rate than another because it has sicker patients and will try to save even high risk cases. Lacking a common starting place, it is hard to judge outputs.

In additions to the assumptions, there are other difficulties. Before tackling those difficulties it will be useful to study the results of a late 1980s survey by the National Research Corporation, which sheds both light and darkness on the matter.

The study asked how quality in health care should be measured. The physicians surveyed offered the following answers: (1) by health outcomes (24 percent); (2) by internal physician review (13 percent); (3) by peer review (13 percent); (4) by patient satisfaction (9 percent); and (5) by mortality rates (9 percent). Only numbers one and five are concerned with what could be objectively measurable outcomes. Numbers two, three, and four really do not tell us how outcomes would be measured, but by whom. These replies miss the whole point. Concentration on process, such as occurs in much peer review and internal physician review, is not very meaningful unless it has been scientifically established that the process improves outcomes. Patient satisfaction may be a poor indicator of quality unless the meaning of patient satisfaction and the manner of ascertaining it are carefully specified. Even health outcomes and mortality, as already noted, are not as easy to ascertain as one might think.

In both health outcomes and mortality measurements, there are problems of definition and of the selection of populations for study. The norm for improvement in health is not a simple thing (Muskin and Dunlop, 1979). Where one group will define it in terms of mortality and expectancy or disability, another will define it in terms of restoration of full functioning, while still others see health only in terms of being able to function as one pleases. This is to say that preference scales must be considered. This is in accord with our idea in Chapter Four that the desires of society and of individuals play a role in the very definition of health and disease. Finally, there are questions of whether the mere relief of pain or the diminution of symptoms are favorable *health* outcomes, even though they are certainly desirable *medical* outcomes.

The mortality criterion poses similar problems. One area may have a higher death rate than another simply because it has a much older population. Merely increasing the amount of medical care may or may not improve health and mortality statistics. Indeed, if health care lowers the mortality rate while leaving us with more suffering old people, it may not have been quality health care at all. Indeed, one may ask if care which decreases human dignity and prolongs human suffering is worthy of even the name health care.

Strangely enough, there is evidence that during the strikes of physicians and other health care workers, the death rate goes down (Rothman, 1983), only to resume its former rate when health care is restored. While the lowering of the death rate may be due to the postponement of elective surgery, it does point up the fact that health care can be damaging to your health. The writings of Illich (1976) and Robin (1984) on iatrogenic (physician-induced) diseases raises similar interesting questions about the relative value of health care.

In all of this, it is well to remember that 70 percent of all conditions which are presented to the primary care physician are self-limiting, that is, will go away by themselves. Treatment may speed up the healing, but it is not always necessary. In any event, it may be hard to say how much of the "cure" is due to health care and how much to Mother Nature or the patient's own activities.

The final difficulty involves the fact that improvements in the health of entire populations as well as of individuals are due to factors other than health care. Environmental factors such as clean air and water and safe working conditions are important for health. Like it or not, genetic endowment also plays a major role in both health and longevity. Finally, cultural and lifestyle factors such as diet, exercise, sleep, the use of tobacco and alcohol, and the safety of one's sexual practices may have more to do with maintaining and improving health than all the health care in the world. It is thus difficult to say what is due to health care and what to other health related factors.

We are left with the conclusion that assessing the quality of health care and the contribution of health care to the well being of society is not an easy task. Yet it is a task that needs to be done. Since the individual practitioner cannot do it, the health care professions and ultimately the society as a whole have an obligation to research the issue and to make public policy in accord with the results of the research.

If the research discovers that much health care is meaningless and should be eliminated, we have discovered one means of easing the problem of distribution which has so often been considered in the course of this book.

THE OBLIGATION TO POLICE

The healing professions, like other full-fledged professions, fulfill needs in society and in return for this are given special privileges, such as a monopoly on certain activities. These professions are also charged with policing their own members in order to protect the clients and the public good. Because special knowledge is required to furnish this protection, the society has frequently given the decisions of professional groups the force of law. Thus, to a large extent, the professions are accountable directly to themselves and only indirectly to the government.

In court, where there is accountability to the public, the health care professions often find themselves more severely judged than when only peers are involved. Indeed, it may be argued that the increasing malpractice judgments against health professionals may indicate that the professions should be more stringent in their self-policing and look to the standards of the public as well as to those of the profession. Self-interest as well as professional obligation call for vigorous self-policing if the professions are to keep their privileges.

The policing includes examinations for licensing and in many cases periodic reexamination, peer review by hospital staffs and supervisory personnel, and, increasingly, review by panels appointed to hear complaints about professional misconduct.

Official Policing

In theory, the State Board of Nursing Examiners or the State Medical Boards are the official policing agencies for their respective professions. Though generally appointed by the governor, the nominations come from the profession, so that these boards can be seen as professional groups backed up with state power. There is, however, debate as to how well the State Medical Boards do their jobs. According to the Federation of State Medical Boards, the number of physicians disciplined in 1985 increased 59 percent over the year before. At the same time an Inspector General of Health and Services had criticized the board for disciplining strikingly few physicians. In practice, many states have legal impediments that block them from disciplining physicians. The variation in legal impediments and zeal may help to explain why disciplining differs greatly from state to state. In 1985 Nevada disciplined 2 percent of all the physicians in the state. Alaska disciplined none. New York with its huge number of physicians revoked only 42 medical licenses. Connecticut revoked no licenses and put only four on probation.

The seeming failure to police vigorously may be a cause of the number of malpractice suits, and the increase in policing may be an attempt to hold down suits by weeding out the bad apples.

The practice acts in the various states generally have provisions about self-policing. The following excerpt from a Pennsylvania law entitled *Impaired Professionals* (63 P.S., 422.4) is an example of the statutory duty to denounce. Note that this act also provides immunity from prosecution for those who blow the whistle in good faith.

Any hospital or health care facility, peer or colleague who has substantial evidence that a nurse has an active addictive disease for which the professional is not receiving treatment, is diverting a controlled substance, or is mentally or physically incompetent to carry out the duties of his license shall make or cause to be made a report to the Board: Provided that any person or facility who acts in a treatment capacity to impaired nurses in an approved treatment program is exempt from the mandatory reporting requirements of this subsection.

While the health care professions recognize a duty to denounce, they are not in agreement as to what should be done and on what basis. Different professions have different requirements. The physical therapists require that even *alleged* unethical, incompetent, or illegal acts be reported. The Pennsylvania proposal requires *substantial evidence*. The ANA requires that the nurses *safeguard* the patient, while the physical therapist is specifically required to report. Even within a profession, there have been substantial shifts in requirements. The 1980 AMA code asks that the physician *strive to expose*, where the 1957 version of the AMA Code called for the physician to "expose without hesitation." In view of these differences, it is necessary to go back and develop a consistent ethics of self-policing and whistle blowing for the health professions.

The Obligation to Report?

The obligation to denounce can arise from both the general ethical principles and from the nature of the health care professions, that is, from the special role that is assigned to the health care provider.

The general obligation to avoid evil unless there is a proportionate reason for permitting or risking it is the root of the obligation to denounce. The nature of the health professions adds additional force as well as specification to the general obligation to avoid evil. All of the health professions involve a commitment to the health of the patient and to the good of the profession. The public considers the commitment to the health of the patient part of the role and so of the contract with the health care professional. Traditionally, physicians have been patient advocates, and the professional nurses have adopted the advocacy role as part of their general professional role. The trust in the promise of advocacy and the good will of the professional further increases the obligation to protect the patient. In short, health care practitioners have not only the general obligation to avoid evil but the specific obligation to prevent evil from happening to patients.

It is not merely an obligation to the individual patient, but to all patients and to the public health that creates the obligation. This is clear from the following positive obligation proposed in the ANA Code (1985):

The nurse works with members of health professions and other citizens in promoting efforts to meet the health needs of the public.

The good of the profession also demands that the individual practitioner and the profession as a whole work for the elimination of harmful practices and the control or removal of practitioners who engage in them. This comes not only from the commitment of the profession but from justifiable self-interest. If a profession does not police itself, the public and society will ultimately demand an accounting. We wonder if the present increase in malpractice suits is not just such a demand for better policing of the professions by the professions. In other words, if the health care professions do not do the job of policing, the public will use whatever means it can to express its disapproval and to punish the professions.

Reporting and the Impaired Professional

The law on impaired professionals cited earlier provides an exception when the health care professional is undergoing rehabilitation. There is great need for such rehabilitation since professionals in health care and physicians in particular have higher than average rates of drug dependence, alcoholism, mental problems, and marital troubles. Health care can be dangerous not only to the patients but to the providers of care.

This rehabilitation exception is justified as long as patients are in no danger during the rehabilitation period. Indeed, granted the protection of patients, health care professionals ought to strive to get impaired colleagues into treatment. This obligation springs not only from the general duty of beneficence, but from a collegial duty to other professionals and the obligation to protect the profession and the patients. In no case, however, should the effort to help an impaired professional be an excuse for risking harm to patients.

The Means of Protecting the Public

To fulfill the obligation to police their own ranks, the professions have a variety of means available. No one of them will cure the problem, but all of them taken together will have an impact. Some protection can be afforded by demanding proof of continuing education. Not all groups and not all specialties inside groups currently demand such proof. Additional protection can be afforded by the quality assurance programs, Professional Review Boards, and even Utilization Review Boards. Unfortunately, these are not designed to detect what happens outside the hospital. Sometimes they are said to be more concerned with the insurance company than with the patient. Experience, however, has shown that these are not sufficient. Among other things, the fear of being sued by fellow doctors puts a damper on peer review. Only in 1986 when the Ninth Circuit Court of Appeals overruled a ruling which had given a judgment of $1.95 million against a peer review panel did physicians begin to breathe a little easier (James, 1986). Physicians' liability insurance did not cover the judgment. Fears of such actions help to explain some of the problems with peer review.

Where there is a chain of command, as in a hospital or other health care facility, dangerous or lax practice should be reported through that chain. Often nothing will happen since even health care agencies are often ruled by principles such as "do not

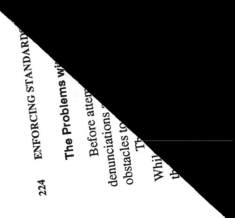

rock the boat," or the even more cynical "to
serious and nothing happens, the health c
methods to remedy the situation.

Public Denunciation or Whistle Blow

Peer review and reporting through the cl
In these cases *public* denunciation or whistle
ment of professional ethics. The obligation t
failed, is grounded in two simple ideas: Fir
Second, the inaction of good people is the mai
harm others.

What Should Be Denounced

In general, anything which violates the rights of the patient or threatens the
physical, psychological, or medico- economic well-being of the patient should be considered for denunciation.

We say that it should be *considered* for denunciation, since it should be obvious
that some threats of harm are so trivial and so infrequent that the harm to the morale
of the health care team will not justify the small good to be obtained by denouncing
them. The morale of the health care team is important and we will return to it below.
The obligation to blow the whistle, then, is *limited to events that are, with rare exceptions, repeated and are of such a nature as to seriously harm patients or the profession.* Something should be done about the physician or nurse who seldom practices
sterile technique, since sooner or later serious harm will result. Something should be
done about the provider who frequently comes to work under the influence of drugs
or alcohol. There may be no need to denounce the isolated instance of drunkenness,
though the provider should be kept temporarily away from patients.

Repeated violations of the patients rights, including those in the *Patients Bill of
Rights* of the American Hospital Association, should also be denounced. Not all of
these rights are equally important, but repeated violations show a contempt for patients
that should not be tolerated. Indeed, since perceived contempt for the patient will
cause more and more malpractice suits, mere self-interest dictates action in this area.

An Important Warning

Although the Physical Therapists Code calls for reporting *alleged unethical, incompetent, or illegal acts,* great care should be exercised. First, if the provider has
not witnessed the offense and its repetition, but has only heard about it, there may be
cause for reporting the rumor to a superior, but there is certainly no grounds for whistle
blowing. Rumor and gossip should be viewed with suspicion here as elsewhere in
life. Second, the supervisor should investigate carefully, looking for evidence, including written and signed descriptions of what was observed. Third, if the investigation
starts to point a guilty finger at a person, the rules for due process given below must
be observed.

th Whistle Blowing

...ipting to answer the questions about when and how and by whom ...re to be made, it is necessary to face the legal, emotional, and social ... whistle blowing.

...e legal obstacles to whistle blowing are important if not always clear-cut. ...e the public might think of a license to practice medicine or nursing as a privilege, ...at license also represents a valuable property right. As such it is guarded by the right to due process. As a result, a health care person who has his license taken away by the licensing board can sue for damages as well as restoration of the license. This has made many boards hesitant to act.

Even if the health care professional whose license has been revoked or suspended does not sue, she has the right to have the case reviewed by the courts. This process can drag on for years. The result is time consuming and expensive for all involved. If the board of licensing lacks funds for good lawyers, they may hesitate to get involved in the cases that may drag on forever.

In some states, the law does not allow for a gradation of penalties. The licensing board in these states may hesitate to take away the license except in the most serious cases. The result is that there is relatively little policing in these cases. Other states that provide not only for revocation and suspension, but for fines and censures and conditions of rehabilitation, have more flexibility and so are less hesitant to use a lesser penalty that may do the job.

The social obstacles to whistle blowing are known to everyone. Nobody likes to be a snitch. There are three reasons for this. First, we are all aware that we are not perfect and so might be the next victim. Second, we all develop loyalty to our group and fellow workers and can see whistle blowing as a violation of that loyalty. Third, we know all too well that the whistle blower may suffer retaliation from the organization as well as from the individual who was denounced.

The awareness of our own imperfection and the fear that we may be next is understandable, but not a valid excuse. If this were an excuse, then we would have an excuse for doing nothing about any evil in the world. A health professional does not have such an excuse when repeated events threaten serious harm to patients. The matter is too serious to permit such general and casual escapes.

Whistle blowing can hurt the credibility and cohesion of the health care team and the health care profession. Loyalty to both makes one hesitate about blowing the whistle. Group and peer loyalty is an important factor since the good of the patient depends on the smooth functioning of the group and this depends on trust and even loyalty to the team. The team, however, is not the goal of health care but only a means, and so the team is subordinated to the good of the patient. To put the team first is to displace goals and to act as if patients existed for the doctors and nurses and not the other way around.

For all that, loyalty does have its claims. Fellow feeling for those with whom one works with and on whom one depends is not only understandable but necessary in health care as in the rest of life. For this reason, among others, we have insisted that it is only when other means have failed and when there is a repeated threat of serious harm to patients that whistle blowing becomes obligatory. Once again, it is a question of a complicated balancing of factors.

The fear of retaliation is not unfounded. People have been fired for blowing the whistle even when they were justified. Whistle blowing can also lead to being black-balled or shunned. In some cases the denunciation provokes countercharges and involves the provider in long and costly litigation. It takes courage to blow the whistle. In line with our general principles, the potential harm to oneself must be part of the calculation of the consequences. The risk to oneself cannot be the sole factor. The good of the profession and the patient and the seriousness of the evil to be avoided have their ethical claims.

In this context, the remarks of Shirley Stoll, a nurse clinician who exposed abuse in a Veterans Administration hospital, are very much to the point. She gives 10 rules based on her experience with whistle blowing. Several are particularly chilling. Rule Four: Expect the worst: the loss of your job at least. Rule Six: Know you will be criticized and humiliated. Rule Nine: Do not expect that your life will ever be the same. It will not. The realization of such truths has made even the brave hesitate to blow the whistle, with the result that much evil continues unabated.

All of these difficulties provide health care workers with so many potential excuses that there is a danger that the good of patients will not be properly protected unless the health care professions unite to protect their members who fulfill their duties to patients. We will return to this when we consider the obligations of the profession as a whole.

No one is obliged to do the impossible. There are cases where the evil is so rooted in the institution that no individual cam remove it. In these cases, there is certainly no obligation to denounce or to do anything except possibly resign when the evil is too monstrous.

Who Shall Denounce?

Those who are formally charged with preventing the evils have the greatest responsibility in this area. Supervisors, chiefs of staff, and ombudsmen are the clearest examples. Because they are formally charged with preventing the evil, we do not believe that they can be excused merely because they might suffer as a result of doing their duty. The board of directors or the trustees of a health care institution, have, of course, the ultimate responsibility for everything in their facilities. They have the obligation to make sure that there is no need for denunciation. One can, however, see cases where individual members would have to blow the whistle on the entire board. This might occur where an institution continuously covers up the incompetence of employees and physicians who are doing serious harm to patients.

Not only those formally charged with preventing the evils but every health care professional also has the *prima facie* obligation to blow the whistle. This obligation disappears only when the good anticipated is outweighed by the evil. Finally, even nonprofessionals who see the evil have some obligation to prevent it. This group generally has less power, and its obligation arises from the general duty to avoid evil and not from professional commitment to the patient. Even the nonprofessional cannot merely stand about mute in the face of fraud and clear incompetence.

When Should One Blow the Whistle?

Denunciation or whistle blowing is a last resort. It should occur only after a whole series of interventions has been attempted. In the first place, the health care professional who witnesses an evil should attempt to intervene personally and discretely with the person at fault. Unfortunately, it is often clear that this will do no good or will involve disproportionate harm to the whistle blower. When this is true, or the intervention has failed, the person should proceed to report the evil through channels. At times this is not feasible, since it may be first-line supervisory personnel who are the guilty parties or are protective of the guilty parties. When either of these conditions exists, going over the heads of supervisors is necessary. Only when all these interventions have failed is the witness of the wrongdoing justified in going first to outside supervisory agencies, such as the Board of Medical Examiners, the State Board of Nursing Licensure, or legislative oversight committees. When these groups fail to respond, the desperate and dangerous appeal to the press and so the general public is in order, at least when we are dealing with extremely serious matters.

Due Process in Handling Denunciations

Those who are denounced have a right to due process, that is, to the protection of a fair procedure. While it is not necessary to have the elaborate procedures of a court system, a certain minimum is required. First, the supervisor should make sure that the charge is clear and specific and described in nonevaluative terms. Dates and places and details are important. Vague charges such as "Everybody knows she is careless" are of little value. In other words, the supervisor should concentrate on what was done or not done, not on what the accuser feels about the event.

Second, the supervisor should demand evidence. Were there other witnesses? What is on the chart? Is the accuser willing to put everything in writing so that there is evidence if the accuser later tries to back out? We note that the need for evidence at this stage pretty well rules out the anonymous whistle blower. Yet, even the anonymous charge should be investigated if it is serious enough. The matter should proceed, however, only when real evidence is discovered.

Third, when the investigation reveals that there is evidence, the supervisor or the appropriate board should allow the accused to answer the charge and to face the accuser and so to defend himself. The meaning of the facts is not always as evident as the facts themselves. The person accused of drunkeness because he was staggering may have been suffering from an inner ear infection. The person accused of striking a patient may have been defending herself. Things are not always what they seem at first glance.

Health care facilities should have due process procedures in place both to protect the accused from unjust allegations and to protect the accuser from their own enthusiasm and lack of experience.

The Obligations of the Professions

It should be obvious that the professions need to set up mechanisms for receiving complaints and for judging them according to the rules of due process. The boards, however, will lack credibility if they are composed only of members of the profession. There is a need for outside members on the boards for several reasons. In the first place, the outsiders should bring to the board a sensitivity to the views of the general public and a critical point of view, which does not simply say, "But that is the way we have always done it." In the second place, the outside members, who are consumers rather than providers of health care, will be less tempted to give too much weight to the good of the profession as opposed to the good of patients and the public. The outside member is also more likely to look critically at the nontechnical aspects of the case, which have much to do with the dignity of the individual. Such critical examination of the human aspects of health care can easily be overlooked by the busy health care professional. In short, outside members should help to reinforce the credibility of the board and, more importantly, should increase protection for the dignity of the patient.

If the boards are to work, then people must not fear retaliation if they report wrongdoing. In practice, that means that some professions, such as nursing and physical therapy, must have more power and be ready and willing to defend their members against retribution. This is particularly important since nurses in particular are the professionals most likely to observe incompetence and fraud in both nurses and physicians. If the nurse abandons her advocacy role because of fear of retribution, the entire health care system suffers.

The last paragraph mentions power, since it is impossible to do good without power, even as power allows some people to continue doing evil. While we insist that might is not right, we also insist that right without might is not practically effective. The problem of power in health care, however, is subject matter for another book.

SUMMARY

There is a professional obligation to improve health care and to report and even denounce those health care professionals who are dangerous to patients. Improving the quality of health care is particularly difficult since we have no easy method of evaluating quality. Eliminating dangerous practitioners is equally difficult. Many of the existing institutions which are supposed to police for both quality and the lack of quality are not particularly effective for a variety of reasons. Loyalty to the patient should, with the rare exceptions of trivial matters, take precedence over all professional loyalties. The various health professions need to organize and demand greater accountability from their members both as regards continuing education and the meeting of professional standards.

Both those who report failures and those who handle the reports should make sure that due process is followed, evidence gathered, and the accused be given a change to rebut the accusations. Mere rumors should not be the basis of denunciations, though they should sometimes be reported for investigation.

CASES FOR ANALYSIS

1. Mrs. Lewis was head nurse on a medical surgical floor in a community hospital of 250 beds. Over the course of six months she noticed that all patients admitted from the Shady Rest Nursing Home had signs of severe injuries other than those connected with the admitting diagnosis. There appeared to be patient abuse in the nursing home. Mrs. Lewis investigated discretely and found no explanation possible except abuse. In accord with the obligations of the law in her state, she reported the matter to the Department of Welfare Bureau of Inspection.

The Welfare Department investigated immediately, found proof of abuse, and threatened to close down Shady Rest if there were any recurrences. Mrs. Lewis was overjoyed until her hospital administrator, bypassing the Director of Nursing, called her in and warned her that she would be fired if she did any more reporting of abuse. Shady Rest sent the hospital a lot of business and good relations should be maintained.

Mrs. Lewis was even more shocked when she discovered that the administrator was a golf partner of the owner of Shady Rest and was doing an old buddy a favor. Mrs. Lewis, despite fears of retaliation, consulted a lawyer, who threatened the hospital with exposure and with the penalties that would follow if one of its employees failed to follow the reporting provisions of the law on abuse in nursing homes.

2. All the nurses in obstetrics and all the physicians on the obstetrics/gynecological service know that Dr. Borracho is an alcoholic. He frequently appears so intoxicated as to be unable to measure the dilation of the cervix. On one occasion he examined a woman and told her she had several hours before delivery. The baby's head appeared before he got out of the room. Up to now there have been no serious injuries to mothers or children because the nurses have been able to stop him from committing really serious mistakes. Of late, however, Dr. Borracho is getting violent when the nurses intercede. The Director of Nursing has been informed and done nothing since Borracho has a lot of influence in the hospital and the Director does not believe in rocking the boat with physicians.

3. Just about half the residents of the small town of Pamplona know that Dr. Cannabis is the equivalent of a drug pusher. He will write you a perscription for just about anything at any time or in any place. You do not have to be his patient and no questions are asked as long as you hand over $10 for the script. Repeated denunciations to the State Board of Medical Examiners have done little good. Dr. Cannabis is a member of the board of directors of the hospital and his group practice is a major supplier of patients to the hospital. What should be done?

4. Ms. Smith, a nurse in the 150 bed community hospital in Ocala (population 50,000), is a shrewd overseer. She has noted that Dr. Coupay does an extraordinary number of hysterectomies on very young women. He does as many as 10 to 15 a week.

While nursing Dr. Coupay's patients, Ms. Smith gets the impression that they were rushed into the operation and did not fully understand what was happening. Through friends in pathology, she hears a rumor that most of these hysterectomies appear to have been unnecessary, since there were no signs of cancer or fibroids and no signs of damage to the uterus. She mentions this to her supervisor, who tells her that the matter is being investigated. Besides, the hospital census is down and those patients help to keep things going. Six months later the situation is unchanged.

5. Dr. Furibund carries a loaded magnum 44 strapped to his leg at all times, including his long hours in the operating room. Dr. Furibund is an obnoxious person and thoroughly disliked. He justifies carrying the gun on the grounds that people are out to get him. The carrying of the gun violates hospital rules and makes his fellow surgeons and the nurses very anxious, especially when he flourishes it in public. The chief of surgery has witnessed Furibund showing his gun in the physician's lounge but has done nothing about it.

Chapter Twelve
THE ETHICS
OF BIOMEDICAL
RESEARCH

INTRODUCTION

Biomedical research involves both human and animal subjects. We will be concerned only with research that utilizes human beings, including the fetus, as subjects. Those interested in the ethics of animal research should consult Tannenbaum and Rowan (1985) for an excellent overview of the problems in this area.

The ethical problems with research using human subjects involve not only the research proper, but the use made of the research. We will, then, examine the ethics of both the researcher and the consumer of research. By the consumer, we mean the health care provider who reads the research and must make a decision as to whether the research may be applied in practice.

It is also useful to draw distinctions between validated clinical practice and experimental clinical practice. A practice is clinically validated when it has been scientifically studied in clinical trials and the results of the study indicate that it meets the criteria for validation. Other clinical practices, whether accepted in practice or not, may be spoken of as nonvalidated.

Experimental practice may be of two sorts. First, it may involve the trial-and-error method of determining what will work for *a particular patient* when validated and/or accepted practices have failed. This sort of experimentation is a part of normal medical practice. In a second sense, the treatment may be experimental practice in that it seeks to find out if this treatment will help *patients in general*. When the treatment is being used to discover generalizable knowledge, we are in the realm of scientific research where tests should involve a carefully drawn hypothesis in an attempt to draw general conclusions. This type of experimental research is the principal concern of the present chapter.

At the very start, it should be clear that human experimentation is necessary for medical progress. Animal testing is useful, but it cannot provide the final word on either safety or efficacy. At the same time, human beings are not mere objects that can be used as the experimenter desires. In the first place, informed consent is even more necessary here than in the case of treatment. This is particularly true when we are dealing with nontherapeutic research, that is, with research that will not directly benefit the subjects. Since research, unlike validated treatment, ventures into the unknown, the risks are greater and harder to estimate, with the result that the calculation of a proportionate reason for the risk becomes very difficult.

THE ETHICS OF THE RESEARCHER

Both governments and professional societies have devoted much attention to the ethics of research. The Nuremberg Code (1949), dating from the trials of the Nazi war criminals, and The Declaration of The World Medical Association of Helsinki (1964, and revised in 1975) are further explicated by the Department of Health, Education and Welfare (now Health and Human Services) Regulations on the Protection of Human Subjects (1978). Professional associations such as the American Psychological Association and the American Medical Association (1984) spell out the obligations of members in conducting both academic and clinical investigations. One provision of the AMA statement is central to all that follows:

> 2.07 (2) In conducting clinical investigation, the investigator should demonstrate the same concern and caution for the welfare, safety, and comfort of the person involved as required of a physician who is furnishing medical care to a patient independent of any clinical investigation.

More than that is required, however. Research on human subjects is not justified unless the benefits to be derived outweigh the risks taken. The mere increase of human knowledge is not a sufficient justification when there are risks involved. We must agree with Robin (1984) that some research is trivial, done more to satisfy some need of the researcher than to bring any real benefit to mankind. The benefits of even important research must, however, be balanced against the human and economic costs. The memory of Nazi atrocities in medical research made this all too clear and led to the following provisions in The Nuremberg Code.

2. The experiment should be such as to yield fruitful results for the good of society, unprocurable by other methods or means of study, and not random and unnecessary in nature.

4. The experiment should be so conducted as to avoid all unnecessary physical and mental suffering and injury.

5. No experiment shall be conducted where there is an *a priori* reason to believe that death or a disabling injury will occur, except, perhaps, in those experiments where the experimental physicians also serve as the subjects.

6. The degree of risk should never exceed that determined by the humanitarian importance of the problem to be solved by the experiment.

In our society, the federal government requires that institutions involved in research have Institutional Review Boards (IRBs) to oversee this aspect of research. The main obligation remains with the researcher. The basic principle is clear: Granted informed consent and granted there is no other way to get the knowledge, the degree of risk to the subjects is to be minimized. Any risk, however, still needs to justified by the humanitarian goods to be obtained from the research. These humanitarian goods are those which promote directly the welfare and dignity of the human person. It should be noted that it is the humanitarian goods and not scientific knowledge which supplies the justification for the risks. In human research, knowledge is not self-justifying and nothing can justify research which disregards the dignity of the human subjects.

Even granted agreement about these points, three different emphases or points of view emerge when actual judgments are to be made (Veatch, 1987). The first point of view stresses protecting the subject from harm; the second point of view emphasizes social concerns; and the third focuses on freedom of choice.

Those who stress protecting the subject from harm use as a rule of thumb: "When in doubt, do what is safest for the subject." This is in line with the very traditional medical dictum: *primum est non nocere* (the first thing is not to injure). The second point of view recognizes that the humanitarian good involves society and patients who are not in the research study. It sees marginal risks justified by the good to this broader group. The freedom of choice approach holds that, granted informed consent, the subject should be able to choose what is most convenient even if it involves risks that a prudent person might not want to take. Each of these competing emphases has merit, and in practice all three points of view need to be considered. For this reason, the decision on the ethical correctness of a given piece of research cannot always be delineated with absolute clarity.

The problem is actually even more complicated than this. Sometimes the risks, say that of radiation, are a matter of public debate and therefore politically and socially controversial (Veatch, 1987). The issue cannot be settled merely on the basis of scientific facts or scientific norms. Society itself must have its say about the ethics of an experiment involving such radiation. In addition, radiation may involve risk to parties not directly involved in the research: offspring, family members, and people who just happen to be in the neighborhood. The authors' practical wisdom approach would call for the consideration of these risks as well as the risks to the subject of the research.

Informed Consent: Information

When we are dealing with therapeutic research, that is, research which may directly benefit the subject, everything required for informed consent in Chapter Two should be revealed to the subject or his surrogate. In both therapeutic research and nontherapeutic research, the subject should also be told the purpose of the research and whether or not random assignment will be used. This is to say the subject must be told the chances that he will end up in a control group with no treatment, a placebo, or with an alternate treatment. The subjects should also be told of prior animal research and their results, with appropriate warnings about overextending the results to human beings. The subject should be told the *possible* therapeutic benefits to himself or others, but should not be given more hope than is justified, especially in desperate situations where a subject is liable to say yes to anything. The Belmont Report (1978) correctly insists that the subject should be informed that it is possible to withdraw from the experiment at any time. The surrogates, moreover, should have a chance to observe the research and to withdraw the subject as the research proceeds.

No fact should be concealed which might cause the particular patient or a reasonably prudent person to refuse participation in the study. For example, if the experiment involves the injection of dead cancer cells, the subject should be told even if the dead cancer cells are harmless. Physicians who failed to give just this sort of information have lost their licenses in the past.

We strongly disagree with *Current Opinions of the Council on Ethical and Judicial Affairs of the American Medical Association* (1986) on therapeutic research, which states:

> 2.07,(3), B.i. In exceptional circumstances and to the extent that disclosure of information concerning the nature of the drug or experimental procedure or risks would be expected to materially effect the health of the patient and would be detrimental to his best interests, such information may be withheld from the patient. In such circumstances, such information shall be disclosed to a responsible relative or friend of the patient where possible.

This statement, which invokes therapeutic privilege in an experimental situation, suffers from all the defects of therapeutic privilege discussed in Chapter Two. It arrogantly assumes that the physician can know the "best interests" of the subject and in general disregards the need for informed consent even from the surrogates. Physicians are not licensed to do clinical investigations on uninformed subjects.

Nondisclosure for Scientific Reasons

Just as physicians sometimes attempt to justify nondisclosure for therapeutic reasons, scientists are tempted to conceal important information for scientific reasons.

In particular, they argue that (1) disclosure would invalidate the research, (2) intentional deception is necessary for the research, and (3) disclosure would cause people to refuse their consent.

Before considering each of these points individually, it should be stated categorically and without any "ifs," "ands," or "buts" that the pursuit of scientific knowledge never justifies violating the rights of people. Knowledge is never superior to the dignity of the individual human being. The needs of the scientist do not and cannot take precedence over the dignity of the individual.

While the pursuit of scientific knowledge does not justify hiding substantial items of information, it is not necessary to disclose every detail. General rather than particular disclosure is sufficient and ethical for an informed consent and need not invalidate the research. Thus, when *particular disclosure,* for example the disclosure of who would be and who would not be in the control group, would invalidate the experiment, a *general disclosure,* that is, the revelation that there will be random assignment to a control group, does not invalidate the experiment. A general disclosure of this sort of information is also ethical and suffices for informed consent.

The argument that intentional deception is necessary for the success of the experiment casts doubt on the ethical correctness of the experiment not only because of the deception, but because of the possible motives for the deception. If the subject is being deceived, lest she refuse consent, the experiment is clearly reprehensible.

Though the authors of the Belmont Report are not quite so strict, they add important considerations and their opinion demands great respect (p. 12).

> A special problem of consent arises where informing subjects of some pertinent aspect of the research is likely to impair the validity of the research. In many cases, it is sufficient to indicate to subjects that they are being invited to participate in research of which some features may not be revealed until the research is concluded. In all cases of research involving incomplete disclosure, such research is justified only if it is clear that (1) incomplete disclosure is truly necessary to accomplish the goals of the research, (2) there are no undisclosed risks to subjects that are more than minimal, and (3) there is an adequate plan for debriefing subjects, when appropriate and for dissemination of research results to them. Information about risks should never be withheld for the purpose of eliciting the cooperation of subjects and truthful answers should always be given to direct questions about the research. Care should be taken to distinguish the cases in which disclosure would destroy or invalidate the research from cases in which disclosure would simply inconvenience the investigator.

Who Pays for Bad Results?

The subject should also be informed of who pays for unforeseen bad results, for example, a crippling or debilitating side effect of the treatment. It is not merely a question of who pays for the treatment of the side effect, but of who pays for the loss of income and enjoyment of life. While it may be argued that, at least in therapeutic research, the risks are the price the patient pays for the hope of a cure, such is not the case in nontherapeutic research. In any event, if the subject and the subject's insurance carrier will bear all the costs, this should be stated and a written agreement obtained at the time the consent is being obtained.

Informed Consent: Competence and Surrogates

All of the factors considered in Chapter One enter into the consideration of the competence of research subjects to give informed consent. In the research context, however, particular attention must be paid to surrogate consent and to the situation of institutionalized subjects.

There are no special problems with surrogate consent to experimentation that is therapeutic. In therapeutic research, the patient can hope to benefit directly from the experiment and so the surrogate may judge that the experiment is for the good of the subject. There may, however, be problems with surrogate consent to nontherapeutic research since, by definition, the patient will receive no direct benefit from this. The problems have their roots in the various principles which the surrogate may use.

You will recalled from Chapter Three that the surrogate may use one of three principles: (1) the substituted judgment principle, (2) the best interests principle, or (3) the rational choice principle.

There is no problem if the substituted judgment is used, since in that case the surrogate is doing what he knows the subject wants or would want in the situation. If the subject would consent to the research, the surrogate can certainly do so.

If the rational choice principle is used there are no additional problems aside from those connected with the principle itself. The rational choice principle, you will recall, includes consideration of the good and evil consequences for others as well as for the patient. The American Medical Association (1984), which invokes the rational choice principle for the surrogate is useful in this context.

> 2.07,(4), Minors or mentally incompetent persons may be used as subjects only if:
> i. The nature of the investigation is such that mentally competent adults would not be suitable subjects.
> ii. Consent, in writing, is given by a legally authorized representative for the subject under circumstances in which an informed and prudent adult would reasonably be expected to volunteer himself or his child as a subject.

There are, however, problems if the best interest principle is applied, since in nontherapeutic research the subject is not going to benefit directly. In this case, participation can hardly be said to be in the interest of the subject, let alone her best interests.

Even when the best interest principle seems to forbid surrogate consent, the following points should be considered. When there is no risk or minimum risk to the subject and considerable good to be obtained from the research, it seems petty to forbid consent. Since minimal risk involves no more than the risk of a routine physical examination or the risks of everyday living, there is no real ethical problem with surrogate consent in this sort of research. If there is more than minimal risk, the best interest principle cannot justify surrogate consent. Of course, the substituted judgment and the rational choice principles may still permit consent.

Consent and the Special Classes of Subjects

The case of institutionalized subjects raises special problems for informed consent. It is argued that the institutionalized live in an inherently coercive environment such that there is always undue influence on their consent. This argument is especially plausible when it is a question of prisoners who will get extra privileges and know that participation may help their case for parole. At the same time, there may be a question of a paternalism which rushes in to protect everyone, whether they need the protection or not. Certainly, the experimenter should be particularly cautious in getting consent from such subjects but, absent legal restrictions, the institutionalized subject need not be universally ruled out of consideration.

Something similar may be said of the objections against research on older people. Granted that there have been abuses, the mere fact that a person is old does not make them incapable of informed consent. If all older people were considered incompetent, then there could be no therapeutic research for the group that most needs medical care. Such paternalism would be both insulting and physically injurious to the older citizen. The experimenter should be extra cautious in dealing with the older subject, especially the institutionalized older person, but there can still be ethical experimentation in these areas.

Justice and the Distribution of Research Risks

It has been argued that the "overuse" of institutionalized persons and the poor constitutes an unjust distribution of research risks. "Overuse," or use out of proportion to their distribution in the population as a whole, does not necessarily constitute an injustice. There is injustice *only if justice demands that the risks be distributed equally.* As we saw in Chapter Four, equality of distribution of health care is not required for justice, and so risk need not be equally distributed.

Risk and burden can never be distributed equally in a society that believes in free choice and protects the right to refuse to contribute, except when overriding social interests requires it by law. In such a society, only two groups of people are likely to accept the burden of being research subjects. The first and smaller group is comprised of extremely altruistic and generous people. The second and considerably larger group is comprised of those who are so deprived that there is some financial or social reward for their participation. As we noted, the prisoner participates in the interest of better living conditions and an improved chance of parole. The poor may participate in exchange for medical care or a fee. While this may not be an ideal situation, it is a situation that must be accepted and worked with under current economic circumstances.

A wider distribution of research risks will come about only if the people come to believe that medical research is so important to them and their society that they feel an obligation to participate and so require it legally. The fact that the general population does not feel as strongly about this as the research establishment is not to condemn the priorities of the general population. After all, there are other goods besides the health care system.

Although there is no overall solution even for a society of good will, certain warnings of the Belmont Report (1978) are still very applicable to justice on the individual level. The report notes that the poor, the institutionalized, and certain minorities should be protected from being used "solely for administrative convenience or because they are easy to manipulate as a result of their illness or socioeconomic condition." In addition, it would be clearly unfair to offer beneficial research to those whom the researcher likes and to select only "undesirable" persons for risky research.

Ethical Problems of Research Methodology

In general, poorly designed research is both unscientific and unethical since it wastes resources. When it is poorly designed, medical research also tends to expose subjects to risks that are unnecessary. Since no good can come of poorly designed research, there is never any proportionate reason which will justify the risks and the waste of resources. Finally, as we will stress in the section on the consumption of research, poorly designed research that gets published creates ethical problems for health care providers who may hurt patients by using poor research in their decision making.

A brief look at some of the basics of scientific research of well-designed clinical research will give some idea of what is involved.

In general, if the results of scientific research are to be generalizable, the subjects should be drawn from the population appropriate to the study. Further, even granted the proper population, the sampling would still have to be random in order to remove bias. A random sample is one in which every member of the population being studied has an equal chance of being studied. This condition would not be verified if researchers gave preference to their own patients who belong to the population being studied. Randomness of selection would also be destroyed if selection from the population were made on the basis of the ability to pay, or the willingness to be a subject for pay, or even on the basis of mere availability. Many studies have been known to violate these basic norms. More often than not, only a subset of the population will be selected and that on the basis of medical criteria. When we are dealing with drug experimentation for such deadly diseases as AIDS, the question of how these subjects are picked becomes crucial. As Macklin and Friedland (1986) suggest, medical criteria may not be value-free. Thus, for example, there might be a temptation to eliminate intravenous drug abusers from a trial for an AIDS drug on the ground that they are less healthy than gay men. This would not only narrow the value of the results but also discriminate against a whole class of persons in need.

In order to assure scientific rigor, medical research needs a base line, generally supplied by a control group to use as a basis for comparison with the experimental group. The control group gets either the standard treatment, no treatment, or a placebo. The experimental group gets the treatment being studied. In order to eliminate bias on the part of the subjects and the researchers, subjects are assigned to each group randomly, that is, by a procedure imitating chance. Just as the entire sample was selected randomly from the population to be studied, the sample is then divided and assigned by a second randomization. This is part of the effort to make sure that the two groups are similar and so truly comparable. They would not be comparable if such factors as social status, influence with the researcher, or place of residence influenced assignment.

To further eliminate bias, the experiment should be double blind, that is, neither the subjects nor the experimenters should know who is in what group. In this way, the patients will not feel better because they have been noticed or just because they have received something new and the researchers will not be tempted to imagine improvements where there are none.

These basic methods give rise to some very basic ethical questions quite aside from the problem of informed consent (Levine, 1979; Marquis, 1983).

The Ethics of Randomized Trials

While the use of randomized trials (studies where the patient is randomly assigned to either the experimental or control group) is scientifically necessary when there is no base line, it poses ethical problems when the *a priori* odds (the odds before the experiment starts) are not approximately equal for both the control and the experimental groups. Let us envisage a case as follows. Historically, there has been no effective treatment for disease Z. With rare exceptions, those who get Z die. This is a historical baseline. A drug Beta has been found effective in animals, safe in humans, and effective in diseases similar to Z. There is thus some probability that it will work in the case of disease Z. The tests of its efficacy in humans are about to begin. Those assigned to the control group will have no chance of recovery, since there is no effective treatment and the disease is generally fatal. Those assigned to the experimental group may have some small hope, since drug Beta worked with similar diseases.

Is it ethical to use a control group? As indicated above, the answer is no, since the best interests of those in the control group are disregarded. That is, the control group is not given a chance of the slight hope that Z will help. In addition, the control group serves no scientific purpose in this case, since a historical base line already existed.

Something similar occurred in the case where the Public Health Service used blacks with untreated syphilis as a control group despite the availability of effective treatments. Neither the good of patients nor sound scientific methodology was respected. The racist selection of patients completed the moral nightmare of that case.

Let us change the examples. In the case of disease Y, there is a standard treatment, and the research involves a new drug which may or may not be an improvement over the standard treatment. In this research, the control group gets a standard treatment while the experimental group gets the new drug. Suppose that halfway through the experiment, it *appears* that drug Beta is vastly superior to the standard treatment. Is it ethical to continue the experiment, or should the test be stopped and all patients given drug Beta?

The answer is not as simple as it seems. If the experiment is not completed, we do not know if the scientific requirements of proof have been met. That is, there is no validation of the drug. There may be an increase in false positives, that is, cases where a cure is seen when there is none. There are cases where the favorable results were due to a poorly designed experiment. Equally serious is the fact that premature termination of the experiment may fail to reveal harmful long-term effects, as well as long-term benefits.

It is our best but by no means unshakable opinion that the experiment should be discontinued in the face of early favorable results under two conditions: first, the good results are certain, statistically significant, or with a high degree of probability due to the treatment; or if the discontinuance has been scientifically planned. It is for these reasons that we speak of the *a priori* odds and not of the interim results as posing the ethical problem. Second, the control group being given a placebo or a standard treatment is suffering from a fatal or seriously crippling disease such that there is no proportionality between their suffering and the information to be gained.

Discontinuance in these cases is warranted by immediate beneficence but leaves us without scientific validation and with all the problems mentioned earlier. In case of doubt, however, the health care professional's first duty is not to science and the future, but to the patient who is present here and now.

There is, in many cases, another solution to the problem of the ethics of random selection. If a cross-over study is employed, the odds of both the experimental and control groups profiting are equalized. In the cross-over design, there is a set point at which the experimental group is changed from the experimental drug to the other treatment or no treatment, while the control group is now given the experimental treatment. Such a methodology may be a viable alternative in some circumstances and so offer an ethical solution to the problem of random assignment.

Problem of the Double Blind

The fact that the experiment is to be double blind (neither the experimenter nor the patient knows who is getting what treatments) raises problems with regard to the deception of subjects and the suppression of the truth in the informed consent procedure. Even when the subjects know that they will be randomly distributed between the control and the experimental group, there can be ethical problems. In the interests of eliminating bias, the double blind also reduces the ability of the health care professionals to respond rapidly to the changing condition of the subject. The subjects cannot be given the best health care in such situations. This aspect should be part of the informed consent process, that is, subjects should be told that they may not get the best medical care in some situations.

Institutional Review Boards

Federal law requires an Institutional Review Board (IRB) in hospitals and educational and research institutions which receive federal research funds. Not all federally funded research must be reviewed by these boards, since exceptions are made for ordinary tests given in educational settings, research involving surveys, interviews or data collection, or the observation of public behavior. The law does not even require informed consent in the case of these exempt areas.

The composition of these boards is to be structured in order to prevent conflicts of interest resulting from a narrow approach to their work. The regulations provide that not all members may be of the same sex or from the institution or from the same professional group. In addition, no one may be a member if a conflict of interest would result. Though these specifications of membership may be well intentioned, they pose problems which will be discussed in a moment.

The IRB reviews and approves, or disapproves, of the proposed research in their institutions in terms of risk benefit analysis. In addition, the board is to make sure that there is written informed consent which contains the necessary information. Without that approval, the research cannot be funded or be permitted to begin.

While these boards are not infallible or always effective, they are an attempt to provide some ethical safeguards in research.

Veatch (1987) raises interesting questions about the effectiveness in terms of the composition of the boards. Those boards which are dominated by professional and institutional members and chosen by the institution may have a systematic bias which causes them to overlook factors of importance to the normal prudent person. On the other hand, the jury model of the board, which is composed of nonprofessionals and so more representative of the community, is more powerful as a representative for the ordinary person and the conscience of the community. A fully representative and randomly chosen board is not really applicable here, since an IRB needs at least some members who understand the complexities of research. The representative model of the IRB contains both experts and representatives of the public. Ideally, such a group would represent all the ethical, moral, and legal interests of society as well as scientific expertise.

Even granted a representative IRB, there may be problems arising from the method of selection, the method of voting, and the balance between institutional and noninstitutional members. If the institution controls the selection of members, it can easily and even unintentionally stack the committee to favor one rather than another perspective. Perhaps outside groups need a right to appoint representatives with specific points of view.

If voting on the committee is by majority, indeed, if anything less than unanimity is required, a significant point of view may be left out of the decision. Thus, a psychologist who votes against a physiological research project because of anticipated psychological problems may be a minority of one, but she still represents a valid and important point of view. The same may be said of the pure layperson, who represents the community point of view and is unimpressed by the scientific justifications of acts that are repugnant to the average person. Once again, a majority vote could disregard this crucial aspect of the ethics of research.

Veatch (1987) argues that the number of noninstitutional members should be increased so that the number of perspectives is enlarged. Even though institutional members might represent a large number of disciplines, their membership in the institution may have narrowed their perspective. Thus the need for an increased number of public members.

Those interested in more details on the nature and structure and functions of the IRB should consult the Code of Federal Regulations 45 CFR 46: Protection of Human Rights, as well as *IRB: A Review of Human Subjects Research*, and the 1978 *Report and Recommendations: Institutional Review Boards and Appendix*, issued by the National Commission for the Protection of Human Subjects (nos. OS 78–0008 and OS 78–0009).

Summary

In biomedical research, subjects must be told everything required for the informed consent of patients (see Chapter Two), plus the nature of the study and such details as might influence the consent of the subject. Particular attention must be paid to the autonomy of institutionalized patients and the elderly as well as to poor who might easily be exploited. Risks must be taken only when necessary and must be minimized as well as requiring justification from the humanitarian and not merely the scientific good results.

Special problems exist in research that uses double blinds and randomized assignment to treatment and control groups.

THE ETHICS OF THE USERS OF RESEARCH RESULTS

The health care professional is obliged to protect patients from harm in so far as possible. This protection involves, among other things, a careful reading of research publications with two purposes in mind. First, the professional will want to be up on the latest in his field. Second, the professional will want to screen the research so that poor work is not used as a basis of health care practice. This second purpose demands a critical and informed reading of professional journals.

Some may object that a critical and informed reading of the journals is not required since the editors and, in the case of the better journals, the referees have read the article critically and in an informed way, culled out the poor articles, and put their seal of approval on those that are published. In short, many professionals rely on the editors and referees. Unfortunately, some of the medical and nursing literature is not subject to peer review. Periodicals supported by advertisements from drug companies often solicit articles. Even in the case of those with peer review, research shows that this reliance is not always well founded. In addition, even in those cases where the reliance is well founded, a critical and informed reading is still required if the health care provider is going to use the information intelligently and safely.

Reliance on the editors and the referee is not an adequate safeguard in science in general, or in medical research in particular. Broad and Wade (1982), Schoolman et al. (1968), and Sabine (1985), all speak to the errors and defects of methodology which regularly get by the editors and referees of even the best journals. Mosteller

(1985) and Patterson and Bailar (1985) have studied the peer review process and the selection of papers and concluded that the reader still needs to proceed with care. Shapiro and Charrow (1985) write of "Scientific Misconduct in Investigational Drug Trials." McDonald (1986) summarizes studies which indicate that as many as 75 percent of the papers examined may be flawed by some scientific misconduct. As many as 25 percent may be marked by *serious* scientific misconduct, such as publishing statements that were known to be misleading. In view of this, it seems clear that the obligation to read critically remains in force.

Kenneth S. Warren's (1981) *Coping with the Biomedical Literature: A Primer for the Scientist and the Clinician* is an attempt to provide the basic tools for such critical reading. Duffy (1985) supplies a checklist for evaluating nursing research reports. *The New England Journal of Medicine* frequently publishes articles on research methodology which will help the critical health care professional. We will not attempt to summarize any of this work, but will illustrate some of the simpler and more obvious points that are so often neglected by readers.

The critical reading of a scientific paper requires that the reader know something about research methodology and the statistical methods used in reporting and analyzing data. The reader, for example, should be aware that you cannot draw generalizable conclusions from a nonrandomized sample. An experiment done on seven volunteers from your medical ethics class would not produce results which you could then apply to all human beings, or even all Americans or all college students. The results might raise some interesting questions, but they would not provide you with any general truths that you could with honesty and safety apply to others.

The mere fact that the researchers fail to inform you of how they randomized the sample should create suspicions about the results. Not all methods which look random are random. For example, methods which involve taking every tenth name from a patient list after you have excluded those too sick to be interviewed is hardly a random process. But if the authors fail to tell the reader the crucial details, careless or unsophisticated readers may treat bad research as if it were well designed and its results significant. In addition, good scientific writing demands that those important details be shared so that the study can be reduplicated. Failure to include pertinent details may thus show ignorance of or contempt for sound methodology.

Even when there is a properly drawn random sample, the results must be properly analyzed. Statistics, after all, do not give us certainty, but only probabilities. The mere fact that one treatment produced better results than the other does not tell us much, unless we know what are the chances that the difference between treatments was due to more than mere chance.

We need to know the confidence level of the differences so that we can know how much weight to give the results. This is to say that we should know the probability that there is a type I error, which occurs when the observed results are attributed to treatment, but are merely due to chance. We would also like to know the probability of a type II error, which occurs when the effect is attributed to chance, but is actually an effect of treatment.

A good piece of research will tell us that P (the probability that the differences are due to chance) is less than a preselected number such as 0.05 or 0.10. The number 0.05 tells us that there is a 5 percent chance or less, that is, one chance in 20 or less, that the results were due to chance. If the number were 0.10, indicating a one out of 10 chance that the results were due merely to chance, a clinician might not want to use the results, or at least would be on his guard against the chance that the results were not valid in a given case. If nothing else, constant attention to the confidence level would keep practitioners aware that they are not dealing with certitude, but only with the odds. If no confidence level is given, beware.

Successful replication of an experiment is supposed to reduce the odds that the results, favorable or unfavorable, were due to chance. When the replication is unsuccessful, that is, gets the opposite results of the original experiment (again with the chance that it too is due to chance), we are left very much in the dark. A classic case is presented in the *New England Journal of Medicine* for October 24, 1986. The *Journal* published two articles on postmenapausal estrogen therapy related to coronary heart disease (Stampfer et al., 1985; Wilson et al., 1985). Each article was based on scientific research that was impeccable, but the results were contradictory. The results of one or both of the studies were due to chance. Neither one of them should be followed in practice until additional research clears up the matter.

Unfortunately, there is not enough replication in medical research, and what replication there is is most often not published since it achieved negative results. In general, scientists do not submit, and scholarly journals do not publish, studies with negative results. As a consequence, valuable negative information is lost, while successful but erroneous or misleading research is accepted, published, and acted on.

The Double Blind

The critical reader of health care research will want to know not only about randomization, confidence levels, and replication, but about the existence or nonexistence of a double blind. Because medical researchers as well as patients are subject to biases, the researcher will want to guard against this by the use of the double blind, a method which assures that neither the researcher nor the subject knows who is getting the experimental treatment. When there is no double blind, the reader will have to be on his guard against all sorts of biases and psychological effects which arise from the patients getting extra attention or believing that they are getting a miracle drug.

All of this comes down to saying that health care professionals need to know statistics and research methodology. If they lack such knowledge, they are not capable of a critical reading of the research and should be both ethically and professionally inhibited from using research they do not really understand.

When There Is No Research

While health care is supposed to be based on scientific study, there are many cases where there is no clinical research to justify the treatment. This is particularly true in the case of surgical procedures. For years male children were routinely circumcised. Research has now shown that there was no necessity for the procedure. Indeed, it exposed male babies to unnecessary risks. At one time tonsils were extracted in a wholesale fashion. Now we know that it should be done only rarely and for very serious reasons. Unfortunately, there is no organized vehicle for detecting such errors and it may take a long time for reform to occur. Even when the error is detected, it takes time for health care providers to unlearn their errors (Robin, 1984).

In view of this sort of situation the health care provider should constantly ask to see the scientific basis and the carefully controlled clinical trials which justify practice and not merely assume that accepted and professional approved practice is justified practice. A critical attitude will save more lives than a blind acceptance of even health care professional group think.

When the Research Is Disregarded

The careless reading of research or the reliance on fads among peers can lead to disastrous results. The best known case involved diethylstilbestrol (DES). From the 1940s to the early 1970s this drug was given to pregnant women. Between four and six million daughters of the women who received the drug have had problems. These range from clear cell carcinomas to benign vaginal conditions associated with, among other problems, various forms of cancer.

The drug was designed for women who had serious medical problems and who had repeatedly miscarried. The research indicated that it did nothing positive for healthy women or even slightly increased their incidence of reproductive difficulties. Despite this, it became a fad and was used indiscriminately, with grave consequences for DES daughters. A critical reading of the research and a resistance to faddish thinking could have saved much heartache and illness. Similar questions have been raised about the use of research on borderline high blood pressure (Guttmacher, 1981) and radical mastectomy (Katz, 1984).

Summary

The health care provider has an ethical obligation to read research critically. This requires a knowledge of statistics and research methodology. In addition, practitioners should beware, lest they follow accepted practice when it is not based on sound clinical trials or worse yet follow professional fads which run counter to the research.

A PROBLEM AREA

Fetal Research

The ethical problems connected with fetal research are particularly thorny not only because such research is often connected with abortion, but because there are so many different types of fetal research it is difficult to generalize. In this section, we will confine ourselves to research on living fetuses using the report of the National Commission for the Protection of Human Subjects as a focal point for the problems.

First, it will help to look at some key, if controversial, definitions of the Commission and the Department of Health Education and Welfare (DHEW), which is now the Department of Health and Human Services (DHHS).

The DHEW definition of the fetus *in the context of fetal research* is extremely broad (1981, Section 46.203c). The fetus is:

> The human from the time of implantation until determination is made following delivery that it is viable or possibly viable.

DHEW defines viability in the context of fetal research (1981, Section 46.203d) as:

> Being able after either spontaneous or induced delivery to survive (given the benefit of available medical technology) to the point of independently maintaining heartbeat and respiration.

Once the fetus is viable, it is considered a premature infant by DHEW. This is, of course, a stricter standard than that of the Supreme Court. The legal and ethical consequences of this stand are obvious. First, the health care team has an obligation to sustain the life of the premature infant if this is medically indicated. Second, the ethics of research given in the previous pages apply. Third, the informed consent of the surrogate is required and the best interests of the premature infant or the viable fetus are to be protected such that in general only therapeutic research will be justified. Because such a premature infant is so fragile, even therapeutic research and non-validated treatments should in general be done only as a last possible means of saving the infant's life.

If the living fetus is not viable, the informed consent of the surrogate is still required. There are, however, additional distinctions to be made. If the nonviable fetus is destined for abortion, DHEW guidelines forbid experimentation involving risks to the fetus, lest permitting such studies encourage abortion. Those who see nothing ethically wrong with abortion will, of course, disagree with this position and argue that the risks are irrelevant. At the same time, the right of the pregnant woman to change her mind and to deliver a healthy child would seem to indicate that the DHEW guidelines are sound even for those who do not oppose abortion. That is, the regulations protect the fetus in case the mother should exercise her right to change her mind and have the child.

When we turn to the problems of nonviable fetuses, we find that the National Commission (1976) followed two sound, though not necessarily uncontroversial, principles. First, there should be equality of protection for all human research subjects including nonviable fetuses. Second, the benefits to the individual and society were to be weighed carefully against the risks.

The first principle seeks to erect a wall which will protect not only all fetuses, but all human subjects from abuse in the name of science. Some who are more trusting of scientists and who see no problem with experimentation on nonviable fetuses will want to put the wall elsewhere. We are, in short, back to the dispute which was so central in the abortion issue: How high an ethical and legal wall should we build around the rights of those who clearly have rights?

The second principle is merely a reemphasis of the principle of proportionality, which applies in this research as elsewhere in health care ethics.

These two principles do not exclude all fetal research. After stressing the fact that the approval of the Institutional Review Board (IRB) is always required and insisting not only on the informed consent of the mother but on the nonobjection of the father, the Commission approved certain areas of fetal research.

First, it approved therapeutic research directed to the good of the fetus. This would include research on fetal surgery to cure obstructive hydrocephalus and obstructive uropathy. Second, it approved therapeutic research directed toward the mother if there were only minimal risks to the fetus. This was changed in the DHEW regulations, so that it approved research when the fetus was placed at risk only to the extent necessary to protect the health of the mother. In any event, the regulations point up the obvious fact that the health of the mother can justify risks to the fetus.

Assuming informed consent of the mother and no objection by the father (this requirement recognizes the fact that the father has a least some minimum rights in the situation), the Commission also approved the following types of more controversial nontherapeutic research:

First, research directed to the fetus in utero when (a) there is no anticipation of abortion, the risks are minimal, and the knowledge can be obtained by no other means, or when (b) there is an anticipation of abortion but the risks are minimal. Second, nontherapeutic research on the pregnant woman if the risks to the fetus are minimal. Third, nontherapeutic research directed to the fetus in utero when (a) abortion is not anticipated, the risks are minimal, and the knowledge is not obtainable in any other way, or (b) there is an anticipation of abortion and the risks are minimal. Fourth, nontherapeutic research directed towards the fetus during the abortion and nontherapeutic research directed toward the nonviable fetus ex utero, provided the fetus is less than 20 weeks gestational stage and no significant changes made in the interests of the research alone are introduced into the process. The DHEW regulations remove the 20–week provision.

Finally, research directed toward a possibly viable fetus is permitted provided there are no additional risks to the infant and that the knowledge cannot be obtained by any other means.

The following questions can and should be raised about these permitted areas. First, does the fact that abortion is anticipated justify doing away with the requirement that the knowledge not be obtainable in any other way? Has the fact of an anticipated abortion suddenly made this fetus less equal? Second, does the fact that the aborted fetus is not viable justify doing away with the condition that the knowledge cannot be obtained in any other way? To put it another way, does the fact that a fetus is doomed, whether by nature or someone's choice, give it a different moral status? The authors do not know the answers to these questions, though they are inclined to answer all of them with a "no." The questions deserve carefully argued answers. There are, however, several important points to be made in the discussion of these questions. The fact that a society, which seems to permit all sorts of abortions, still limits research on the fetus indicates that we are still groping our way towards a consensus about the moral status of the fetus. The limits on research certainly indicate a sense that great harm could result if everyone were free to do with what he wanted in this area.

SUMMARY

Ethical research must not only be competent, lest resources be wasted, but must produce a good proportionate to the evils risked or permitted. Problems of informed consent are particularly delicate since whole classes of potential subjects live in coercive environments and may be exploited as research subjects out of proportion to their numbers in the population. Scientific method can pose ethical problems when the *a priori* odds of success for the control and experimental group are not equal.

In addition, the health care provider who uses the results of research has an obligation to read research critically. The user of biomedical research cannot simply rely on the editors of journals, but needs enough basic knowledge of statistics and research methodology to understand more than the mere conclusions of research. In addition, the health care personnel should be aware of the fact that much validated practice is not based on scientific research and cannot simply be followed with good conscience. Critical thinking is required even there.

Such critical areas as fetus research are not simply matters of a black-or-white morality, but require careful distinctions to be made.

CASES FOR ANALYSIS

1.   (NOTE: This is based on James J. McCarthy, "Encephalitis and ARA-A: An Ethical Case Study," *The Hastings Center Report*, vol. 8, 6 (December), 1978, pp. 5–7 and a letter from the researchers in *Hastings Center Report*, vol. 9, 4 (August), 1979, pp. 4, 46 and the reply of McCarthy, pp. 46–47.)

Herpes simplex viral encephalitis has a rapid onset. It is a severe clinical disease during the acute phase. There is a high percentage of seizures regardless of age. Seventy percent of those who contract it die, many of the survivors are left with neurological deficits and some have to be institutionalized. The researchers, however, say that the studies indicate mortality rates varying from 13 to 70 percent.

The definitive diagnosis requires a brain biopsy with culturing of the sample. The biopsy, however, can miss the focus point of the involvement and give false negatives, that is, the test can indicate there is no disease when the disease is actually present.

The research in question sought to discover if the experimental drug ARA-A (adenine arabinoside, brand name Vira A) would be an effective treatment. ARA-A had already proved effective in the treatment of herpes simplex infections and disseminated herpes simplex infections in newborns. It had also been approved by the FDA for the treatment of herpeskeratitis, a localized infection which produces inflammation of the cornea. Within the antiviral dosage range there was no demonstrated hepatic, renal, or hematologic toxicity. The researchers note that there had been no controlled studies demonstrating this and, further, that ARA-A could be very toxic and cause bone marrow depression and damage to the liver and kidneys.

The research involved a controlled, double blind clinical trial with the subjects randomly assigned. There were 28 subjects with a positive biopsy. The biopsy-positive subjects received either ARA-A for 10 days or a placebo. The biopsy-negative subjects got either ARA-A for 5 days or a placebo.

The subjects were not told that the disease was 70 percent fatal, nor of the effectiveness of ARA-A in the case of the other herpes simplex infections. They were not told that the biopsy involved making a hole in the scalp and taking tissue from the brain. Nor were they told why a brain biopsy was necessary for this clinical trial. The researchers note that they changed the consent form after the first years of the test and used oral presentation. They do not, however, specify the changes.

Of the 18 biopsy-positive cases who were on ARA-A for 10 days, 5 (27.9 percent) died, 7 (38.8 percent) recovered to lead normal lives. Of this last group 4 (22.23 percent of the 18) recovered completely. Six (33.3 percent) had serious drug or brain damage, perhaps because the treatment was started too late. Of the 10 biopsy-positive subjects who were on the placebo, 7 (70 percent) died while 2 (20 percent) recovered to lead a reasonably normal life. The study was stopped when the deaths in this placebo control group reached the normal mortality figures for the disease.

2.   (NOTE: This is a very simplified case based on the famous Willowbrook case. It has been edited to promote discussion and does not purport to be a report of the original case.)

Shadowbrook was an institute for the mentally retarded near a major metropolitan area. It had grown rapidly from 200 patients in 1950 to 6,000 in 1965. Four thousand of the patients were severely retarded, with IQs of less than 20. Over half of the patients were not toilet trained and had to be diapered. The institution was understaffed and it was difficult to change diapers. As a result the patients often sat in their own fecal matter for hours. Since hepatitis is spread by the anal-oral route, this lead to nearly every patient getting hepatitis within the first six to twelve months at Shadowbrook. This was particularly true for those patients who were in the three- to ten-year-old range.

The study in question artificially exposed the subjects to the mild Shadowbrook strain of hepatitis both to achieve a better understanding of the disease and to develop methods of immunization.

Even when regular admissions to Shadowbrook had been stopped because of overcrowding and understaffing, patients were still admitted to a special hepatitis unit with the written permission of the parents. The parents had been informed by letter or by personal interview or in groups. Children who were wards of the state were not included.

Many of the parents were desperate to have their child admitted because they could no longer care for the child due to either the seriousness of the child's needs or their own inability to cope.

In the special ward children were also protected from other infectious diseases and often developed immunity to hepatitis. The research had been approved by various local, state, and federal agencies.

Over the years, including the years when regular admissions had been stopped, approximately 800 out of 10,000 admissions were involved in the research project.

3.   (NOTE: This is a simplified case inspired by the sophisticated case by Peter Sordillo and Kenneth Schanffner, "Case Studies: The Last Patient in a Drug Trial," *Hastings Center Report*, (1981) Vol. 11, 6 pp. 21–23.)

An experimental design calls for a test to end after the nineteenth patient. The drug being tested has proved ineffective in the first 18 cancer patients used as subjects. The drug has caused the usual side effects: nausea and vomiting for about 48 hours after taking it. Some patients developed sores and nearly all have had temporary, but severe, decreases in their blood counts. John De Nobili, on whom all other treatments for this cancer have failed, is admitted to the hospital conducting the research. If John is used, they can, *unless John responds favorably,* conclude the experiment with a clearly negative conclusion. John is desperate and wants to be treated.

What are the experimenters obliged to tell John?

5.   Bill, who holds an E.D., and has taken the advanced course in therapeutic touch, wishes to study the effect of therapeutic touch on patients with persistent headaches. He gets volunteers from the clinic in which he works. The sample is largely female and largely composed of people who are on welfare. There are also a disproportionate number of blacks and Hispanics in the sample. He randomly assigns them to a test group and a control group. The test group is given the therapeutic touch. With the control group, the experimenter goes through the motions of therapeutic touch but withholds the intention of transferring energy, which is the soul of therapeutic touch. His results show that the experimental group reported a significant reduction in the severity of their headaches and that the difference between the two groups has a 95 percent confidence level, that is, that there is only a 5 percent chance that the results are due to chance. On the basis of this research he applies therapeutic touch to all patients with headaches.

6.   As part of a nontherapeutic research, Drs. Laboure and Cortona intend to inject dead cancer cells into seriously ill patients. There is no danger from the dead cancer cells other than the minimal danger of infection at the injection site. They feel that if they reveal the nature of the injection, patients and their surrogates will refuse consent. Even the word cancer creates fear in most people. As a result they do not reveal the nature of the injection on the consent form. They justify this on the ground that there was no real danger to the patients and that the research is aimed at gaining knowledge that ultimately might help thousands of people.

7.   The Canisius Drug Company wants to test drug Q as a relief for high blood pressure. Tests have shown that the drug is not toxic in the doses required by the research protocol. Animal tests indicate that drug Q has fewer undesirable side effects than the existing treatments. Drug Q works by opening up the veins and uses a chemical compound produced by the heart itself. It promises to be far superior to present treatments because it uses a chemical natural to the body.

All of this, including the side effects, has been explained to the prospective subjects, who understand that they will be randomly assigned to one of three groups. Some will receive drug Q, some an accepted treatment, and some a placebo. They are also informed that this will be a double blind experiment.

The results show that drug Q is more effective than the accepted treatment and has fewer side effects, but the significance of this is not clear, since the probability that the difference is to due to chance is less that 10 percent and the researchers had originally decided on 5 percent as the cut-off figure. Despite this, they publish the article concealing the difference in probabilities by just not mentioning it.

REFERENCES

ABROMOWITZ, SUSAN (1984). "A Stalemate on Test-Tube Baby Research," *Hastings Center Report*, 14, no. 1, pp. 5–9.

ACKERMAN, TERRENCE F. (1982). "Why Doctors Should Intervene," *Hastings Center Report*, 12, no. 4, pp. 14–17.

AIKEN, WILLIAM, and HUGH LAFOLLETTE (Eds.) (1980). *Whose Child?: Children's Rights, Parental Authority, and State Power*. Totowa, N. J.: Littlefield, Adams and Co.

AMERICAN BOARD OF INTERNAL MEDICINE (1983). "A Guide to Awareness and Evaluation of Humanistic Qualities in the Internist," *Annals of Internal Medicine*, 99, no. 5, pp. 720–724.

AMERICAN COLLEGE OF PHYSICIANS (1984). "Ethics Manual," *Annals of Internal Medicine*, 101, pp. 129–137, 263–274.

AMERICAN HOSPITAL ASSOCIATION (1985). *Values in Conflict: Resolving Issues in Hospital Care: Report of the Special Committee on Biomedical Ethics*. Chicago: American Hospital Association.

AMERICAN MEDICAL ASSOCIATION, Council on Ethical, and Judicial Affairs (1986). *Current Opinions of the Judicial Council of the American Medical Association*. Chicago: American Medical Association.

AMERICAN NURSES ASSOCIATION (1985). *Code for Nurses with Interpretive Statements*. Kansas City, Mo.: American Nurses Association.

ANDREWS, LORI B. (1986). "My Body, My Property," *Hastings Center Report* (October), 16. no. 5, pp. 28–38.

ANNAS, GEORGE J. (1986). "The Baby Broker Boom," *Hastings Center Report*, 16, no. 3, pp. 30–31.

——— (1984). "Redefining Parenthood and Protecting Embryos: Why We Need New Laws," *Hastings Center Report*, 14, no. 4, pp. 50–52.

——— (1981). "Contracts to Bear A Child," *Hastings Center Report*, 11, no. 2, pp. 23–24.

——— (1975). *The Rights of Hospital Patients: The Basic ACLU Guide to a Hospital Patient's Rights*. New York: Avon Books (A Discus Book).

ANNAS, GEORGE, LEONARD H. GANTZ, and BARBARA F. KATZ (1982). *The Rights of Doctors, Nurses and Allied Health Professionals: A Health Law Primer*. Cambridge, Mass.: Ballinger Publishing.

APFEL, ROBERTA J., and SUSAN M. FISHER (1984). *To Do No Harm: DES and the Dilemmas of Modern Medicine*. New Haven, Conn.: Yale University Press.

APPLEBAUM, PAUL S., ET AL, (1987). "False Hopes and Best Data: Consent to Research and the Therapeutic Misconception," *Hastings Center Report* (April), 17, no. 3, pp. 20–24.

APPLEBAUM, PAUL S., CHARLES W. LIDZ, and ALAN MEISEL (1987). *Informed Consent: Legal Theory and Clinical Practice*. New York: Oxford University Press.

ARNEY, WILLIAM RAY, and BERNARD J. BERGER (1984). *Medicine and the Management of Living: Taming the Last Great Beast*. Chicago: University of Chicago Press.

ASHLEY, BENEDICT M., and KEVIN D. O'ROURKE (1978). *Health Care Ethics: A Theological Analysis*. St. Louis, Mo.: Catholic Health Care Association of the United States.

BAILLIE, HAROLD (1988). "Learning the Emotions," *The New Scholasticism*, Vol. LXII, No. 2, pp. 221–227.

BAKER, ROBERT (1983). "On Euthanasia," in James M. Humber and Robert F. Almeder (Eds.), *Biomedical Ethics Reviews*. Clifton, N.J.: Humana Press, pp. 5–28.

BARON, CHARLES H. (1985). "Fetal Research: The Question in the States," *Hastings Center Report*, 15, no. 2, pp. 12–16.

BATTIN, M. PABST (1982). *Ethical Issues in Suicide*. Englewood Cliffs, N.J.: Prentice-Hall.

BAUMRIN, BERNARD, and BENJAMIN FREEDMAN (Eds.) (1983). *Moral Responsibility and the Professions*. New York: Haven Publications.

BAYLES, MICHAEL D. (Ed.) (1978). *Medical Treatment of the Dying: Moral Issues*. Cambridge, Mass.: Schenkman.

BAYLES, MICHAEL D. (1984). *Reproductive Ethics*. Englewood Cliffs, N.J.: Prentice-Hall.

BEAUCHAMP, TOM L., and LAURENCE B. MCCULLOUGH (1984). *Medical Ethics: The Moral Responsibilities of Physicians*. Englewood Cliffs, N.J.: Prentice-Hall.

BEAUCHAMP, TOM L., and SEYMOUR PERLIN (Eds.) (1978). *Ethical Issues in Death and Dying*. Englewood Cliffs, N.J.: Prentice-Hall.

BEIS, EDWARD B. (1984). *Mental Health and the Law*. Rockville, Md.: Aspen.

BELL, NORA K. (Ed.) (1982). *Who Decides?: Conflicts of Rights in Health Care*. Clifton, N.J.: Humana Press.

Belmont Report: Ethical Guidelines for the Protection of Human Subjects of Research (1978). Washington, D.C.: The National Commission for the Protection of Human Subjects of Biomedical and Behavioral Research. DHEW Publication no. (OS) 78–0012.

BERNAT, JAMES L., CHARLES M. CULVER, and BERNARD GERT (1982). "Defining Death in Theory and Practice: The Report of the President's Commission," *Hastings Center Report*, 12, no. 1, pp. 5–8.

BioLaw, Vol. II: Updates and Special Sections (1987). Frederick, Md.: University Publications of America.

BLAKISTON (1972). *Blakiston's Gould Medical Dictionary*, (3rd ed.). New York: McGraw Hill Book Company.

BLASSAUER, BELA (1986). "In Hungary, the Old Medical Ethics Meet the New," *Hastings Center Report*, 16, no. 3, pp. 25–27.

BOK, SISSELA (1984). *Secrets: On the Ethics of Concealment and Revelation*. New York: Vintage Books.

——— (1979). *Lying: Moral Choice in Public and Private Life*. New York: Vintage Books.

BONDESOR, WILLIAM B. H., TRISTRAM ENGLEHARDT, JR., STUART F. SPICKER, and DANIEL H. WINSHIP (Eds.) (1983). *Abortion and the Status of the Fetus*. Boston: D. Reidel Publishing, p. 267.

BRAHAMS, DIANA (1987). "The Hasty British Ban on Commercial Surrogacy," *Hastings Center Report*, 17, no. 1, pp. 16–19.

BRANDT, R.B. (1975). "The Morality and Rationality of Suicide," in Seymour Perlin, (Ed.), *A Handbook for the Study of Suicide*. New York: Oxford University Press.

BRENNAN, THOMAS A. (1986). "Ethics in Health Care: Do-Not-Reuscitate Orders for the Incompetent Patient in the Absence of Family Consent," *Law Medicine and Health Care*, 14, no. 1, pp. 13–19.

BROAD, WILLIAM, and NICOLAS WADE (1982). *Betrayers of Truth: Fraud and Deceit in the Halls of Science*. New York: Simon and Schuster.

BRODY, BARUCH (1975). *Abortion and the Sanctity of Human Life: A Philosophical View*. Cambridge, Massachusetts: MIT Press.

——— (1987). *Life and Death Decision Making*. New York: Oxford University Press.

BURSZTAJN, HAROLD, RICHARD I. FEINBLOOM, ROBERT M. HAMM, and ARCHIE BRODSKY (1981). *Medical Choices, Medical Chances: How Patients, Families, and Physicians Can Cope With Uncertainity*. New York: Merloyd Lawrence Book.

CALIFANO, JOSEPH, JR. (1986). *America's Health Care Revolution*. New York: Random House.

CALLAHAN, SIDNEY, and DANIEL CALLAHAN (Eds.) (1984). *Abortion: Understanding Differences*. New York: Plenum Press.

CAMUS, ALBERT (1955). *The Myth of Sisyphus and Other Essays*. (Justin O'Brien, trans.). New York: Alfred A. Knopf Inc.

CAPLAN, ARTHUR L. (1986). "Baby Jesse and Beyond," *Ethics Center Update*, 2, no. 3 (July), pp. 1–2.

——— (1985). "Some Reflections Regarding Organ Transplants," *Ethics Center Update*, 1, no. 3 (Spring), pp. 3–6.

——— (1983). "Organ Transplants: The Cost of Success," *Hastings Center Report*, 13, no. 3, pp. 23–32.

CAPRON, ALEXANDER MORGAN (1987). "Anencephalic Donors: Separate the Dead from the Dying," *Hastings Center Report*, 17, no. 1, pp. 5–8.

——— (1984). "Current Issues in Genetic Screening," in James M. Humber and Robert F. Almeder (eds.), *Biomedical Ethics Reviews*. Clifton, N.J.: Humana Press, pp. 121–149.

CARLTON, B. CHAPMAN (1984). *Physicians, Law and Ethics*. New York: New York University Press.

CARLTON, WENDY (1978). *In Our Professional Opinion. . . .The Primacy of Clinical Judgment Over Moral Choices*. Notre Dame, Ind.: University of Notre Dame Press.

CHILDRESS, JAMES F. (1982). *Who Shall Decide?: Paternalism in Health Care*. New York: Oxford University Press.

CHRISTIE, RONALD, and C.B. HOFMASTER (1985). *Ethical Issues in Family Medicine*. New York: Oxford University Press.

CHRISTOPHERSON, LOIS K. (1982). "Heart Transplants," *Hastings Center Report*, 12, no. 1 (February), pp. 18–21.

COHEN, BARBARA (1984). "Surrogate Mothers: Whose Baby Is It?," *American Journal of Law and Medicine*, 10, no. 3, (Fall), pp. 243–286.

CONGREGATION FOR THE DOCTRINE OF THE FAITH (1987). *Instruction on Respect for Human Life in its Origin and on the Dignity of Procreation: Replies to Certain Questions of the Day*. Vatican City.

CONNERY, JOHN R. (1977). *Abortion; Development of the Roman Catholic Perspective*. Chicago: Loyola University Press.

CORNFORD, RONALD E. (1982). "Brain Death and the Persistent Vegatative State," in A. Edward Doudera and J. Douglas Peters (Eds.) *Legal and Ethical Aspects of Treating Critically and Terminally Ill Patients*. Ann Arbor, Mich.: AUPHS Press, pp. 63–76.

COWDREY, MICHAEL L. (1984). *Basic Law for the Allied Health Professional*. Monterey, California: Wadsworth Health Sciences.

CRANFORD, RONALD E. (1988). "The Persistent Vegetative State: The Medicial Reality (Getting the Facts Straight)." *The Hastings Center Report*, 18, no. 1, pp. 27–32.

CULVER, CHARLES M., and BERNARD GERT (1982). *Philosophy in Medicine: Conceptual and Ethical Issues in Medicine and Psychiatry*. New York: Oxford University Press.

CUSHING, MAUREEN (1984). "Wrong Rights in Nursing Homes," *American Journal of Nursing* (October), pp. 1213–1218.

DANIELS, NORMAN (1985). *Just Health Care*. London: Cambridge University Press.

DAVIS, IWAN (1985). "Contracts to Bear Children," *Journal of Medical Ethics*, 11, pp. 61–65.

DEPARTMENT OF HEALTH, EDUCATION AND WELFARE (1981). *Rules and Regulations: 45 CFR 46*. Printed in the *Federal Register*, 46, no. 16, (Monday, January 26, 1981).

DEPARTMENT OF HEALTH, EDUCATION AND WELFARE (1983). Guidelines on Fetal Research, *Code of Federal Regulations*, 45/cfr 46, (March 8).

DEPARTMENT OF HEALTH AND HUMAN SERVICES (1985). *Organ Transplantation: Questions and Answers*. Rockville, Md.: Superintendant of Documents no. HE 20.9002: Or 3.

DEPARTMENT OF HEALTH AND HUMAN SERVICES (1985). "Baby Doe Rule," 45 CFR Part 1340, *Federal Register* (April 15), pp. 14878–14901.

DEPARTMENT OF HEALTH AND HUMAN SERVICES (1986). *Report of the Task Force on Organ Transplantation, Organ Transplantation: Issues and Recommendations*. U.S. Government Printing Office, HE20.9002: OR3/2.

DEVINE, PHILIP E. (1978). *The Ethics of Homicide*. Ithica, N.Y.: Cornell University Press.

DOUDERA, A. EDWARD, AND J. DOUGLAS PETERS (Eds.) (1982). *Legal and Ethical Aspects of Treating Critically and Terminally Ill Patients*. Ann Arbor, Mich.: AUPHS Press.

DUCANIS, ALEX J., AND ANNE K. GOLIN (1979). *The Interdisciplinary Health Care Team*. Germantown, Md.: Aspen Systems Corporation.

DUFFY, MARY E. (1985). "A Research Appraisal Checklist for Evaluating Nursing Research Reports," in *Nursing and Health Care*, 6, no. 10 (December), pp. 539–547.

DUNCAN, RONALD, AND MIRANDA WESTON-SMITH (Eds.) (1984). *The Encyclopedia of Medical Ignorance: Exploring the Frontiers of Medical Knowledge*. Oxford, England: Pergamon Press.

EIDELMAN, ARTHUR L. (1986). "Caring for New Borns: Three World Views: In Israel Families Look to Two Messengers of God," *Hastings Center Report*, 16, no. 4 (August), pp. 18–19.

ELSTEIN, ARTHUR, ET AL. (1978). *Medical Problem Solving: An Analysis of Clinical Reasoning*. Cambridge, Mass.: Harvard University Press.

ENGELHARDT, H. TRISTAM, JR. (1973). "Viability, Abortion, and the Difference between a Fetus and an Infant," *American Journal of Obstetrics and Gynecology*, 116, pp. 432.

——— (1985). *The Foundations of Bioethics*. New York: Oxford University Press.

ENGLISH, JANE (1975). "Abortion and the Concept of a Person," *Canadian Journal of Philosophy*, 5, pp. 233–243.

ENNIS, BRUCE J. (1978). *The Rights of Mental Patients*. New York: Avon.

FABREGA, HORACIO, JR. (Ed.) (1980). "Social and Cultural Perspectives on Disease," *Journal of Medicine and Philosophy*, 5, no. 2, pp. 145–68.

FADEN, RUTH R., and TOM L. BEAUCHAMP, IN COLLABORATION WITH NANCY M.P. KING (1986). *A History and Theory of Informed Consent*. New York: Oxford University Press.

FEINBERG, JOEL (Ed.) (1984). *The Problem of Abortion*, 2nd edition. Belmont, Calif.: Wadsworth Publishing.

——— (1975). "Legal Paternalism," in *Today's Moral Problems*, Richard Wasterstrom, (Ed.). New York: MacMillan.

FEINBERG, KEITH S., ET AL. (1984). *Obstetrics/Gynecology and the Law*. Ann Arbor, Mich.: Health Administration Press.

FELIU, ALAFRED G. (1983). "The Legal Side: Thinking of Blowing the Whistle," *American Journal of Nursing*, (November), pp. 1541–1542.

FLETCHER, JOHN C., JOSEPH D. SCHULMAN, AND CHARLES H. BARON (1985). "Fetal Research: The State of the Question," *Hastings Center Report*, 15, no. 2, pp. 6–11.

FORTESS, ERIC E., AND MARSHALL B. KAPP (1985). "Medical Uncertainy: Diagnostic Testing and Legal Liability," *Law, Medicine and Health Care*, 13, no. 5 pp. 213–218.

GALLAGHER, JAMES (1985). "Reflections Regarding William Bartling: Siding with Life," *Ethics Center Update*, 1, no. 2 (Winter), pp. 3–4.

GARRETT, THOMAS (1963). *Ethics in Business*. New York: Sheed and Ward.

GAYLIN, WILLARD (1982). "The Competence of Children—No Longer All or None," *Hastings Center Report*, 12, no. 2 (April), pp. 33–38.

GIBSON, JOAN, AND THOMASINE KIMBROUGH KUSHNER (1986). "Will the 'Conscience of an Institution' Become Society's Servant?," *Hastings Center Report*, 16, no. 3, (June), pp. 9–11.

GIERTZ, GUSTAV (1980). "The Ethics of Randomized Clinical Trials," *Journal of Medical Ethics*, no. 6, pp. 55–57.

GLAZER, MYRON PERETZ, and PENINA MIGDAL GLAZER (1986). "Whistleblowing," *Psychology Today*, (August), 20, no. 8, pp. 36–43.

GOFFMAN, ERVING (1963). *Stigma: Notes on the Management of the Spoiled Identity*. Englewood Cliffs, N.J.: Simon and Schuster.

GOLDMAN, ALAN H. (1980). *The Moral Foundations of Professional Ethics*. Totowa, N.J.: Rowman and Littlefield.

GOODMAN, MADELEINE J., AND LENN E. GOODMAN, (1982). "The Overselling of Genetic Anxiety." *Hastings Center Report*, 12, no. 5 (October), pp. 20–27.

GOROVITZ, SAMUEL (1982). *Doctor's Dilemmas: Moral Conflict and Medical Care*. New York: Macmillan.

GOULDEN, PAULA, AND BENJAMIN NAITOVE (Eds.) (1984). *Medical Science and the Law*. New York: Facts on File Publications.

GRABER, GLENN C., ET AL. (1985). *Ethical Analysis of Clinical Medicine*. Baltimore: Urban and Schwarzenberg.

GREENBERG, DAVID F. (1974). "Interference with a Suicide Attempt," *New York University Law Review*, 49 (May–June), pp. 227–269.

GREENLAW, JANE (1980). "On Concealing Mistakes," *Nursing Law and Ethics*, 1, no. 9 (October), pp. 5–6.

GROBSTEIN, CLIFFORD (1982). "The Moral Use of 'Spare' Embryos," *Hastings Center Report*, 12, no. 3, pp. 5–6.

GUTTMACHER, SALLY, ET AL. (1981). "Ethics and Preventative Medicine: The Case of Borderline Hypertension," *Hastings Center Report*, 11, no. 1 (February), pp. 12–20.

HANSEN, HUGH J., SAMUEL R. CAUDILL AND JOE BOONE, (1985). "Crisis in Drug Testing: Results of CDC Blind Study," *Journal of the American Medical Association*, 253, no. 16 (April 26), pp. 2382–2387.

HASTINGS CENTER (1987). *Guidelines on the Termination of Life-Sustaining Treatment and the Care of the Dying*. Briarcliff Manor, N.Y.: The Hastings Center.

HLATKY, MARK A. (1986). "Evaluation of Diagnostic Tests," *Journal of Chronic Diseases*, 39, no. 5, pp. 357–358.

HULL, RICHARD T. (1985). "Informed Consent: Patient's Right or Patient's Duty?," *Journal of Medicine and Philosophy*, 10, no. 2 (May), pp. 182–197.

HUMBER, JAMES M., AND ROBERT T. ALMEDER (Eds.) (1984). *Biomedical Ethical Reviews*. Clifton, N.J.: Humana Press.

——— (1983). *Biomedical Ethics Reviews*. Clifton, N.J.: Humana Press.

HUMPHREY, DEREK (1984). *Let Me Die Before I Wake: Hemlock's Book of Self Deliverance for the Dying*. Los Angeles: Hemlock Society.

ILLICH, IVAN (1976). *Medical Nemesis: The Expropriation of Health*. New York: Bantam Books.

INGELFINGER, JOSEPH A. ET AL. (1981). "Reliability of the Toxic Screen in Drug Overdose," *Clinical Pharmacology and Therapeutics*, 29, no. 5 (May), pp. 570–575.

JAMES, FRANK E. (1986). "Peer Review Among Doctors Receives Boost," *Wall Street Journal* (October 20), p. 31.

JONAS, STEVEN, ET AL. (1981). *Health Care Delivery System*, 2nd ed. New York: Springer Publishing.

JONSEN, ALBERT R., MARK SIEGLER AND WILLIAM J. WINSLADE (1986). *Clinical Ethics: A Practical Approach to Ethical Decisions in Clinical Medicine*, 2nd ed. New York, Macmillan Publishing Co.

JORDAN, KENNETH G. (1987). Let's Replace "Do Not Resuscitate" with "Care for the Dying," *Ethics Center Update*, 3, no. 2, pp. 4–6.

JORDAN, SHANNON M. (1985). *Decision Making for Incompetent Persons: The Law and the Morality of Who Shall Decide*. Springfield, Ill.: Charles C. Thomas.

KANT, IMMANUEL (1963). *Lectures on Ethics*, Louis Infield (trans.). New York: Harper and Row, pp. 147–154.

KASS, LEON R. (1983). "Professing Ethically: On the Place of Ethics in Defining Medicine," *Journal of the American Medical Association*, 249, no. 10, pp. 1305–1310.

KATAYAMA, K. PAUL, AND MARK R. ROESLER (1986). "Five Hundred Cases of Amniocentesis Without Bloody Tap," *Obstetrics and Gynecology*, 68, no. 1 (July).

KATZ, JAY (1984). *The Silent World of Doctor and Patient*. New York: The Free Press.

KLEIMAN, DENA (1985). "Hospital Care of the Dying: Each Day, Painful Choices," *New York Times*, January 14, pp. A1, B4.

KOLATA, GINA BARI (1980). "Mass Screening for Neural Tube Defects," *Hastings Center Report*, 10, no. 6 (December), pp. 8–10.

KRIMMEL, HERBERT T. (1983). "The Case Against Surrogate Parenting," *Hastings Center Report*, 13, no. 5, pp. 35–39.

KUHSE, HELGA (1986). "The Case for Active Involuntary Euthanasia," *Law, Medicine & Health Care,* 14, no. 3–4 (September), pp. 145–148.

LANKTON, JAMES W., BARRON M. BATCHELDER, AND ALLAN J. OMINSKY (1977). "Emotional Responses to Detailed Risk Disclosure for Anesthesia, A Prospective, Randomized Study," *Anesthesiology,* 46, pp. 294–296.

Lancet (1984). "Review of Mortality Results in Randomized Trials in Early Breast Cancer," 2, no. 8414, Nov. 24, p. 1205.

LEVINE, CAROL (1984). "Questions and (Some Very Tentative) Answers about Ethics Committees," *Hastings Center Report,* 14, no. 3 (June), pp. 9–12.

LEVINE, CAROL, JOYCE BERMEL, AND PAUL HOMER (Eds.) (1987). "Biomedical Ethics: A Multinational Review, Special Supplement," *Hastings Center Report,* 17, no. 3 (June), p. 36.

LEVINE, ROBERT J. (1979). "Clarifying the Concepts of Research Ethics," *Hastings Center Report,* 9, no. 3 (June), pp. 21–26.

LEWIS, CHARLES E., RASHI FEIN, AND DAVID MECHANIC (1976). *A Right to Health: The Problem of Access to Primary Health Care.* New York: John Wiley and Sons.

LO, BERNARD (1987). "Promises and Pitfalls of Ethics Committees," *New England Journal of Medicine,* 317, no. 1 (July 2), pp. 46–49.

LOEWY, ERICH H. (1986). *Ethical Dilemmas in Modern Medicine: A Physician's Viewpoint.* Lewiston, N.Y.: The Edwin Mellen Press.

LOMBARDO, PAUL A. (1981). "Consent and Donations from the Dead," *Hastings Center Report,* 11, no. 6, pp. 9–11.

LYNN, JOANNE (1986). *By No Extraordinary Means.* Bloomingdale, Ind.: Indiana University Press.

LYNN, JOANNE, AND JAMES F. CHILDRESS (1983). "Must Patients Always Be Given Food and Water?," *Hastings Center Report,* 13, no. 5 (October), pp. 17–21.

MACINTYRE, ALASDAIR (1979). "Ethical Issues in Attending Physician-Resident Relations: A Philosopher's View," *Bulletin of the New York Academy of Medicine,* 55, no. 1 (January), pp. 57–61.

MACKINTOSH, DOUGLAS, R. (1978). *Systems of Health Care.* Boulder, Colo.: Westview Press.

MACKLIN, RUTH, AND GERALD FRIEDLAND (1986). "AIDS Research: The Ethics of Clincal Trials," *Law, Medicine and Health Care,* 14, no. 5–6 (December), pp. 273–280.

MAHOWALD, MARY B., JERRY SILVER, AND ROBERT A. RATCHESON (1987). "The Ethical Options in Transplanting Fetal Tissue," *Hastings Center Report,* 17, no. 1, pp. 9–15.

MAPPES, T. A., AND G.S. ZEMBATY (Eds.) (1980), *Biomedical Ethics,* 2nd Ed. New York: McGraw Hill.

MARQUIS, DON (1983). "Leaving Therapy to Chance," *Hastings Center Report,* 13, no. 4 (August), pp. 40–47.

MASSACHUSSETTS TASK FORCE ON ORGAN TRANSPLANTS (1984). *Report of the Task Force.* Boston: Department of Public Health reprinted in *Law, Medicine and Health Care,* 13, no. 1 (February 1985), pp. 8–26.

MAY, DAVID (1986). "The Concept of Rational Suicide," *Journal of Medicine and Philosophy,* 11, no. 2 (May), pp. 143–155.

MAY, WILLIAM F. (1983). *The Physician's Covenant: Images of the Healer in Medical Ethics.* Philadelphia: The Westminster Press.

MAYER, KLEMENS B., AND STEPHEN G. PAUKER (1987). "Screening for HIV: Can We Afford the False Positive Rate?" *New England Journal of Medicine,* 317, no. 4, July 23, pp. 238–240.

MCCARTNEY, JAMES J. (1980). "The Development of the Doctrine of Ordinary and Extraordinary Means of Preserving Life in Catholic Moral Theology Before the Karen Quinlan Case," *The Linacre Quarterly*, (August), pp. 215–224.

MCCORMICK, RICHARD A. (1984). "Ethics Committees: Promise or Peril?," *Law, Medicine and Health Care*, 4, no. 4 (September), pp. 150–155.

———— (1981a). *How Brave a New World: Dilemmas in Bioethics*. Garden City, New York: Doubleday.

———— (1981b). *Notes on Moral Theology 1965–1980*. Washington D.C.: University Press of America.

MCDONALD, KIM (1986). "Misconduct by Scientists Said to Be More Common than Many Believe in Scholarship," *The Chronicle of Higher Education*, (May 21), pp. 7, 10.

MCGOVERN, MARGARET M., JULES D. GOLDBERG, AND ROBERT J. DESNICK (1986). "Acceptablility of Chorionic Villi Sampling for Prenatal Diagnosis," *American Journal of Obstetrics and Gynecology*, 155, no. 1 (July), pp. 25–29.

MECHANIC, DAVID (1986). *From Advocacy to Allocation: The Evolving American Health Care System*. New York: The Free Press.

Medical Letter on Drugs and Therapeutics (1987). "Serum Cholesterol Determinations," 29, no. 738, April 24, pp. 41–42.

MENDELSOHN, ROBERT S. (1981). *Male Practice: How Doctors Manipulate Women*. Chicago: Contemporary Books.

———— (1979). *Confessions of a Medical Heretic*. Chicago: Warner Books.

MENZEL, PAUL T. (1983). *Medical Costs, Moral Choices: A Philosophy of Health Care Economics in America*. New Haven: Yale University Press.

MONAGLE, JOHN F., AND DAVID C. THOMASMA (1987). *Medical Ethics: A Guide for Health Care Professionals*. Frederick, Md.: Aspen.

MORRISSEY, JAMES M., ADELE D. HOFFMANN, and JEFFREY C. THORPE, (1986). *Consent and Confidentiality in the Health Care of Children and Adolsescents: A Legal Guide*. New York: The Free Press.

MOSKOP, JOHN C. (1987). "The Moral Limits to Federal Funding for Kidney Disease," *Hasting Center Report*, (April), 17, no. 2, pp. 11–15.

MOSTELLER, FREDERICK (1985). "Selection of Papers by Quality of Design, Analysis, and Reporting," from Kenneth S. Warren (Ed.), *Selectivity in Information Systems: Survival of the Fittest*. New York: Praeger, pp. 98–116.

MURPHY, CATHERINE, AND HUNER HOWARD (1983). *Ethical Problems in the Nurse-Patient-Relationship*. Boston: Allyn and Bacon.

MURPHY, PATRICIA (1980). "Dilemmas in Practice: Deciding to Blow the Whistle," *American Journal of Nursing*, (September), pp. 169–62.

MURRAY, THOMAS H. (1987). "Gifts of the Body and the Needs of Strangers," *Hastings Center Report*, 17, no. 2 (April), pp. 30–38.

———— (1985). "The Final, Anticlimactic Rule on Baby Doe," *Hastings Center Report*, 15, no. 3, pp. 5–9.

MUSKIN, SELMA J., AND DAVID W. DUNLOP (Eds.) (1979). *Health: What Is it Worth?* New York: Pergamon Press.

NATIONAL COMISSION FOR THE PROTECTION OF HUMAN SUBJECTS OF BIOMEDICAL AND BEHAVIORAL RESEARCH (1976). *Report and Recommendaions: Research on the Fetus*, DHEW Publication, no. 0S, 76–127.

———— (1977). *Research Involving Children: Report and Recommendations*. Washington, D.C.: U.S. Government Printing Office.

——— (1978a). *The Belmont Report: Ethical Guidelines for the Protection of Human Subjects of Research.* Washington, D.C.: DHEW, no. OS, 78–0012 and *Appendixes A and B,* no. OS, 78–0013–14.

——— (1978b). *Report and Recommendations: Institutional Review Boards* and *Appendix.* Washington, D.C.: Department of Health and Human Services, nos. OS 78–0008 and OS 78–0009.

——— (1978c). *Report and Recomendations: Research on the Fetus.* Washington, D.C.: Department of Health and Human Services, DHEW Publication, no. OS 76–127.

NEW YORK STATE TASK FORCE ON LIFE AND THE LAW (1986). *Do Not Resuscitate Order: The Proposed Legislation.* Albany, N.Y.

NOONAN, JOHN T. (Ed.) (1970). *The Morality of Abortion: Legal and Historical Perspectives.* Cambridge, Mass.: Harvard University Press.

NUMBERS, RONALD L., AND DARREL E. AMUNDSEN (Eds.) (1986). *Caring and Curing: Health and Medicine in the Western Religious Traditions.* New York: Macmillan.

OPPENHEIMER, GERALD M., AND ROBERT A. PADUG (1986). "AIDS: The Risk to Insurers, the Threat to Equity," *Hastings Center Report,* 16, no. 5 (October), pp. 18–27.

ORSHER, STUART I. (1979). "Ethical Issues in Attending Physician-Resident Physician Relations," *Bulletin of the New York Academy of Medicine,* 55, no. 1 (January), pp. 52–56.

OZAR, DAVID T (1985). "The Case Against Thawing Unused Frozen Embryos," *Hastings Center Report,* 15, no. 4, pp. 7–12.

PANNER, MORRIS J., AND NICOLAS A. CHRISTAKIS (1986). "The Limits of Science in On-the-Job Screening," *Hastings Center Report,* 16, no. 6 (December), pp. 7–12.

PARKER, P. (1983). "Surrogate Mothers' Motivations: Initial Findings." *American Journal of Psychiatry,* 7, p. 153.

PATTERSON, KAY, AND JOHN C. BAILAR III (1985). "A Review of Journal Peer Review," from Kenneth S. Warren (Ed.), *Selectivity in Information Systems: Survival of the Fittest.* New York: Praeger, pp. 65–82.

PELLEGRINO, EDMUND D. (1979a). *Humanism and the Physician.* Knoxville, Tenn.: University of Tennesse Press.

——— (1979). "Toward A Reconstruction of Medical Morality," *Journal of Medicine and Philosophy,* 4, no. 1 (March), pp. 32–56.

PELLEGRINO, EDMUND D., AND DAVID THOMASMA (1987). *For the Patient's Sake.* New York: Oxford University Press.

——— (1981). *The Philosophical Basis of Medical Practice: Toward an Ethic of The Healing Profession.* New York: Oxford University Press.

PENA, JESUS J., ET AL. (1984). *Hospital Quality Assurance: Risk Mangement and Program Evaluation.* Rockville, Md.: Aspen.

Perspectives: The Blue Cross and Blue Shield Magazine. (1985). "Second Surgical Opinions: Struggles to Get Out of a Political Box," (Fall), pp. 19–25.

PETERS, DAVID A. (1986). "Protecting Autonomy in Organ Procurement Procedures: Some Overlooked Issues," *The Milbank Quarterly,* 64, no. 2, pp. 241–270,

POLONOFF, DAVID B., AND MICHAEL J. GARLAND (1979). "Oregon's Premarital Blood Test: An Unsuccessful Attempt at Repeal," *Hastings Center Report,* 9, no. 6 (December), pp. 5–6.

PORTWOOD, DORIS (1983). *Common Sense Suicide: The Final Right.* Los Angeles: Hemlock Society.

POST, JOSEPH (1979). "Changing Staff-Attending Staff Relations," *Bulletin of the New York Academy of Medicine,* 55, no. 1 (January), pp. 46–51.

POTTS, MALCOLM, PETER DIGGORY, AND JOHN PEEL (1977). *Abortion.* New York: Cambridge University Press.

PRESIDENT'S COMMISSSION FOR THE STUDY OF ETHICAL PROBLEMS IN MEDICINE AND BIOMEDICAL AND BEHAVIORAL RESEARCH (1981). *Defining Death: Medical, Legal and Ethical Issues in the Determination of Death.* Washington D.C.: U.S. Government Printing Office.

——— (1982). *Making Health Care Decisions: The Ethical and Legal Implications of Informed Consent in the Patient-Practioner Relationship.* I, Report, Washington, D.C.: The President's Commission.

QUINN, CARROLL A., and MICHAEL D. SMITH (1987). *The Professional Committment: Issues and Ethics in Nursing.* Philadelphia: W.B. Saunders.

RAMSEY, PAUL (1978). *Ethics on the Edges of Life: Medical and Legal Intersections.* New Haven, Conn.: Yale University Press.

RAWLS, JOHN (1971). *A Theory of Justice.* Cambridge, Mass.: Belknap Press of Harvard University Press.

REGAN, TOM (Ed.) (1980). *Matters of Life and Death: New Introductory Essays in Moral Philosophy.* New York: Random House.

——— (1983). "Nursing Complaints: Going Public is Risky," *The Regan Report on Nursing Law,* (September), 24, no. 4, p. 1.

——— (1984). *The Case for Animal Rights.* Berkeley: University of California Press.

RHODEN, NANCY K. (1986). "Treating Baby Doe: The Ethics of Uncertainty," *Hasting Center Report,* 16, no. 4, (August), pp. 34–42.

ROBERTSON, JOHN A. (1983). "Surrogate Mothers: Not So Novel After All," *Hastings Center Report,* 13, no. 5, pp. 28–34.

ROBIN, EUGENE D. (1984). *Medical Care Can Be Dangerous to Your Health: A Guide to the Risks and Benefits.* New York: Harper and Row.

ROBINSON, WADE L., AND MICHAEL S. PRITCHARD (Eds.) (1979). *Medical Responsibility: Paternalism, Informed Consent and Euthanasia.* Clifton, N.J.: Humana Press.

RODES, NED D., ET AL. (1986). "The Impact of Breast Cancer Screening on Survival: A 5– to 10–Year Follow Up Study," *Cancer* vol. 57, pp. 581–585.

ROE VS. WADE, U. S. 113 (1973).

ROSENFELD, ALBERT (1984). "At Risk for Huntington's Disease: Who Should Know What and When," *Hastings Center Report* 14, no. 3 (June), pp. 5–8.

ROSENTHAL, CAROLYN J., ET AL. (1980). *Nurses, Families and Patients.* New York: Springer.

ROSOFF, ARNOLD J. (1981). *Informed Consent: A Guide for Health Care Providers.* Rockville, Md.: Aspen.

ROSOVSKY, FAY A. (1984). *Consent to Treatment, A Practical Guide.* Boston: Brown, Little and Co.

ROTHMAN, DAVID J., AND SHEIL M. ROTHMAN (1980). "The Conflict Over Children's Rights," *Hastings Center Report,* 10, no. 3 (June), pp. 7–10.

ROTHMAN, WILLIAM (1983). *Strikes in Health Care Organizations.* Owings Mill, Md.: National Health Publishing.

SABINE, JOHN R. (1985). "The Error Rate in Biological Publication: A Preliminary Survey," in *BioScience,* 35, no. 6 (June), pp. 358–363.

SACKETT, DAVID L. (1981). "Evaluation: Requirements for Clinical Application," in Kenneth S. Warren (Ed.), *Coping with the Biomedical Literature: A Primer for Scientist and the Clinician.* New York: Praeger, pp. 123–157.

——— (1980). "The Competing Objectives of Randomized Clinical Trials," *New England Journal of Medicine*, 303, no. 18, pp. 1059–1060.

SARTORIUS, ROLF (Ed.) (1983). *Paternalism*. Minneapolis: University of Minnesota.

SASS, HANS-MARTIN (1983). "Justice, Beneficence or Common Sense?: The President's Commission's Report on Access to Health Care," *Journal of Medicine and Philosophy*, (November), 8, no. 4, pp. 381–388.

SCHAFFNER, KENNETH F. (Ed.) (1986). "Ethical Issues in the Use of Clinical Controls," *Journal of Medicine and Philsophy*, (November), 11, no. 4.

SCHARTZ, ROBERT, AND ANDREW GRUBB (1985). "Why Britain Can't Afford Informed Consent," *Hastings Center Report*, 15, no. 4, pp. 19–25.

SCHOEMAN, FERDINAND (1985). "Parental Discretion and Childrens's Rights: Background and Implications for Medical Decision Making," *Journal of Science and Medicine*, 10, no. 1 (February), pp 45–61.

SCHOOLMAN, HAROLD M., JACK M. BECKTEL, WILLIAM R. BEST, AND ARTHUR F. JOHNSON Hines, III (1968). "Clinical and Experimental Statistics in Medical Reserach: Principles Versus Practices," in *The Journal of Laboratory and Clinical Medicine*, 71, no. 3, (March), pp. 357–367.

SHAPIRO, MARTIN F., AND ROBERT P. CHARROW (1985). "Special Report: Scientific Misconduct in Investigational Drug Trials," *New England Journal of Medicine*, 312, no. 11, pp. 731–736.

SHAW, MARGERY W., AND A. EDWARD DOUDERA (1983). *Defining Human Life: Medical, Legal and Ethical Implications*. Ann Arbor, Mich.: AUPHA Press.

SHELP, EARL E. (Ed.) (1985). *Virtue and Medicine: Explorations in the Character of Medicine*. Boston: D. Reidel Publishing.

SIEGLER, MARK (1986). "Ethics Committees: Decisions in Bureaucracy," *Hastings Center Report*, 16, no. 3, pp. 22–24.

SINGER, PETER (1985). "Making Laws on Making Babies," *Hastings Center Report*, 15, no. 4, pp 5–6.

SMITH, HARMON L., AND LARRY R. CHURCHILL (1986). *Professional Ethics and Primary Care Medicine*. Chapel Hill, N.C.: Duke University Press.

SMITH, SHERI (1980). "Three Models of the Nurse Patient Relationship," in Stuart F. Spicher and Sally Gadow (Eds.), *Nursing Images and Ideals: Opening Dialogue with the Humanities*. New York: Springer, pp. 176–188.

SORDILLO, PETER P., AND KENNETH F. SCHAFFNER (1981). "The Last Patient in a Drug Trial," *Hastings Center Report*, 11, no. 6 (December), pp. 21–23.

SPECTOR, RACHEL E. (1985). *Cultural Diversity in Health and Illness*, 2nd Ed. Norwalk, Conn.: Appleton-Century-Crofts.

STAMPFER, MEIR J., ET AL. (1985). "A Prospective Study of Postmenopausal Estrogen Therapy and Coronary Heart Disease," *New England Journal of Medicine*, (October), 313, no. 17, pp. 1044–1049.

"Standards and Guidelines for Cardiopulmonary Resuscitation (CPR) and Emergency Cardiac Care (ECC)" (1986). *Journal of the American Medical Association*, 255, no. 21, (June), pp. 2905– 2985.

STARR, PAUL (1982). *The Social Transformation of American Medicine*. New York: Basic Books.

STARZL, THOMAS E. (1985). "Will Live Organ Donations No Longer Be Justified?," *Hastings Center Report*, 15, no. 2, p. 5.

STEINBOCK, BONNIE (1983). "The Removal of Mr Herber's Feeding Tube," *Hastings Center Report*, 13, no. 5 (October), pp. 13–16.
——— Ed. (1980). *Killing and Letting Die*. Englewood Cliffs, N.J.: Prentice-Hall.
STEINBROOK, ROBERT (1986). "In California: Voluntary Mass Prenatal Screening," *Hastings Center Report*, 16, no. 5 (October), pp 5–7.
——— (1980). "Unrelated Volunteers as Bone Marrow Donors," *Hastings Center Report*, 10, no. 1, pp. 11–14.
STEWART, W.W., AND NED FEDER (1987). "The Integrity of the Scientific Literature," *Nature*, 325 (January), pp. 207–214.
SZASZ, THOMAS (1977). *The Theology of Medicine: Political-Philosophical Foundations of Medical Ethics*. New York: Harper and Row.
TANNENBAUM, JERROLD, AND ANDREW N. ROWAN (1985). "Rethinking the Morality of Animal Research," *Hasting Center Report*, 15, no. 5, pp. 32–45.
TARANTO, RICHARD B. (1986). "The Psychiatrist-Patient Privilege and Third Party Payers: Commonwealth v. Korbin," *Law, Medicine and Health Care*, 14, no. 1, pp. 25–29.
TAUB, SHEILA (1985). "Surrogate Motherhood and the Law," *Connecticut Medicine*, 49, no. 10 (October), pp. 671–674.
THOMPSON, J., ET AL. (1987). "Retaining Rights of Impaired Elderly," *Journal of Gerontological Nursing*, 13, no. 3 (March), pp 2–25.
THOMSON, JUDITH JARVIS (1971). "A Defense of Abortion," *Philosophy and Public Affairs*, 1, no. 1, pp. 47–66.
TOOLEY, MICHAEL (1972). "Abortion and Infanticide," *Philosophy and Public Affairs*, 2, pp. 137–65.
UHLMANN, RICHARD F., ET AL. (1987). "Medical Management Decisions in Nursing Home Patients," *Annals of Internal Medicine*, 106, pp. 879–885.
UNIFORM LAW COMMISSIONERS, (1985). *Uniform Rights of the Terminally Ill Act*. Chicago: National Conference of Comissioners on Uniform State Laws.
VANDERPOOL, HAROOD Y., AND GARY B. WEISS (1987). "False Data and Lost Hopes: Enroling Ineligible Patients in Clinical Trials," *Hastings Center Report*, 17, no. 2 (April), pp. 16–20.
VANDEVEER, DONALD (1986). *Paternalistic Intervention: The Moral Bounds on Benevolence*. Princeton, N.J.: Princeton University Press.
VAN SCOY-MOSHER, MICHAEL (1982). "An Oncologist's Case for No-Code Orders," in A. Edward Doudera, and J. Douglas Peters (Eds.). *Legal and Ethical Aspects of Treating Critically and Terminally Ill Patients*. Ann Arbor, Mich.: AUPHS Press, pp. 14–18.
VEATCH, ROBERT M. (1987). *The Patient as Partner: A Theory of Human-Experimentation Ethics*. Bloomington, Ind.: Indiana University Press.
——— (1986). "DRG's and the Ethics Allocation of Resources," *Hastings Center Report*, 16, no. 3 (June), pp. 32–40.
——— (1981a). *A Theory of Medical Ethics*. New York: Basic Books.
——— (1981b). "Nursing Ethics, Physician Ethics and Medical Ethics," *Law Medicine and Health Care*, 9, no. 5 (October), pp. 17–19.
——— (1978). "Defining Death Anew: Technical and Ethical Problems," in Tom L. Beauchamp and Seymour Perlin (Eds.), *Ethical Issues in Death and Dying*. Englewood Cliffs, N.J.: Prentice-Hall, pp. 18–38.
——— (1972). "Models for Ethical Practice in a Revolutionary Age," *Hastings Center Report*, 2, no. 3 (June), pp. 5–7.

WAITZKIN, HOWARD (1983). *The Second Sickness: Contradictions of the Capitalist Health Care System.* New York: The Free Press.

WARREN, KENNETH S. (ed), (1981). *Coping with the Biomedical Literature: A Primer for the Scientist and the Clinician.* New York: Praeger.

WARREN, MARY ANNE (1973). "On the Moral and Legal Status of Abortion," *The Monist* 57, no. 1, pp. 43–61.

WASS, DEBBIE M., ET AL. (1986). "Chorionic Villus Sampling: Clinical Experience in 50 diagnostic cases," *The Australian and New Zealand Journal of Obstetrics and Gynaecology,* 26, no. 65, pp. 65–70.

WEINER, HERBERT (1977). *Psychobiology and Human Disease.* New York: Elsevier North Holland.

WILSON, PETER W.F., ET AL. (1985). "Postmenopausal Estrogen Use, Cigarette Smoking and Cardiovascular Morbidity in Women over 50: The Framingham Study," *New England Journal of Medicine,* (October), 313, no. 17, pp. 1038–1043.

WINSLADE, W.J. (1981). "Surrogate Mothers—Right or Wrong?," *Journal of Medical Ethics,* 40, no. 1.

WINSLADE, W.J., AND JUDITH WILSON ROSS (1986). *Choosing Life or Death: A Guide for Patients, Families and Physicians.* New York: The Free Press.

WOLF, SUSAN M. (1986). "Ethics Committees in the Courts," *Hastings Center Report,* 16, no. 3 (June), pp. 12–15.

INDEX

E

Economics of health care, 93
Egalitarian justice, 76
Embryo
frozen, 168
transfer, 167
Emergencies, 37
Emotions and ethics, 11
Enforcement of standards, 220–27
Engelhardt, H. Tristam, Jr., 50n, 53, 142
Engineering model of medicine, 16
Entitlement theory of justice, 77
Ethical diversity and health care, 24–25,
    83–86
Ethics
applied, 11
and law, 1, 139
and organ donation, 178
professional, 13
and religion, 1, 139
theories of, 2–11
and unity of procreation and love, 169
Ethics committees, 40, 63, 132
Ethics of the patient, 58–59
and suicide, 115–18
Euthanasia, 128, 137n
Evil
and causal influence of the agent, 55,
    57–58
certitude of, 56
impossibility of avoiding all, 52
levels of, 55
Exploitation in research, 236

F

Faden, Ruth R., 30, 32, 34
Fairness as justice, 77
Family
and confidentiality, 107
and distribution of health care,
    91–92
and organ donation, 185–86
place in death and dying, 133
Family physician, 20
Feinberg, Joel, 50n
Fetus
definitions, 141, 245
fetal research, 244–47
fetal tissue transplant, 180
moral status, 141, 146
Freedom, 27

G

Genetic screening, 209
Goffman, Erving, 208
Good
certitude of, 56
impossibility of doing all, 51–52
levels of, 55
proportionate, 125
Gorovitz, Samuel, 36

H

Harm
and the medical indications principle, 59
Health
defined, 83–84
Health care
and ethical diversity, 24
humane, 88
limits, 85
not always a good, 86
purpose, 14–15, 86–88
and social power, 90
versus public health, 88
Health care professions
purpose, 14
Homicide, 125–26
Hospital records
confidentiality, 108
Hydration, 129

I

Identified lives, 15
Impaired professionals, 220–21, 222
Individualism, 4
Informed consent (see also Paternalism;
        Therapeutic privilege)
children and adolescents, 40
and the courts, 39
criteria, 29
difficulties with, 35
emergencies, 37
exceptions, 32, 38
incompetence, 31
nonemergency exceptions, 38
possibility of, 35
and research, 233, 235–36
responsibility to provide, 45
surrogates, 44
and testing, 206